Pickleball

by Mo Nard, Reine Steel, Diana Landau, and Carl Landau

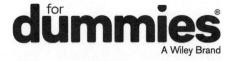

for
dummies®
A Wiley Brand

Pickleball For Dummies®

Published by: **John Wiley & Sons, Inc.**, 111 River Street, Hoboken, NJ 07030-5774, www.wiley.com

Copyright © 2022 by John Wiley & Sons, Inc., Hoboken, New Jersey

Media and software compilation copyright © 2022 by John Wiley & Sons, Inc. All rights reserved.

Published simultaneously in Canada

For general information on our other products and services, please contact our Customer Care Department within the U.S. at 877-762-2974, outside the U.S. at 317-572-3993, or fax 317-572-4002. For technical support, please visit https://hub.wiley.com/community/support/dummies.

Wiley publishes in a variety of print and electronic formats and by print-on-demand. Some material included with standard print versions of this book may not be included in e-books or in print-on-demand. If this book refers to media such as a CD or DVD that is not included in the version you purchased, you may download this material at http://booksupport.wiley.com. For more information about Wiley products, visit www.wiley.com.

Library of Congress Control Number: 2022944050

ISBN: 978-1-119-89513-8 (pbk); ISBN 978-1-119-89514-5 (ebk); ISBN 978-1-119-89515-2 (ebk)

SKY10036907_101722

Contents at a Glance

Table of Contents

PART 2: GETTING INTO THE SWING OF THINGS 97

Introduction

I t doesn't matter whether you love pickles or don't care for them one bit. Pickles have nothing to do with pickleball — no vinegar, brine, or cucumbers are involved. We're hoping you aren't disappointed, but if so, we highly recommend *Canning and Preserving For Dummies* as your next book purchase.

If you are here for pickleball, be assured that just about anyone can play it, and we want you to enjoy this sport as much as we do. Pickleball is good for both your mind and body. Going beyond the studies showing that exercise improves physical and mental health, pickleball offers the added psychological benefit of being a highly social sport. If you're ready to make dozens of new friends, get in better shape, and challenge yourself with some casual (or serious) competition, you've come to the right sport — and the right book to help you get the most out of it.

Pickleball is serious fun. People all over the world are discovering the joy of play again. Why should recess have to end just because you're an adult? You've probably heard the buzz about celebrities getting hooked on the game and building pickleball courts in their backyards. Fortunately, you don't need to be a millionaire to go all-in on pickleball. It's an inexpensive and accessible sport. Pickleball is the people's game!

This book is for beginners, intermediate players wanting to improve, and advanced players looking for new strategies to add to their toolbox. *Pickleball For Dummies* is one of the most comprehensive resources you can find about everything pickleball. As you play more and more, this book will serve as a guide to your ongoing development and improvement.

About This Book

All you need to get started playing pickleball are a paddle, some balls, good shoes, and a court to play on. Although the game is easy to learn, it's full of nuanced strategies to master if you want to advance to higher levels. In this book, we take you through every aspect of the game, with detailed explanations, diagrams, and photographs to help you understand the more complex points.

Pickleball For Dummies starts with an overview of the sport, the rules, various body mechanics involved, and how to "think before you dink." We go on to explain all the different shots and strategies used in pickleball, as well as how to prevent possible injury. After you've mastered the fundamentals, this book can continue to serve as a helpful resource for advanced strategies in both doubles and singles. We also cover ways to boost your mental game, find the right coach or clinic, understand the world of tournament play, find ways to volunteer, and much more. At the end of the book, we've included a glossary of terms and expressions that you'll read in this book and hear people using on the court (with our own "spin" on some of them, just for fun).

This book also covers etiquette on the court, where to find places to play, and ideas for organizing your own fun events. One of the best features of *Pickleball For Dummies* is that we address all skill levels, because this sport is played by kids and grandparents, professional athletes, and everyone in between. We're certain you'll discover something practical and invaluable in the following pages.

Note: We apologize in advance for the frequent use of the word "fun." It's because, well, it's the best word to describe playing pickleball! (Sorry, not sorry.)

Foolish Assumptions

Although pickleball is a sport for people of all ages and athletic abilities, we did have to make some assumptions about you while we were writing this book. Here's what we came up with:

>> You've either never played pickleball or you want to take your play to the next level, improve your skills, and learn the finer points of pickleball strategy.

>> You've seen advanced players hit dazzling shots and may want to know how to play just like them!

>> You understand that practice is the only way to get better in any sport, so you're ready to practice on your own or with friends, or to seek more training.

Conventions Used in This Book

We use the following conventions throughout the book:

>> All web addresses appear in monofont in the print book and as live links in the e-book. (Note that we haven't inserted any extra punctuation if an address breaks across a line.)

>> New terms appear in *italics* and are closely followed by an easy-to- understand definition.

>> **Boldface** is used to highlight the action parts of numbered steps and keywords in bulleted lists.

As a final note on the convention front, we recognize that every player is different, and we kept that in mind when writing this book. For example, even though we may seem to tell a right-handed player to do pretty much the reverse of what we tell a lefty, we often provide the instructions for both right-handed and left-handed folks.

Icons Used in This Book

Throughout this book, you find icons in the left margins that alert you to information you need to know. You find the following icons in this book:

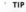
TIP

Text marked with this icon includes suggestions for different things you can do to improve your game. The tips are practical and easy to implement.

REMEMBER

If you take nothing else away from *Pickleball For Dummies* but the information marked by this icon, you will still have a solid foundation for years of pickle-ball fun.

WARNING

When you see a paragraph marked with this icon, pay attention because you're about to absorb something you need to know, both to avoid making mistakes and to stay safe and healthy while you play.

Beyond the Book

In addition to the material in the print or e-book you're reading right now, this book also comes with some access-anywhere goodies on the web. Check out the free Cheat Sheet by searching this book's name at www.dummies.com. The Cheat Sheet offers an at-a-glance reference for scoring, serving, and what you can (and can't) do in the kitchen.

Where to Go from Here

If you don't have a thorough understanding of pickleball yet, you may enjoy starting with Chapter 1 and reading your way through the book, from cover to cover. Or feel free to go straight to the topics that interest you and flip around to areas you want to focus on. Chapter 2 covers all the rules of the game, for example, and Chapter 3 tells you about the equipment you need. Chapter 12 covers intermediate and advanced strategies.

We designed this book to be a resource for you throughout your development as a pickleball player. No matter where you start reading this book, you'll find practical advice to inspire you to get to the courts and play your best!

1
Starting Out: Let the Dinking Begin!

Chapter **1**

Welcome to Your New Favorite Sport

Before coauthor Reine discovered pickleball, she was your typical work-from-home programmer leading a boring, sedentary lifestyle. Some weeks, she wouldn't leave the house for several days in a row. She felt isolated, depressed, and out of shape. Clearly, she needed a hobby! After failing to find much interest in knitting, hot yoga, soap making, or matchstick model building, something new in the adult learning class catalog caught her eye: pickleball! This sounded right up her alley. From day one of starting to play, she was hooked. She not only enjoyed the game but was also meeting a lot of interesting, fun-loving people and laughing more than she had in years. In a very short time, pickleball brought joy back into her life, transformed her health and self-confidence, and led to many close friendships.

This story is not unique to Reine. We've heard variations countless times, told by people from all walks of life. Former athletes are discovering pickleball and competing again for the first time in decades, igniting a spark they once thought was lost. Lonely folks are finding themselves immediately welcomed into a community of people who share a passion for this quirky, addictive game. Those struggling with various health issues are finding pickleball to be a safe, accessible option for getting more fresh air and exercise (definitely way more fun than using an elliptical.) The list goes on and on. Can pickleball save the world? Probably not, but there's no doubt it's saving lives.

Who's Playing Pickleball? Everyone!

Why, you may ask, would you want to get off of your comfy, custom-indented spot on the couch and go running around a tiny court chasing a plastic ball? Here's why: It's *fun!* Pickleball is pure joy. Despite its silly name, it's an amazing game. It has action, patience, surprises, athleticism, power, finesse, strategy, trash talk (all in good fun), and so much more.

The rules of the game have made it perfect for players of all ages. Does your shoulder no longer allow you to hit an overhead serve? No problem — the serve is underhand! Do you suffer from some abdominal swelling (a.k.a. overeating), or dislike running long distances? This sport is typically played as doubles on a small court, so you don't need to train for a marathon. It's not uncommon to see players of three different generations on the same court enjoying the game together, as you can see in Figure 1-1.

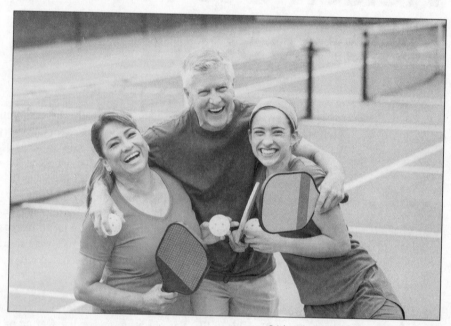

FIGURE 1-1: Pickleball is fun for everyone, young and old!

© John Wiley & Sons, Inc./Courtesy of Getty Images

The learning curve is short in pickleball, but you can spend a lifetime trying to master it. You can pick it up in less than an hour and enjoy the challenge indefinitely because there is always more to learn. Therein lies the joy for many of us. People play the game at swanky country clubs as well as small city parks, schools, and prisons. It's the same game, no matter where you play it.

Now, don't get us wrong; this sport can definitely be physically challenging, and is played by elite athletes at the highest levels. Multiple professional pickleball tours take place with amazing players who constantly push the limits of the sport. This game will continue to grow and change. One thing we can say with certainty is that pickleball is here to stay. Welcome to your new healthful addiction! (It's like having broccoli as your passion. "Pickleball" has a better ring to it than "broccoliball," though.)

In this book, we cover why people love to play pickleball, how and where to play, and the proper body mechanics for safe and effective play. We take you through all the different shots, the fine art of "dinking," and how to strengthen the mental part of the game. If you choose to advance into intermediate levels, we take you on a deep dive through improving, training, and even playing in tournaments. Pickleball is quite social, offering many different opportunities to meet new friends. This comprehensive book on the game of pickleball can serve as a handy reference tool for anything you want to know about the sport as you begin to play, play more often, possibly get addicted as so many others have, and more.

In this chapter and the rest of Part 1, you dip just briefly into the origins of this wonderful sport and then get to know the basic rules and scoring. We also cover the burgeoning world of pickleball equipment, gear, and fashion. We give you the low-down on the different kinds of courts, where to find them, and how to find people to play with. Are you a former soccer star or tennis ace? If so, you'll want to read Chapter 5 for some help with transitioning from other sports. Part 1 gives you all the information to get started in your new pickleball life.

Pickleball in a Nutshell

Created in 1965, pickleball is a hybrid of tennis, table tennis, and badminton. You play the game on a court with a three-foot high net, and the aim is to hit a perforated plastic ball over the net with a paddle (about twice the size of a table tennis paddle) in a way that prevents your opponents from returning it. At first glance, it looks a lot like tennis on a miniature court. It involves less running than tennis, which is great if your knees don't like that sort of thing. Pickleball has unique rules that place a high emphasis on precision and strategy. The sport, which has a multigenerational following, can be fast-paced and competitive. Pickleball is a fast-growing sport all over the world, with more than 5 million players and counting.

Fun and accessibility were at the heart of pickleball from the very start. It was designed to be a game that everyone could play. After players are introduced to the sport, they often find that they can't stop smiling. It's so easy to become addicted! You may find yourself waking up in the morning, looking forward to playing pickleball, possibly after dreaming about it all night. You will start looking for pick-up games anywhere you can find them — a gym, local park, tennis club — you name it. You'll start recruiting all your friends to play so that you can keep talking about pickleball nonstop without seeing them roll their eyes so much. Then you'll probably want to learn more and improve. *Pickleball For Dummies* is for anyone with the enthusiasm to step on the court, understand the rules and fundamentals, perhaps move on to more advanced strategies, and, of course, have a blast playing.

Getting Everyone in on the Act

Joel Pritchard (shown in Figure 1-2) was a congressperson from Seattle who spent summers with his family and friends on Bainbridge Island, Washington. One summer in 1965, the kids were complaining of boredom. Joel and his friend, Bill Bell, felt there must be a way to get kids and parents to play together, so Joel set out to create a new game. Failing to find enough tennis rackets, he tried four table tennis paddles and a wiffle ball. The table tennis paddles didn't work so well, so the dads crafted some larger wooden paddles to use. They started to play on the old badminton court in the yard, and the kids lowered the net to waist height. Soon there was laughter, some shrieking, and a lot of rallying back and forth. They introduced the game to another friend, Barney McCallum, and made up some rules and a scoring system (with some inspiration from badminton). From there, the game has continued to evolve to this day.

We've encountered more than one version of how the sport's unique name came about. One story from Barney McCallum claims that the game was named after Pritchard's dog, Pickles. Peggy Pritchard, Joel's daughter, points out that the dog came later, however. She says that her mother, Joan Pritchard (a competitive rower in college), came up with the name, loosely derived from the term *pickle boats* that college rowing teams use for the "odds and ends" members of their team. The "odds and ends" were much like the random pieces of equipment Pritchard had grabbed to play the new game. Whichever story rings true, the quirky name is as fun as the sport itself.

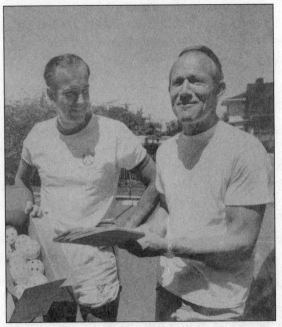

FIGURE 1-2: Pickleball pioneer and U.S. Congressperson Joel Pritchard (left) with Dan Evans, Governor of Washington (right).

Here's a quick timeline of pickleball's evolution:

» **1965:** Pickleball is created by Congressperson Joel Pritchard and his friends.

» **1967:** The first "official" pickleball court is built on Bainbridge Island, Washington.

» **1972:** A corporation is formed for the new sport.

» **1975:** Articles begin being published about "America's newest racquet sport."

» **1976:** The first known pickleball tournament in the world is held at South Center Athletic Club in Tukwila, Washington.

» **1982:** The United States Amateur Pickleball Association (USAPA) is organized to encourage the growth and advancement of pickleball on a national level, and the first official rule book is published two years later.

» **1990:** Growing exponentially each year, pickleball is now played in all 50 states.

» **1999:** The first pickleball website is launched.

» **2001:** Pickleball is introduced for the first time at the Arizona Senior Olympics.

» **2008:** The first mass-media exposure of the sport appears on ABC's *Good Morning America,* which airs a live, in-studio segment on pickleball that includes a brief demonstration.

- **2009:** The first USAPA National Tournament for players of all ages is held in Buckeye, Arizona.

- **2014:** The Pickleball Channel is launched.

- **2016:** USAPA reports 17,000 members and over 4,600 places to play.

- **2019** The Sports Fitness Industry Association 2019 report indicates that pickleball continues to be one of the fastest-growing sports in the U.S. as participants reached 3.3 million.

- **2021:** Pickleball is featured on NBC's *The Today Show,* CNBC, BBC News, and *Live with Kelly and Ryan.* Stories are published in top-rated publications including the *New York Times, Vanity Fair, Forbes, Allure,* the *Boston Globe,* the *Economist, USA Today, Sports Illustrated, Parade,* and *Axios.*

- **2022:** More than 5 million people are playing pickleball all over the world. Washington State's Governor Jay Inslee signs a bill into law that makes pickleball the official state sport of Washington.

As the preceding timeline shows, the sport of pickleball has grown gradually and steadily over the decades. As baby boomers started to retire, it grew faster, and then the pandemic hit in 2020 — and *boom!* The sport exploded. *U.S. News and World Report* said that pickleball "encouraged recreational opportunities closer to home, with participation surging by nearly 40% between 2019 and 2021." Each year, more and more people are playing pickleball all over the world.

Discovering the Benefits of Pickleball

One of the reasons we wrote this book is to set the record straight. For example, many people assume that pickleball is played only by retirees and older people. Not true! People aged four to 100 are playing pickleball. About a third of players are under the age of 25, and this number is growing steadily. Pickleball is being integrated into many schools' Physical Education programs, and a whole new generation of kids is growing up loving the game.

The many good reasons to play pickleball start with its impact on body and mind. The health benefits of regular exercise are obvious, and pickleball is a relatively low-impact sport yet provides a great workout. Your body releases endorphins while you play, improving your mood. Keeping score and devising strategies to win are enough to keep your brain engaged for hours. The significant social aspect of the sport means that it's easy to meet lots of new people — and the truth is, making new friends as an adult can be hard! Your mental, physical, and emotional well-being are all connected, and pickleball checks every box.

Here are some of the top benefits to playing pickleball:

>> **It's easier to start playing than most sports.** Sure, the scoring seems kind of quirky at first, but the barrier to begin playing is very low. Chapter 2 tells you everything you need to know to start playing real games your first time on a court.

>> **It's available year-round.** You can play the sport indoors or outdoors, in any season.

>> **You can find many places to play.** As Chapter 4 describes, you can already find courts in many parks, gyms, athletic clubs, and community centers, and many cities are busy converting basketball and tennis courts to pickleball this very minute. Resorts and residential communities are also actively adding more pickleball courts for their residents.

>> **You can easily find other players.** User-friendly online resources and handy apps help you find people to play with wherever you are, as you find out in Chapter 4.

>> **The sport is affordable.** No fancy gear is required — you just need a paddle, a ball, and a positive attitude. Playing is often free in places like public parks.

>> **You can improve your fitness.** The multidirectional movement in pickleball improves strength, balance, and agility. Quick bursts of play action provide interval-like training to boost your cardio fitness.

>> **The matches are often played quickly.** Pickleball is great for short attention spans, young and old. With quick games and rotating players, it's constant fun.

>> **It's a multigenerational sport.** Family and friends of all ages can play together. Hello, bonding!

>> **It improves social skills and boosts confidence**. Newbies are warmly welcomed onto the court to play. "We all started just like you!" can be heard on pickleball courts everywhere.

>> **You get to use your brain.** Strategy and placement rule over raw athletic speed and strength, so you can work on your pickleball game even while waiting in line at the grocery store or commuting to work.

>> **You get to channel your inner-kid.** Playing pickleball is so much *fun!* Everyone needs more fun in their lives.

This chapter gives you many great reasons to start playing pickleball right now, so read on to find out how to play. A good place to start is Chapter 2, "Playing by the Rules," which, in addition to the rules, tells you about the layout of the court, how to serve, and a few basics to get you going.

IN THIS CHAPTER

» Staying safe on the courts

» Learning the layout of the court and basic rules

» Understanding doubles, singles, and rally-style scoring

» Making fair and accurate line calls

» Diving deeper into the rule book

Chapter 2

Playing by the Rules

Have you ever arrived at a party and wished you'd read the invitation a bit more closely? First you realize it's a potluck and you've brought nothing to share. Then you begin to see that it's quite obviously *not* a costume party. Worst of all, you talked about the party earlier in the day with the birthday girl, and now everyone is hiding behind the couches, ready to yell, "Surprise!" Oopsy.

This chapter is like the fine print on the invitation. It tells you the things you need to know to be safe, understand the court and its markings, how to keep score, and a few other essentials. After reading this chapter, you can arrive at the courts calm, cool, and collected because you'll know everything you need to start playing. Time to party!

Don't wear out the pages on scoring by nervously reading them over and over again. Scoring takes a little bit of practice, and the best way to learn is by trying it. Don't stress! We have full faith and belief in you that you will learn to keep score just fine. When you get on the courts and start playing, you'll quickly get the hang of it. We typically count on the other players on the court to help us figure out the score. In fact, you'll often hear it called out as a question rather than a statement. (We once saw a player declare, "There's a score out there somewhere" and then serve the ball.) Close enough! Pickleball players are all here to help each other and enjoy playing the game together.

First Things First: Safe Pickleball Is No Accident!

In our totally unbiased opinion, pickleball is *the* most fun sport in the world. But nothing ruins the fun as quickly as an unexpected injury. The good news is that pickleball is considered a fairly safe sport. Plastic balls, lightweight paddles, and smaller courts make for a kinder, gentler way to play, for the most part. And although we don't see players falling very often, the court surface can feel pretty darn hard if you do take a tumble.

Here are some safety tips you should know before stepping onto the court:

>> **Protect your peepers.** Pickleballs are made of hard plastic and fly at very fast speeds. Getting hit with a pickleball probably won't result in more than a small bruise for most parts of your body, but your delicate eyeballs are another story. Please keep them covered at all times. Regular sunglasses or prescription glasses work just fine, or you can buy clear safety glasses at a sporting goods or hardware store. (You can find more information on protective eyewear in Chapter 3.)

>> **Wear court shoes.** Court shoes are built to provide lateral stability and movement. Running or walking shoes are designed for moving forward. There is a big difference! We get into more detail on different types of court shoes in Chapter 3.

>> **Warm up properly.** To avoid muscle pulls and cramping, always stretch before you play, and do your full warm-up routine. Chapter 10 goes into more detail on how to warm up properly and avoid injuries.

>> **Never run backward.** Not only is backpedaling a terribly inefficient way to move to the ball, it's one of the leading causes of injuries in pickleball. If you do decide to chase down the ball, turn and run in the direction it's heading (see Chapter 12 for more detailed instructions on lob retrieval). Or you can always just say "Nice shot." (If a ball is sailing high over your head, yell "YOU!" before your partner does — now you're off the hook!)

>> **Don't play on wet courts.** When testing a court to see whether it's dry, check the lines first — they are typically the slickest part of the court. Be aware of damp, shadowed areas.

>> **Call the ball.** If the ball is coming to the middle between you and your partner, be sure to communicate with each other. Yell out "Mine!" or "Yours!" Calling the ball prevents you and your partner from hitting each other while swinging simultaneously at the ball.

>> **Alert others when a stray ball goes on their court.** If you or someone on your court hits a ball that goes astray and is stealthily endangering a neighboring group of players who could step on it, please yell "Ball On!" repeatedly, until play stops. Failing to do so is not only dangerous but also a huge breach of pickleball etiquette that will earn you some wicked side eye.

>> **Know where the first-aid kit and nearest AED (Automatic External Defibrillator) are located.** Take a CPR/first-aid class and encourage other players to join you. Learn to use an AED machine, and have a plan for dealing with different types of emergency situations.

>> **Stay hydrated and know your limits.** No question about it: Pickleball is addictive. Even when you're already exhausted, you may feel the urge for just one more game. This is usually one game too many! Drink plenty of water, and consider supplementing with electrolytes if you perspire a lot or are prone to cramping.

Looking at the Layout of the Court

The pickleball court is laid out the same for both singles and doubles. It's a rectangle (ugh, who knew there'd be geometry in this book?) that measures 44 feet long by 20 feet wide. This is the same size as a doubles badminton court, or roughly one third the size of a tennis court. Along the outside boundaries of the court, you'll find the *sidelines* on the long ends and the *baselines* on the shorter ends.

The court is divided (ugh, more math?) in the middle by a net, or as we like to call her, "Annette." A real heartbreaker, Annette's measurements are 36-34-36 — she's 36 inches tall at the sidelines and 34 inches at the center. Although a pickleball net is actually 2 inches lower than a tennis net, the height relative to the size of the court can make Annette a lot like a bad ex — hard to get over!

On each half of the court is a 7-x-20-foot area directly in front of the net called the non-volley zone (NVZ), more commonly known as *the kitchen.* As the name non-volley zone implies, players aren't allowed to hit a volley (a shot hit before the ball has bounced) while in this zone. We go into much more depth on these rules later in this chapter. Historians aren't sure how the kitchen got its nickname, but one theory claims that the term was borrowed from shuffleboard.

The court between the kitchen and the baseline is divided lengthwise into two service boxes by the *centerline.* (Historians haven't spent any time researching that one.) The line that divides the kitchen from the service boxes is known as the *non-volley zone line,* or the *kitchen line.* Figure 2-1 shows the names and locations of the lines and zones on the court.

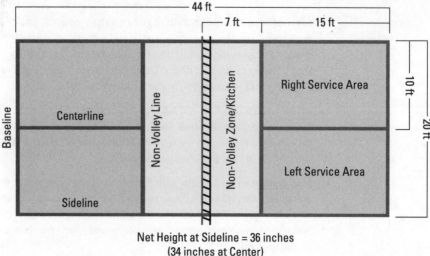

44 ft

7 ft — 15 ft

Baseline

Centerline

Sideline

Non-Volley Line

Non-Volley Zone/Kitchen

Right Service Area

Left Service Area

10 ft

20 ft

FIGURE 2-1:
The names and
locations of the
lines and zones of
the court.

Net Height at Sideline = 36 inches
(34 inches at Center)

Order on the Court: Learning the Basic Rules

As a general rule, you should learn the basic rules of a game before you attempt to play. An official pickleball rule book currently runs about 75 pages, but you don't need to commit all that to memory. The rules summary in this section helps you get out on the court and play your first few games today. Pickleball is a very social sport, so even if you don't know all the rules yet, there's probably another player on the court (or three) who are willing to help you. They were all beginners once, too, so don't be shy!

In this section, we assume that you're playing doubles, which is by far the most popular format. Later in this chapter, we explain how singles scoring differs from doubles.

Serving things up

You can't start playing a game of pickleball until somebody serves the ball. Here are the basic rules you need to know to get started serving:

>> **You must serve diagonally (crosscourt) into the service box.** Your serve must clear the kitchen and bounce in the service box that's diagonal from you, on the opponent's side of the court. If it lands on the sideline, baseline, or

centerline, the serve is considered in. If it lands on the kitchen line, it's a fault. Figure 2-2 shows the path of a serve into the correct service box.

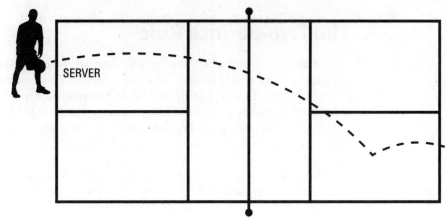

© John Wiley & Sons, Inc.

FIGURE 2-2: The path of a serve into the correct service box.

>> **The ball must go over the net.** If your serve goes into the net without going over, it's a fault. If your serve glances off the top of the net but still lands in the service box, it's good and must be played. If it touches the top of the net and lands out of bounds or in the kitchen, it's a fault.

>> **You must strike the ball below the level of your waist with a low-to-high motion.** You must serve underhand in pickleball, contacting the ball below your waist with an upward swing path. In addition, no part of your paddle may be higher than your wrist. Chapter 7 goes into more detail on service-motion rules.

>> **If serving off the bounce, you may not add force to the bounce.** You can choose to hit the ball out of the air, before it bounces, by either tossing or dropping the ball with your non-paddle hand. Or you may choose to hit it off a bounce, but in this case you cannot apply any upward or downward force to the ball. This is called the drop serve, and you can find out more details about it in Chapter 7.

>> **You must stand behind the baseline and between the imaginary extensions of the centerline and the sideline.** At the moment you strike the ball, neither foot can be inside the court boundaries, and at least one foot must be touching the ground behind the baseline (both feet can't be in the air). You can't stand way off to the side when you serve; you must be standing in the area behind the service box on your side of the court. Figure 2-2, shown previously, shows where you must stand to legally serve.

>> **You get only one service attempt.** You get just one chance to hit your serve in. If your serve goes into the net or out of bounds, you lose your serve and do not get to try again.

The Two-Bounce Rule

After a player serves the ball, the receiver must let the serve bounce before they are allowed to hit it. (Otherwise, the world would be left wondering whether that serve was going to land in bounds.) When the receiver returns the ball to the serving team, that team must also let it bounce before they can hit. After those first two shots have been allowed to bounce, any player can legally *volley*, which means to hit the ball out of the air before it bounces.

The Two-Bounce Rule is one of the genius ideas that makes pickleball great. It prevents the "serve and volley" strategy commonly used in tennis, keeping players from blasting a huge serve and immediately running up to the net to volley the next ball. For this reason, in pickleball the serving team is not considered to be at an advantage at the start of each rally.

TIP

If you have trouble at first remembering to observe the Two-Bounce Rule, just count the bounces in your head: "One . . . two . . . game on!" Another way to think about this rule is that the ball must bounce *on each side of the court* before players may volley. So after you've watched the ball bounce on your side of the court, either on the serve or return, you can forget worrying about counting those darn bounces.

Starting positions

The server is the only player required to stand in any particular place on the court when the point begins. (Actually, there is a rule stating that you must stand on your own team's side of the net, but we can't imagine why you wouldn't choose to do so). However, the Two-Bounce Rule clearly influences where the other three players should stand at the start of the point. Figure 2-3 shows the typical positions of each player when one player is serving.

Here's the breakdown for each player:

>> **The server must stand behind the baseline.** The rules state that the server must serve from behind the baseline and between the imaginary extensions of the centerline and sidelines.

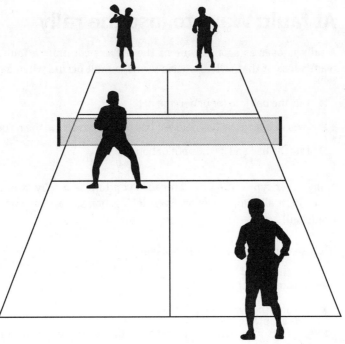

FIGURE 2-3:
The typical
positions of the
players when
starting a point.

© John Wiley & Sons, Inc.

» **The server's partner should also stay behind or near the baseline.** Again, the Two-Bounce Rule requires the serving team to let the return bounce before they can hit it. In case the return is hit deep (as we recommend in Chapter 7), both members of the serving team will want to stay back as far as possible so that they won't have to backpedal to hit the ball.

» **The receiver stands behind the baseline.** The Two-Bounce Rule requires the receiver to let the serve bounce before they can return the serve. The receiver should also stay well behind the baseline in order to more easily deal with a deep serve.

» **The receiver's partner stands up at the kitchen line.** Because the Two-Bounce Rule affects only the serving team and the receiver, the receiver's partner doesn't worry about the Two-Bounce Rule and instead focuses on being in the most offensive position at the kitchen line, ready to volley the next ball that comes to them. We go into strategy more in Chapter 11.

TIP

If you're not sure where you're supposed to be standing, remember that all players should ideally stand behind the baseline at the beginning of the point, except for the person standing directly across from the server. Also remember that when it's your partner's turn to serve, they need you back there with them. It's their big moment! Stay back and support your partner when they're serving. Only the receiver's partner should be up at the kitchen line.

At fault: Ways to lose the rally

A rally is over as soon as one of the players commits a fault, resulting in their team's loss of that rally. In basic terms, a fault occurs when a player

>> Hits the ball into (or under) the net

>> Fails to return the ball before it has bounced twice on their side

>> Hits the ball and it lands out of bounds

Many other types of faults can cause you to lose a rally, and these authors have done them all! Don't worry: Even losing points can be tons of fun — it's still pickleball!

It's also considered a fault if a player

>> Violates any of the serving rules

>> Violates the Two-Bounce Rule

>> Contacts the ball with anything other than the paddle or the hand that is holding the paddle

>> Serves or returns as the incorrect player, or from the incorrect side (see "Knowing the Score," later in this chapter)

>> Violates any of the kitchen rules (explained in the upcoming section "Non-volley zone: It's hot in the kitchen!")

>> Touches the net, net posts, or the opponent's side of the court. This rule applies to your paddle and clothing as well, which is why we've stopped playing in hoop skirts and parachute pants.

There are a few even less common ways to lose a rally, such as taking too long to return from a time-out in tournament play, but the faults in the preceding list are the main ones to worry about during recreational play.

Non-volley zone: It's hot in the kitchen!

The non-volley zone (NVZ), a.k.a. *the kitchen*, is another genius idea that makes pickleball great. If players could just lean over the net and spike the ball directly into your face, that may impede your ability to enjoy this great pastime. The kitchen makes it so that players have to stay at least seven feet away from the net if they want to hit the ball out of the air (a shot known as a *volley*).

If you think of the kitchen as its technical name, the non-volley zone, it tells you exactly what it is — a zone where you cannot volley. To be more specific, you cannot have any contact with the ball before it has bounced while you're in this zone. If anything about your volley starts, finishes, or takes place while you're in the kitchen, it's a fault. Note that the kitchen is a two-dimensional surface, not a three-dimensional space. In other words, it's perfectly legal to lean in and hit the ball out of the air from the area above the kitchen, as long as you are not touching its surface. The kitchen line and bordering sidelines are considered part of the kitchen. The out-of-bounds area adjacent to the kitchen is not.

TIP

If you see that a ball is going to bounce short in the kitchen and you can't reach it without going in, by all means *go!* You don't have to wait for the ball to bounce before you can go in — that's a common misconception. After you have gone in and made your shot, try to get back out of the kitchen as quickly as possible. Otherwise, your opponent may flick the ball right at you, forcing you to illegally contact it before it has bounced.

REMEMBER

Because the kitchen is unique to pickleball and the rules are frequently misunderstood, many new players are petrified of being anywhere near the kitchen. We urge you to let go of this irrational fear because it will only hinder your development as a player. Remember: The kitchen is not hot lava! Not only are you allowed to go in there, you will absolutely *need* to go in there sometimes to retrieve the ball. The only similarity between the kitchen and your average lava field is that you don't want to camp out in there like the player in Figure 2-4.

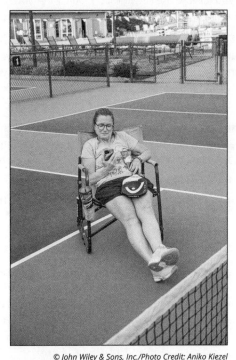

FIGURE 2-4:
Don't hang out in the kitchen!

© *John Wiley & Sons, Inc./Photo Credit: Aniko Kiezel*

WARNING

You may hear pickleballers advising each other to "Stay out of the kitchen!" Although it's a cute turn of phrase, this advice is not entirely accurate. Instead of hanging signs in the kitchen that say "Keep Out," we'd prefer more helpful signs that say, "No Loitering."

So now you know there's only one thing you can't do in the kitchen: contact the ball before it bounces. That doesn't sound so complicated, right? The confusing part for many players is understanding what qualifies as being "in" the kitchen, and in what situations it applies.

The rules define a kitchen violation (fault) as occurring when

>> **You hit a volley while any part of your body is contacting the kitchen.** Remember, the kitchen surface includes the kitchen line and adjoining sidelines. Even if just your pinky toe (the one that went "wee wee wee" all the way home) touches the very back of the kitchen line, it's a fault.

>> **You hit a volley and your momentum carries you into the kitchen.** If you initially strike the ball outside the kitchen but the momentum from the shot makes you step inside it, it's considered a fault. There is no time limit on this rule; that is, it doesn't matter if your opponents have already made their next shot (or three), or your partner smashes the next ball for a gold-medal, match-ending winner. If you haven't yet regained your balance from your earlier volley and you fall into the kitchen, it's a fault. After you have reestablished your balance, it is no longer considered part of the same shot, and you can go into the kitchen as you please.

>> **You hit a volley and touch the kitchen with your paddle.** If you lose your balance after hitting a volley and fall forward, try to avoid using your paddle to steady yourself. If your paddle makes contact with the kitchen during or after your shot, it's a fault.

>> **You hit a volley and your hat, glasses, or other gear falls into the kitchen.** If you hit a volley and your dentures fall into the kitchen, it's a fault for a variety of reasons (and one that your fellow players are unlikely to ever forget).

>> **You hit a volley and in the process knock your partner into the kitchen.** By contacting your partner in the midst of your shot, you made them a part of that shot. Nothing that you touch during the act of volleying can come in contact with the kitchen until after you have reestablished yourself outside it.

>> **After legally going into the kitchen, you hit a volley before reestablishing both feet outside the kitchen again.** This one's a little tricky to visualize, so imagine that you've stepped into the kitchen to retrieve a short, bouncing ball — knowing that you're perfectly safe because the kitchen is not hot lava — and you are contacting the ball after it has bounced. You return the

ball, but as you are in the process of hustling back out of the kitchen, your opponent hits the ball right back at you. Unless you have managed to touch both feet outside the kitchen again, you may not contact the ball out of the air. Figure 2-5 shows examples of legal and illegal volleying.

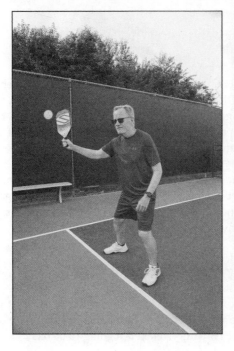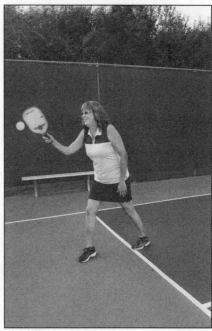

FIGURE 2-5:
A legal volleying example (left) and illegal volleying example (right).

REMEMBER

The kitchen is a flat surface defined by its boundary lines and does not include the "air space" above it or the out-of-bounds area next to it. It's legal to volley while stepping or leaping over the corner of the kitchen, as long as your feet do not touch the in-bounds surface. This is called an *Erne*. (It's actually pronounced like "Ernie," and people may suspect you're a rookie if you don't pronounce it correctly.) If you want to show off, just tell them it's named after Erne Perry. The Erne is an advanced move, so don't worry if you can't hit one just yet — you'll at least win pickleball trivia night. We discuss the finer points of hitting the Erne (and his best friend, *the Bert*) in Chapter 14.

TIP

Be honest when you break the kitchen rules. Kitchen violations in recreational play are typically called by the player who made the violation, or by their partner. The call usually sounds something like, "Oh wait, no, stop. Stop stop stop stop stop. I was in the kitchen." This declaration is often paired with a sheepish look, or in some cases a big smile, because smashing a ball from the kitchen feels really great — until you realize it didn't count! In tournaments with referees, the referees will call the kitchen violations. If you've been cheating a bit in recreational play, you will suffer in tournaments because referees are very good at spotting kitchen faults.

Knowing the Score

We won't try to sugarcoat it: Learning to keep score in pickleball can be a bit challenging at first. Although you may feel discouraged at first, we've never met anyone who quit the game because they couldn't keep score. You can do this! Scoring is a bit dry on paper but gets much easier when you start actually playing. It becomes second nature in no time.

TIP

At least one other person is always on the court. If you don't know the score, they may! Even at the most advanced levels, players frequently forget the score and have to ask their partner or opponents. Don't ever be embarrassed about losing track of the score. If anything, it will help you fit right in!

Doubles scoring: Easy as 0-0-2

In doubles, the score consists of three numbers. We know what you're thinking. "Wait, wait, wait! The score has three numbers? But there are only two teams! This is crazy. I give up!" Breathe. Relax. It's going to be okay.

The first two numbers keep track of each team's score. Easy enough, right? The third number will always be either a 1 or a 2, and it keeps track of the player who is currently serving. Each team has two players and they each get chances to serve. That third number in the score is helpful for remembering whether you're the *first server* (1) or the *second server* (2) on your team because the server keeps changing throughout the game. Now that you're breathing again, we can get into exactly how this works.

Only the serving team can score points. At the opening of the game, the first team to serve is decided by chance. In recreational play, it's typically based on a venue's house rule (such as the team standing on a particular side of the court). In tournament play, the first team to serve is usually determined by guessing a number written on the back of the scorecard.

After the first team to serve has been determined, the player on that team who is standing on the right side of the court (when facing the net) becomes the first server. This player continues to serve as long as their team is winning the rallies (meaning that the other team is the first to commit a fault and end the rally).

When the serving team wins a rally, they earn a point. When you win a point, you and your partner trade sides of the court (right and left). You never serve in the same direction (or to the same opponent) twice in a row. To remember this, just think, "When you win, you switch." It's like a do-si-do in square dancing. (We assume you're an avid square dancer, so that analogy should hit home for you.)

When the serving team commits a fault and loses the rally, the first server no longer gets to keep serving. Now it's their partner's turn to serve. (This rule has one big exception, which we introduce a little later in this section. For now, just roll with it.) This player is naturally referred to as the second server. Because the serving team didn't just win a point, however, the partners don't trade places but instead stay put. ("When you lose, you linger.")

The second server continues serving, alternating sides, until their team loses another rally. That team has now run out of chances to serve. It's the other team's turn to serve and try to win some points. Whenever the serve transfers from one team to the other, it's known as a *sideout*.

When a sideout occurs, the player who is standing on the right side of the court for the new serving team begins serving. They continue serving and winning points until their team commits a fault and loses the rally. Then their partner starts serving (from whichever side they happen to be standing on) until their team commits a second fault, resulting in a sideout back to the other team.

It is a rule that before you can serve, you must call all three numbers of the score. Call your own team's score first, your opponents' score second, and either a "one" or a "two", depending on whether you're the first or second server for that round. You'll often hear players asking each other, "Am I the 'one' or the 'two'?" This is just shorthand for asking, "Am I the first server or the second server?" If your team is ahead, be sure to call the score extra loudly for all to hear. If your team is behind, just mumble it under your breath.

REMEMBER

The first server is always the player standing on the right side of the court when the ball comes back over to that team to serve again. Just because you were the first server (the "one") a minute ago doesn't mean that you'll stay the "one" for the entire game. Don't get married to your number! It will change constantly throughout the game.

Just when this was all starting to make sense, we must also tell you that the pickleball powers-that-be decided to create an exception to the aforementioned rules, just to drive pickleball instructors (and book authors) crazy. Remember that at the opening of the game, the first team to serve was chosen at random. To make things more fair, that team gets only one chance to serve for that round, rather than the usual two. This rule prevents them from racking up a ton of points before the other team has had an opportunity to serve and score. For this reason, the opening score of a pickleball game is actually 0–0–2, not 0–0–1. As soon as the original serving team commits a fault, it's a sideout, and the other team gets to serve. From that point on, both teams get two chances to serve on every round.

Games are typically played to 11, but you must win by two points. So if it's 11–10, the game continues until someone wins by a margin of two points. We've seen games end at 20–18! In some tournament situations, games are played to 15 or even 21, but in recreational play, games to 11 are the norm.

TIP

When a game ends, players customarily come to the net and gently tap paddles, saying, "Good game!" This is an important part of pickleball etiquette, so always strive to be a good sport, whether you win or lose. See Chapter 4 for more details on pickleball etiquette.

A play-by-play example of scoring in doubles

In this section, we take you through a play-by-play demonstration of how scoring works in doubles. Figure 2-6 shows the players' positions at the very beginning of the game, with the players labeled as A, B, C, and D. The scoring seems tricky at first, but don't get discouraged. After you learn it, scoring will be a breeze. Also, as mentioned earlier, players and teams commonly ask each other what the score is because the game moves fast. When in doubt, just ask!

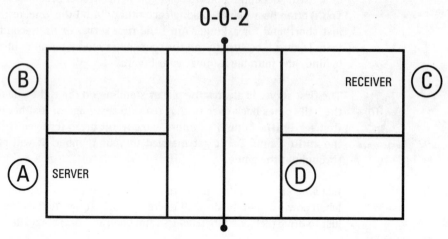

FIGURE 2-6: Note the player positions at the start of a game.

© John Wiley & Sons, Inc.

Team AB starts the game as the serving team, and Team CD is the receiving team. The game begins at 0–0–2:

>> 0 is the serving team's score.

>> 0 is the receiving team's score.

>> The "2" part of the score represents that the serving team has only one chance to serve because of that funny rule, the opening-score exception, that we mention in the preceding section. (It's as if the first serve just disappeared into thin air!)

The player on the right side of the court for the serving team (Player A) is the first server and announces the score as 0–0–2.

Player A serves the ball to Player C and a rally begins. Player D hits the ball out of bounds — and that's a point for the serving team! Player A continues to be the server, but Players A and B switch places (do-si-do) in celebration of winning a point (but also because it's the rule). Figure 2-7 shows where the players are now that the serving team has won a point.

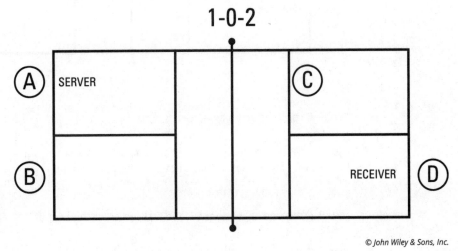

1-0-2

FIGURE 2-7: Player positions and serving direction after the first rally.

© John Wiley & Sons, Inc.

Player A now calls the score as 1–0–2:

>> 1 is the serving team's score (they just scored a point!).

>> 0 is the receiving team's score.

>> 2 represents that Player A is still considered the second server for this very first round in the game.

Player A serves again, this time from the left side of the court, to Player D. The rally begins, and Player B hits the ball into the net. Because Player A was considered the second server, or the "2," their team has run out of chances to serve. Players A and B don't trade places because they did not just win a point. No celebratory square dancing allowed!

It's now a sideout, with the serve going next to Player C, who is standing on the right side of the court for Team CD. (See Figure 2-8.)

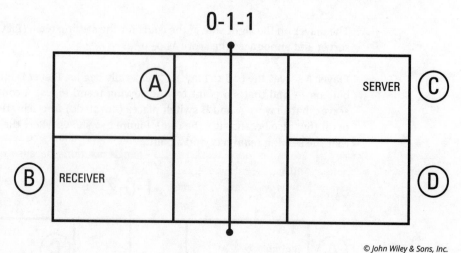

FIGURE 2-8:
Player positions and serving direction after the second rally.

Player C calls the score as 0–1–1:

>> 0 is the serving team's score. (You win points only when your team is serving, so winning that last rally did not earn this team a point.)

>> 1 is the receiving team's score.

>> 1 represents that Player C is the first server for this round.

Player C serves the ball to Player B and a rally ensues. Player A hits the ball out of bounds, which earns a point for Team CD. Players C and D switch places (do-si-do), as you can see in Figure 2-9.

Player C calls the score as 1–1–1:

>> 1 is the serving team's score. (They just scored a point!)

>> 1 is the receiving team's score.

>> 1 represents that Player C is still the first server.

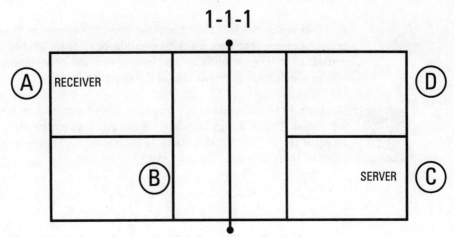

1-1-1

FIGURE 2-9:
Player positions
and serving
direction after the
third rally.

Player C serves the ball into the net. Drat! All hope is not lost, because Player C was the "1," meaning that Team CD still gets one more chance to serve, with Player D as "2." None of the players should change positions because nobody scored a point. Figure 2-10 shows how player positions stay the same but the serving direction now changes.

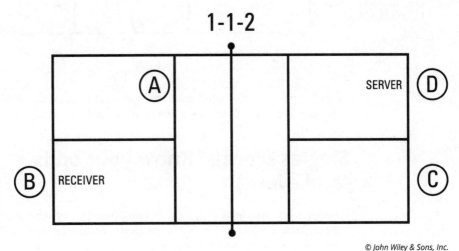

1-1-2

FIGURE 2-10:
Player positions
and serving
direction after the
fourth rally.

Player D calls the score as 1–1–2:

>> 1 is the serving team's score.

>> 1 is the receiving team's score.

>> 2 represents that Player D is the second server for this round.

Player D serves the ball from the right side of the court to Player B, who hits a smoking return that whizzes right past Player C. Team CD has lost the rally and run out of chances to serve. It's a sideout, with the serve now going to Player B, who is standing on the right side of the court.

Just because Player A served first the last round doesn't mean Player A will always serve first. Player B was standing on the right when the sideout happened, so Player B is now the "1" and starts as the server, as Figure 2-11 shows. Player B calls the score as 1–1–1.

1-1-1

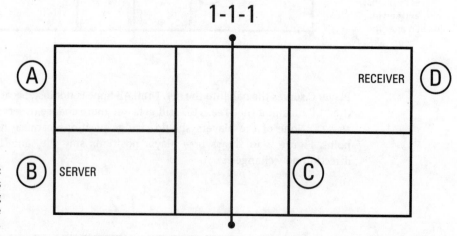

FIGURE 2-11:
Player positions
and serving
direction after the
fifth rally.

© John Wiley & Sons, Inc.

Play continues like this until one team has reached 11 points or however many are necessary beyond 11 to win by a two-point margin.

Singles scoring: Know your odds (and evens)

Keeping score in singles is quite a bit easier than doubles because the third number (explained in the previous two sections) no longer applies. Whew! However, singles scoring does require you to know the difference between an odd number and an even number. (There's that darn math again!)

The game starts at 0–0, with the starting server on the right side of the court (facing the net). The right side is known as the *even side*. Because the server's score is 0, the server should be standing on the even side.

If the server wins the rally, their score becomes 1. Because this is an odd number, the server must switch to the left side, or *odd side* of the court, and serve from there. They continue switching sides as long as the server is serving and winning.

Unlike doubles, a "team" gets only one chance to serve, which is why you can ditch the third number altogether. If the server commits a fault, it's automatically a sideout and their opponent now gets to serve. The new server should begin serving from either the even or odd side, depending on whether their own score is even or odd. The receiver should line up diagonally from the server regardless of their current score.

So if you're serving and the score is 7–2, you will be serving from the odd side of the court. Your opponent will line up to receive serve from their odd side as well. If you lose the rally and it's a sideout, your opponent will begin serving from their even side (because their score is 2) and you'll line up diagonally from them.

Just as in doubles, singles games are typically played to 11 points and you have to win by two, but the game can sometimes be played to 15 or 21 in tournaments, depending on the format.

Rally scoring: Perhaps coming to a court near you

Much debate occurs these days about possibly changing pickleball over to a scoring system called *rally scoring*, which has every rally ending with a point scored, regardless of which team served. If your team wins the rally, you get a point, plus you get to serve next. If you were already serving, you just switch places with your partner and keep serving.

If the serving team's score is an odd number, they must serve from the odd side of the court, and vice versa for an even score. When a sideout occurs, the player standing on the side that matches their team's score (meaning either even or odd) will be the server. Similar to singles scoring, the score would have only two numbers, not three.

This system has both pros and cons. Most people agree it would be simpler for new players to learn. However, the main reason for the consideration of rally scoring is that it makes match times more predictable, which helps with scheduling and televising matches. Of course, television coverage means more advertising money and attention coming to the sport. That makes for bigger pro tours, more prize money, and better odds of getting pickleball into large international events like the Olympics.

Rally scoring does make games tend to go a bit faster, which can be considered a pro or a con, depending on your point of view. However, many people feel it takes away some of the strategic nuances of the game. For instance, with traditional scoring, a first server may decide to take bigger risks, knowing their partner has a chance to serve if they make a mistake. The main argument against rally scoring seems to be that it defies tradition and erases some of the uniqueness of the sport. Change is always hard, especially with a game so beloved for its many quirks.

TIP

If you want to watch a nasty argument unfold on social media, bring up rally scoring on any pickleball forum. There are certainly some strong opinions on both sides!

Making Line Calls

Calling the ball "in" or "out" as accurately as possible is very important in pickleball. When you call lines honestly, you help to improve the integrity of this great sport.

It's both your right and your responsibility to call the balls landing on your side of the court. Your opponents must call the balls on their side of the court. Even in refereed matches in professional tournaments, the players are responsible for making line calls. (Referees are primarily there to keep score and watch for foot faults. They will provide opinions on line calls only if asked, and most of the time they choose not to overrule the original call.) Spectators are not allowed to make line calls.

Here's the golden rule for line calls: "If in doubt, you can't call it out!" In other words, if you didn't clearly see the ball land out of bounds, it's considered in. See Figure 2-12 for balls called both in and out. You need to be able to clearly see space between the line and the ball in order to call it out.

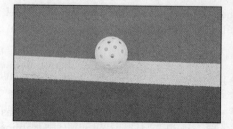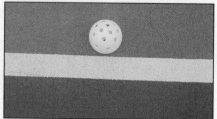

FIGURE 2-12:
A ball that should be called in (left), versus a ball that can be called out (right).

© John Wiley & Sons, Inc./Photo Credit: Aniko Kiezel

If two partners disagree on a call, the ball is considered in. The benefit of the doubt should always go to your opponent. If you ask your opponents for their opinion, you must abide by it. However, if you're so unclear that you're asking for third and fourth opinions, it means enough doubt exists that you cannot call it out. (Remember the golden rule.)

REMEMBER

If the ball lands on any line, it is in, except when the serve lands on the kitchen line. Because the kitchen line is technically part of the kitchen, the rule states that the serve must completely clear the kitchen, including the kitchen line.

You don't need to audibly call the ball in while the ball is in play. Just keep on playing and don't say anything. If it lands out, yell "out!" or signal that it was out by pointing your finger straight up in the air. *Note:* The index finger is preferred for "out" calls; the middle finger sends a completely different message.

Call the lines as promptly as possible, but not until the ball has actually bounced. Calling a ball before it bounces is considered player communication, rather than a line call, and you'll want to choose different words so as not to cause confusion. See Chapter 11 for more suggestions on player communication. It's fine to call a ball out after you've already hit it, but be sure to call it before your opponents hit their next shot. It's extremely poor form to say, "Hey, remember that shot from five minutes ago? That was actually out. Looks like I won after all!"

It's in the Rule Book! More Rules to Know

Every year, USA Pickleball (USAP) puts out a new version of their official rule book. The rules committee makes revisions each year, and keeping up with the latest changes is important. We think it's quite exciting to be part of such a young sport that continues to evolve each year! The proposed changes always generate a lot of lively discussion among players.

TIP

We recommend that you carry an up-to-date rule book in your bag at all times. To purchase an official rule book, visit USAPickleball.org. Read it all the way through at least once (preferably before bed, if you're having trouble sleeping) to familiarize yourself with how it's organized. Then hang on to it for reference in case you ever need to settle a rule dispute among friends. It's a great investment in your game, plus it supports the governing bodies of our sport.

Here are some more interesting rules you should know about as you dive deeper into the game. Some of these situations sound strange, but almost all of them will eventually happen to you as you play more:

>> **You are allowed to strike the ball twice on one hit (known as a carry), as long as it is unintentional and is one continuous motion.**

» **You can switch the paddle between hands when you're playing.** You can also hit the ball with both hands on your paddle. However, you can play with only one paddle at a time, so don't step out onto the court with a paddle in each hand!

» **Your paddle must be in your possession when it strikes the ball.** No throwing your paddle at the ball!

» **If your serve hits the receiver's partner before the ball bounces, it's your point.** This is sometimes called a "Nasty Nelson," after one particularly colorful player who was known for doing it intentionally. Hitting the receiver's partner with your serve is considered very poor sporting conduct, and lest you develop your own "nasty" reputation, we don't encourage doing it on purpose.

» **The ball has to bounce to be considered out, so don't catch balls mid-air that you believe are flying out.** Doing so will be considered a fault on your team.

» **It's legal to hit the ball around the net post without the ball actually going over the net.** This is called an Around the Post (ATP) shot. We tell you how to hit an ATP in Chapter 14.

» **If the ball bounces on your side of the court, but a strong wind (or heavy spin) causes it to fly back over the net to your opponent's side of the court, you must touch the ball before it bounces again or you lose the point.** You may reach over the net to hit the ball, as long as you don't touch the net. If you're extremely clever, you'll reach over and hit the ball straight into your opponent's side of the net to win the rally!

» **Some portable nets have a horizontal crossbar along the bottom of the net.** If your shot goes over the net and hits the crossbar on your opponent's side of the net before it bounces in the court, the point must be replayed. (If it hits the crossbar on your own side of the net, it's a fault as usual.)

» **If the ball hits the net post, ceiling, basketball hoop, or other permanent fixture before bouncing, it is considered out of bounds and is a fault on the team who hit it.**

» **A ball passing through the net cords (between the net and the post) is a fault on the player who hit it.** The ball must either go over the net or around the side of the net post to count.

» **Deliberately distracting your opponent while they are trying to hit, such as by yelling, stomping your feet, or waving your arms, is not allowed.** Although pickleball courts are rarely silent — laughing, trash talking, and strange grunts and noises are expected — there's a clear line between having fun and being a jerk.

Chapter **3**

Shifting into Gear: Equipment and Apparel

When coauthor Reine first caught the pickleball bug, she immediately went online to see what kind of pickleball "merch" was available. At the time, the choices were quite limited. Only a handful of online retailers specialized in pickleball, and no local stores carried equipment. (If you had walked into a sporting goods store and asked for the pickleball section, the clerk would have responded, "What's pickleball?") This was probably a good thing for Reine's wallet. Desperate to flaunt her burgeoning love for her new hobby, she ended up designing her own hat and t-shirts with cute pickleball puns.

Fast-forward six years, and the retail landscape looks very different. There are now countless paddle brands, clothing lines, and gadgets for pickleball enthusiasts. Almost every major sports manufacturer and retailer has jumped into the pickleball market. In this chapter, we guide you through the aisles of the pickleball retail scene. We discuss how to choose your first (and second) paddle, what types of balls to buy, and what other accessories are worth buying. Read on for the very best in pickleball retail therapy!

You Can't Take the Court without a Paddle

Without question, your most important piece of equipment when taking to the pickleball court is your paddle. Although it may feel unfamiliar the first time you pick one up, you're about to form a close relationship with this inanimate object. (Some haters may even call it inappropriately close; we choose to ignore them.) It could turn out to be a beautiful, long-term relationship — love at first smash — or a love-hate relationship if things go sour. Perhaps you've never been great at commitment and would prefer to sample everything that's out there before settling down. You do you. No judgment here.

Beginners often ask more experienced players, "Which paddle should I buy?" This is a lot like asking someone else to pick out eyeglasses or shoes for you. It all comes down to finding "the one" for you (until something newer and better looking comes along).

WARNING

We know we just said we wouldn't judge, but friends don't let friends play with wooden paddles. They are terrible for your arm and your game. They do make excellent kindling for your pickleball club's next bonfire.

Paddle standards: The long and the short of it

This section guides you toward choosing your first paddle, and in case things don't work out between you two, your next paddle (or five) as well.

You can find hundreds of paddle models out there. To help narrow down things slightly, we recommend you that purchase only a USA Pickleball–approved paddle. All approved paddles must conform to certain technical and quality standards. These standards were primarily created to ensure fairness in tournament play. Even if you don't plan to compete in tournaments, you want a paddle that maintains the integrity of the sport by conforming to the standards. You'll also be comforted knowing it has passed tests for consistency and overall quality.

When determining whether a paddle meets their approval standards, USA Pickleball looks at the following characteristics:

>> **Material:** Paddles must be made of rigid, noncompressible material. Rubber-like materials aren't allowed. The paddle can't have any moving parts, springs, electrical, electronic, or mechanical features of any kind.

>> **Surface:** The paddle's hitting surface can't have any bumps, holes, or rough sandpaper-like textures designed to add extra spin on the ball, nor can the paddle have any reflective surfaces that could affect an opposing player's vision.

>> **Length and width:** The paddle length can't exceed 17 inches, including the handle. The combined length and width of the paddle can't exceed 24 inches. So if your paddle is especially long, it has to be a bit narrower, and vice versa.

>> **Thickness:** There are no restrictions on paddle thickness.

>> **Weight:** There are no restrictions on paddle weight.

Understanding paddle technologies

As pickleball explodes in popularity, new models are being released every week. Comparing paddle features can be difficult because most brands use proprietary technologies, often with cryptic names and marketing language inevitably guaranteeing "More spin! Greater touch! Increased power! Six-pack abs! Financial independence in 90 days!"

Be careful of the hype. An expensive paddle won't magically take you from novice to pro, but the right combination of features can certainly make playing more enjoyable. It all comes down to trying different things and deciding what feels right for you.

One material we don't recommend at all is wood. When pickleball was first invented, the paddles were made of wood. We're guessing you wouldn't try to play tennis in the 21st century with a wooden racquet — and the same goes for pickleball. "Beginner sets" made of wood are a waste of money, unless you're buying them for the grandkids to destroy, which sounds fun.

The paddle's core

The first major factor to consider when testing paddle technologies is core construction. The *core* refers to the middle part of your paddle that is sandwiched between the two hitting surfaces. Cores can be solid or use a honeycomb structure. Honeycomb is popular because it provides strength while remaining lightweight (see Figure 3-1). Turns out bees really know what they're doing. Solid cores offer a greater sense of touch, but they don't tend to have the same amount of "pop" (rebound), which some players prefer.

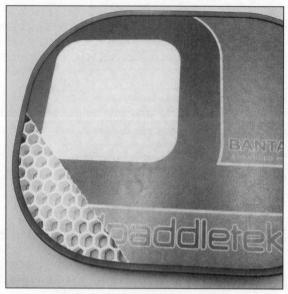

FIGURE 3-1:
Cut-away view of
a honeycomb
paddle core.

Here are the three most common types of core materials used:

>> **Nomex:** A type of cardboard dipped in resin, Nomex was the first material ever used in composite paddles and remains popular today. You get plenty of power and pop because this material is extremely hard, but it can make your shots a bit unruly.

>> **Aluminum:** Aluminum does not provide as much power but is preferred by some players for increased control and touch. One drawback is that aluminum paddles can dent easily.

>> **Polymer:** These cores are made from a plastic blend that is very durable. They tend to feel a bit softer and have a more solid hitting sensation. Polymer strikes a good balance between power and touch, and many new paddles coming out on the market today utilize this type of core.

The paddle's surface

The second factor to consider is the hitting surface. Just as with paddle cores, each type of surface has its own pros and cons. You currently have three main options when choosing a paddle surface:

>> **Graphite:** An enduringly popular choice, graphite paddles are thin, light, and stiff. The stiffness offers a lot of feel down through your hand, and this increased sense of touch is why many players prefer them. The downside of

graphite is that the sweet spot tends to be smaller, and this surface can crack or chip easily.

» **Composite/Fiberglass:** Composite paddles are softer than graphite and typically heavier. They do usually offer a larger sweet spot than graphite paddles and are more forgiving for beginners. Composite paddles are generally durable but can be prone to developing dead spots over time.

» **Carbon Fiber:** Carbon fiber is much stiffer than fiberglass and much more durable than graphite. Its high deflection rate can give you more precise control when aiming the ball. In addition, the "weave" of the fibers offers enhanced spin. Unfortunately, these paddles tend to be the most expensive.

You can also check out a few other technical features while shopping for a paddle:

» **Edgeless paddles** offer more hitting area because they lack the protruding protective edge guard that most paddles have around their outside rim. As you may have guessed, the edge guard is there to protect the paddle from chips and cracks, so you need to be a bit more careful not to drop your prized possession.

» **Unibody paddles** consist of a single molded piece of material rather than a separate paddle face and handle glued together. They offer increased feedback down through your hand, and high durability.

» **Vibration-dampening technologies** claim to reduce the risk of tendonitis by absorbing some of the shock of the ball hitting your paddle.

Picking your perfect paddle shape and grip

After you've settled on your ideal core construction and hitting surface, think about the shape of your paddle. Within the USA Pickleball equipment standards, you can still find plenty of variety in paddle sizes and shapes. (Figure 3-2 shows some different kinds of paddle shapes.)

» **Standard:** A paddle measuring approximately 16 inches long and 8 inches wide is considered to be standard shape. This shape offers a nice balance between reach and control, with an average-sized sweet spot located just above the center of the paddle face. Within this standard category, you see some variation in how the corners are shaped — squared off, rounded, or angled — that affect its aerodynamics.

» **Wide Body:** A wide-body paddle is any paddle wider than the standard 8 inches. Consequently, the length will be shorter by the same amount. Wide-body paddles can be great for beginners because they provide a large, forgiving sweet spot. They won't feel very quick or aerodynamic in your hand, though.

>> **Elongated:** A paddle with a length greater than 16 inches is considered an elongated paddle. To have extra length, you have to sacrifice the equivalent width, which means a narrower sweet spot. Elongated paddles are popular with singles players because they provide added reach.

>> **Blade Shape:** An extreme version of the elongated paddle, blades can be as narrow as 6 inches wide. To use one, you have to be pretty confident in your ability to strike the ball accurately in the center of your paddle every time. Some advanced players feel that the lever-like properties of this paddle help them to "whip" the paddle head at faster speeds.

>> **Oval:** Oval-shaped paddles are designed to mimic the shape of a tennis racquet. They have an aerodynamic feel and a centralized sweet spot. You may find you miss shots by not having any corners on your paddle, because sometimes hitting off the corner is the best you can manage!

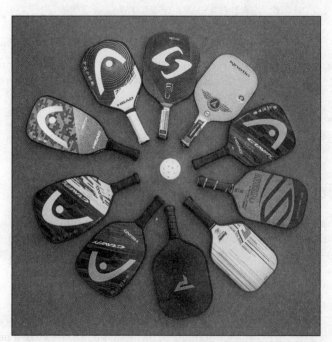

FIGURE 3-2:
Some different
paddle shapes.

© John Wiley & Sons, Inc./Photo Credit: Aniko Kiezel

Just as important as the shape of your paddle face is the size and shape of the handle (which we refer to from now on as the *grip*). We can't think of anything worse for your game than playing with a paddle that feels uncomfortable in your hand. If you pick up a paddle for the first time and it doesn't feel comfortable, immediately put it back down!

Choosing the right size and shape of grip can also help prevent stress injuries to your hand or elbow. The wrong-sized grip, either too small or too large, can cause you to resort to improper technique. (See Chapter 6 for more information on grip technique.) If you're purchasing your first paddle and want to err on the side of caution, go for a smaller-size grip. You can always replace the grip wrap with a thicker one (described later in this chapter).

When looking at grips, keep these four factors in mind:

- » **Size (Circumference):** When referring to a grip's size, manufacturers are talking about the circumference. Most grips are between 3⅞ inches and 4½ inches in circumference. You should select one based on the size of your hand. (Figure 3-3 illustrates how to measure your hand.) Measure from the tip of your ring finger to the middle crease in your palm, and choose a grip that matches this length. Again, this measurement is just a general guideline; the most important gauge is that it feels comfortable in your hand.

- » **Length:** Paddles with elongated faces have proportionately shorter handles, and vice versa. If you use a two-handed backhand, you'll likely want a paddle with an extra-long handle.

- » **Shape/Bevel:** Grip shapes vary from more flat and rectangular to more square to more rounded-off beveling. Some paddles have a larger "butt" at the end to anchor the bottom of your hand against. As far as shape, it's entirely a matter of personal preference.

- » **Wrap:** Paddle handles are typically wooden, so a rubberized wrap is added for comfort (who wants splinters?) and to help prevent your hand from slipping. Some are made from thin, smooth material, some are extra thick for added cushioning, and some have ridges (known as a contour grip) for your fingers to settle into. If you don't like your paddle's original grip wrap, you can always swap it out; see the "Grasping at grips, gloves, and overgrips" section, later in this chapter, for more on replacement grips.

Weighing your options

By now, attempting to select the perfect paddle may feel like a heavy burden. We don't mean to make light of your struggle, but we do have one more topic to weigh in on, and it's an important one: paddle weight. Here's the good news: The difference between the lightest and heaviest paddles out there is only around 2 ounces. That's about the same as 12 pieces of paper, or two AA batteries, or a large egg.

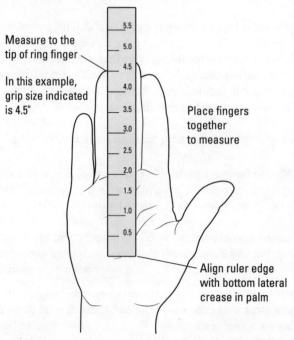

Measure to the
tip of ring finger

In this example,
grip size indicated
is 4.5"

5.5
5.0
4.5
4.0
3.5
3.0
2.5
2.0
1.5
1.0
0.5

Place fingers
together
to measure

Align ruler edge
with bottom lateral
crease in palm

FIGURE 3-3:
How to measure
your hand for the
right paddle grip.

© John Wiley & Sons, Inc.

Although the weight of an egg is hardly going to make or "break" your pickleball career, many players do have a clear preference in paddle weight. Before you shell out your hard-earned money for a new paddle, consider the following weight categories:

» **Lightweight paddles fall in the range of 6.0–7.2 ounces.** They are slightly quicker at the net and offer good control. However, you will struggle to get a lot of power when swinging a light paddle. Many beginners like to use a light paddle until they build up their strength.

» **Midweight paddles range from 7.3–8.3 ounces.** This is the most popular weight range because it offers a balance of control and power.

» **Heavyweight paddles are above 8.4 ounces.** You'll get tons of power swinging one of these beasts, but they are harder to control and can be fatiguing for your arm.

Individual paddles of the same make and model will have slight discrepancies in weight due to the manufacturing process. The difference typically equates to about the weight of three pennies. Only highly advanced players would be able to detect such a difference. In case you're the Goldilocks type, some manufacturers offer a "guaranteed weight" option when ordering.

Choosing your first paddle

Armed with all the information in the previous section, you may feel both empowered and overwhelmed. Spending weeks exploring every possible option before purchasing your first paddle is not realistic. You have to start somewhere, and it's completely normal to purchase your first paddle with plans to upgrade in a few months. As you develop your personal preferences, the choices will start to narrow. Or, most likely, you'll demo a friend's shiny new paddle one day and develop an acute case of Paddle Envy. At that point, you've made up your mind — nothing else will do!

Here are some tips for choosing your first "starter" paddle:

>> **Try some demo paddles, if possible.** By far the best way to choose a paddle is to test different models and pick the one you like the best. Paddle demo programs are often available through local pickleball/tennis shops, paddle brand reps, and online retailers.

>> **Don't assume that expensive is better.** The price of a paddle can be influenced by a lot of things, and not all them reflect its playability. You may end up hating everything about your pricey paddle and be stuck with it while you save up for a new one.

>> **Match the paddle to your personality.** Are you an aggressive competitor who enjoys pushing the limits of strength and speed? You may gravitate toward the power game. Are you a thoughtful, strategic person who prefers to be patient and wait for your moment? You may enjoy more of a controlled, soft game. Choose a paddle accordingly.

>> **Avoid extremes.** As a new player, you'd be smart to start with a midweight, standard-shaped paddle. That will give you a baseline to work from so that you'll have an easier time deciding which direction to explore next — heavier, lighter, softer, stiffer, and so on. The other advantage is that you can customize your very "average" paddle to test different characteristics. For example, adding lead tape to the outside edge will increase the overall weight and change the paddle dynamics.

>> **Make comfort your first priority.** As a newbie, you can expect to develop a few blisters and feel sore in muscles you forgot you had — no need to add to the pain by using a paddle that isn't comfortable to hold.

Choosing your next paddle

Your first paddle will always hold a special place in your heart, but it's rare for players to stick with one kind of paddle throughout their entire career. After a few months of playing, you'll have more data to work with in terms of your individual playing style and preferences. You will hopefully have had a chance to try out a few of your friend's paddles for comparison as well.

The average life of a paddle is about a year, depending on how often you play. You may start to notice dead spots on the paddle, or a sense of lifelessness. This is the perfect excuse to start thinking about your next paddle purchase.

Here are some tips for when it's time to upgrade:

>> **Take your time.** You already have a paddle, so there's no need to rush into things. Start doing some research on what's currently out there. Ask friends if you can try their paddles for a game or two. Demo the latest models, if possible. Enjoy the decision process.

>> **Match the paddle to your playing style.** By now you should have a better idea of your playing style. Are you all about powerful drives and smashes, or do you prefer dinking and the soft game? Although we advised against extremes earlier, now is the time to consider trying some specialized paddles that are just as unique as you are.

>> **Identify your shortcomings.** If your serves and drives are weak, perhaps you need a heavier paddle to give you a little extra "oomph." If you're popping the ball up too much, a softer, less reactive paddle may help calm things down. If you're consistently missing the sweet spot, perhaps you need a paddle with a larger one, or one that is placed in a slightly different spot. Of course, it's always better to fix your technique than to "buy" your way out of a problem, but none of us uses a perfect technique all the time. As your skills progress, nothing is wrong with letting your gear help, rather than hinder, your game.

>> **Consider spending a bit more.** Again, we aren't suggesting that you automatically purchase the most expensive paddle you can find. But by this time, you've probably become addicted to pickleball and are thoroughly enjoying your new, healthful pastime. Pickleball is a relatively cheap endeavor — the main expenses are shoes, balls, and club fees. If spending a few extra dollars every year on a paddle you truly love allows you to enjoy your time on the court even more, go for it. (Also be sure to tell your loved ones that paddles make great birthday, anniversary, Valentine's Day, Christmas, and Arbor Day gifts.)

Pickleball Is Nothing without Pickleballs

In describing the game to the uninformed, you may say that it uses a plastic ball with holes in it, similar to a wiffle ball. When the game was first invented, it did in fact use a wiffle ball. However, a modern pickleball is quite different, from the shape of the holes down to the type of plastic.

Ball standards: It's not a wiffle ball!

Pickleballs are highly engineered and must conform to strict standards to be USA Pickleball–approved. Manufacturers have spent a lot of money on research and development to try to come up with the perfect pickleball.

An approved pickleball must have between 26 and 40 holes. It's made of plastic that's molded with a smooth surface and free of texturing. It must be one uniform color except for identification markings. The most common colors are yellow, neon green, white, and orange. In recreational play, players typically write their name or initials on their balls with permanent marker.

To receive the USA Pickleball Approved stamp of approval, balls must weigh between 0.78 and 0.935 ounces and measure between 2.87 and 2.97 inches in diameter. This is just slightly larger than a tennis ball. Bounce height and compression are also important because these greatly affect playability, and they are measured under highly specific conditions.

Counting the holes: Indoor versus outdoor balls

Balls are manufactured a little bit differently for indoor play versus outdoor play. (See Figure 3-4 for a look at both.) When playing outdoors, you have to deal with wind and more abrasive court surfaces, usually asphalt or concrete. (Indoors, we still try to blame our mistakes on the wind, but everyone knows that's lame.) Indoor courts are typically very smooth, wooden gymnasium floors. These tend to absorb more energy from the ball.

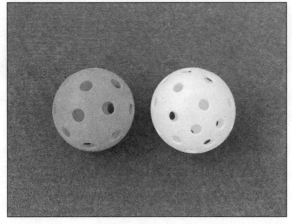

FIGURE 3-4: An indoor ball (left) versus an outdoor ball (right).

© John Wiley & Sons, Inc./Photo Credit: Aniko Kiezel

Some indoor venues, such as indoor tennis courts, have outdoor surfaces. In those venues, the outdoor balls usually perform better than the indoor balls.

The main differences between indoor and outdoor balls are the number of holes, type of plastic, and total weight. Table 3-1 explains these and other differences between indoor and outdoor balls.

TABLE 3-1   ## Comparing Outdoor and Indoor Balls

Outdoor Balls	Indoor Balls
Slightly heavier (~0.9 oz)	Slightly lighter (~0.8 oz)
Slightly larger in diameter	Slightly smaller in diameter
Harder plastic	Softer plastic
Smaller holes, and more of them (usually 40)	Larger holes, and fewer of them (usually 26)
Easier to hit hard	More difficult to hit hard
Harder to control	Easier to control
More painful when it hits you (duck!)	Less painful when you take a shot to the body
More breakable; prone to going out of round	Less breakable
Noisier	Quieter

WARNING

Don't store your pickleball gear, especially balls, in your garage or car. They are very affected by temperature. Heat can cause them to melt slightly and go out of round. Severe cold makes the balls brittle. To be safe, just sleep with all your pickleball gear in your bed, snuggled with you, as we do.

Getting touchy feely: Hard versus soft balls

Some pickleballs are harder than others. The past decade has seen a great debate about using harder, less forgiving balls versus softer, easier-to-control balls. Some high-level players find that the slicker, harder, faster ball makes the game more challenging. Other players prefer the slower pace and extra "touch and feel" provided by softer balls.

Here are examples of "hard" outdoor balls currently on the market:

- Franklin X-40
- Dura Fast 40
- TOP
- CORE
- Selkirk SLK Competition
- Engage Tour

Examples of "soft" outdoor balls currently on the market:

- Penn 40
- ONIX Fuse G2
- ONIX PURE 2
- Wilson TRU 32
- Selkirk SLK Hybrid

Deciding which balls to buy

Pickleballs typically cost between $2 to $4 each. You have many brands of balls to choose from, with more coming out all the time, but don't feel overwhelmed! The easiest answer is to just purchase the same ball the players around you are using. If everyone at your club uses the Penn 40 and you show up with Dura Fast balls, things could get awkward. Indoor venues often provide the balls, but this isn't always the case, so be prepared with at least one indoor ball in your bag.

If you want to purchase your ideal ball for recreational play, choose a ball that pairs nicely with your style of play. If you struggle to control the ball, or enjoy slower-paced games, you may want to pick a softer ball. If you enjoy faster-paced rallies, choose a hard ball. If you're on a tight budget, consider purchasing softer balls because they will last longer. Many players in cold climates purchase harder balls in the summer and softer balls in the winter because the cold temperatures cause the hard balls to break easily.

WARNING

We strongly recommend that you buy only balls that have been tested and approved by USA Pickleball. Many cheap imitations out there just won't bounce right or stay round for more than a game or two.

TIP

If you're getting ready to compete in a tournament, find out ahead of time what ball it will be using so that you can practice with that brand.

Pickleball Fashion (an Oxymoron?)

There are no strict guidelines for pickleball fashion, and further in this section we go into that wacky world. Safety and comfort are a must, of course. But first, a little story. The first-time coauthor Carl set out to play pickleball, his loving wife blocked him from going farther down the stairs. She did this in the name of decency, or so she says. He happened to be wearing his very favorite, perfectly broken-in t-shirt. (So what if the t-shirt had 11 holes and perspiration stains?) His wife mentioned he may want to wear clean, suitable clothing for his pickleball debut. He did not have to be a fashionista, but come on! Carl sighed, grudgingly changed his shirt, tied his shoes properly, and set off. Crisis averted.

From the catwalk to the courts

Although celebrities are playing and falling in love with pickleball in growing numbers, we really don't see Anna Wintour of *Vogue* promoting the fashion of the sport anytime soon. The beauty of pickleball lies in its simplicity, and that principle also applies to "What do I wear to play?" As with any sport, it's important to wear clothing with safety in mind.

Pickleball apparel has two requirements: 1) comfort and 2) climate-appropriateness. In addition to t-shirts and shorts, you often see tennis or golf-style clothing and other athletic wear with wicking properties. Hats, visors, and sweatbands can complete your ensemble. If it's cold, sweatpants, sweatshirts, light jackets, and puffy vests are totally acceptable. In tournament play, doubles teams often wear matching outfits. This is meant as an intimidation tactic to make you think, "That team really has it together!" It's also just fun to be matchy-matchy with your buddy.

REMEMBER

A rule we're glad to see incorporated into the rule book is Rule 2.G.2, which states, "Depictions, graphics, insignias, pictures, and writing on apparel must be in good taste." Remember, courtesy is important.

In addition to the apparel basics, get ready for the wide, wacky, and wonderful world of pickleball fashion. This is a world where crazy t-shirt puns, bright shoes, silly socks, and zany visors are fairly common. Just imagine neon shorts with bright-green pickleballs all over them, paired with a t-shirt that says *Pickleball Ninja*, topped off with a tie-dyed bucket hat (ninjas love tie dye) and, well, you get the idea. (We think the editor of *Vogue* will cringe, but she'll have to "dill" with it.) One of our favorite t-shirts says "Adulting can wait. Let's play pickleball!" Figure 3-5 shows just a few examples of the many fashion statements in pickleball land.

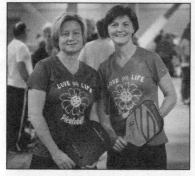
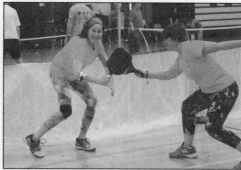
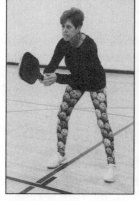
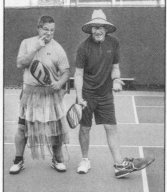
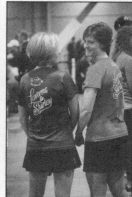

FIGURE 3-5: Players expressing their individuality and creative pickleball spirit!

© John Wiley & Sons, Inc./Photo Credits: David Tedoni (bottom center: Aniko Kiezel)

As you can see from the previous "fashion" examples, pickleball is all about playing safely, comfortably (okay, maybe not the rainbow tutu), and then hitting the courts and having tons of fun! Pickleball and humor go together like green eggs and ham.

Sliding into suitable shoes

How well you move on the court is directly related to the shoes you wear. A well-fitting, quality court shoe will help you glide effortlessly across the court. All court shoes offer heightened durability, stability, and comfort compared to a typical athletic shoe like training or running shoes. Proper court shoes are stiffer, more stable, and specifically designed for those tricky lateral moves that are inherent to pickleball play.

Running shoes are designed to only go in one direction — forward. Attempting to zigzag around the court in running shoes can cause you to roll an ankle or otherwise trip and fall. Never, ever play in sandals, knobby-soled shoes such as hiking boots, or bare feet.

The soles of court shoes are designed to grip court surfaces better, which is useful for quickly taking off in any direction. Speaking of soles, make sure that you get indoor court shoes if you're playing on wooden gymnasium floors. Indoor court shoes usually have a beige gummy sole that helps grip ultra-smooth floors. Unfortunately, those gummy indoor soles wear down very quickly on abrasive outdoor courts. So if you play on both types of surfaces, you should definitely consider getting dedicated pairs of indoor and outdoor shoes.

If you're playing indoors on a wooden floor, you'll find that the dust on the floor can build up on the soles of your shoes. The way to make them grippy again is to moisten them. If you aren't a dainty type, just wipe your sweaty palm on your soles and they will immediately become grippy. If you are more refined, keep a lightly damp towel courtside.

For outdoor play, look for tennis, pickleball, or outdoor basketball shoes. Suitable indoor court shoes may be sold as badminton, racquetball, indoor basketball, or volleyball shoes. Don't assume that the brand you bought last year still fits exactly the same this year; manufacturers constantly change sizing and fit.

Headwear for form and function

Pickleball headwear ideally needs to be lightweight, breathable, and washable. Many styles include wicking for maximum comfort while you're sweating out your big match. Some players prefer visors over hats, but either way, headwear is primarily about protecting your eyes from the glare of the sun (or indoor court lighting). If you're playing on a sunny day without sunglasses or a hat, you're basically wearing a sign that says, "Please lob me!"

Hats and headbands are also useful for keeping hair and sweat out of your eyes when playing. Windy days are bad enough for pickleball without your hair repeatedly whipping across your face. Then there's the dreaded "sunscreen-induced blindness" caused by sweating off the sunscreen you so responsibly applied to your forehead that morning.

Please, if you're without hair on top of your head, choose a hat over a visor or headband. Skin cancer is no joke.

GETTING THE MOST OUT OF YOUR PICKLEBALL SHOES

If you want to get the most out of your pickleball shoes, wear them only for pickleball. If you wear them for yard work and then traipse through mud to get to the courts, you drag dirt onto the court. (We don't want you to end up with the nickname "Pigpen.") Even worse, you're rapidly wearing down your shoes by making them do a job they weren't designed to do. This is especially true for your indoor court shoes. Dirty indoor soles cause slip-and-fall injuries. No bueno! If you really want to keep your indoor shoes pristine, wear different shoes from your house to the gym, and change into your pickleball shoes after you're inside.

Shoes are probably one of the biggest expenses in this affordable sport. You'll need to replace them about every 6–12 months, depending on how often you play and how rough the courts are. Some manufacturers guarantee their shoes for a certain length of time, so if you're playing a ton or are particularly rough on your shoes, look for brands that come with a warranty.

Here are some signs that it's time to purchase a new pair of shoes:

- The tread has completely worn down in one or more spots.
- The leather has holes or splits. (This typically occurs on the sides, where the upper and lower parts of the shoe are glued together.)
- Your feet hurt more than usual after you play.
- You find yourself slipping and sliding on the court.
- Your shoes smell so bad that your roommate makes you keep them outside.

If the tread on your shoes still looks good but you find that your shoes aren't quite as comfy as they used to be, you can replace the insoles with a quality aftermarket pair for about $30–$50. This should extend the life of the pair for a couple more months, but don't push your luck too long or you could end up with an injury.

You'll see hats in every color of the rainbow, or even the whole rainbow on one hat. Baseball caps, bucket hats, beanies, and floppy sun hats are all very common. Headwear is a great way to create a signature look that makes you recognizable everywhere you play. We've even seen sombreros on the court, but you have to be pretty darn confident in your skills to pull that off. Pro tip: Use the chin strap if you play in the sombrero. Learn from our mistakes.

Protective eyewear: Still cheaper than your co-pay

Wearing protective eyewear while playing should be nonnegotiable. We've seen people get hit in the eye and have permanent damage because of it. We can't think of anyone who wants to impair their vision. Typically, it's not a ball hit directly by your opponent, but one ricocheting off your own (or your partner's) paddle that finds its way to your face.

To avoid injury, simply cover your eyes with protective eyewear, sunglasses, or corrective glasses. Sporting goods stores sell athletic eyewear in the racquetball, pickleball, or shooting sections. Some come as a set with interchangeable lenses in different tints. If you're on a really tight budget, you can pick up safety glasses from a hardware store for under $5. Any kind of sunglasses, from cheap drugstore ones to designer frames, will protect you as well. Just keep those eyeballs covered!

If you wear prescription lenses, eyewear manufacturers offer custom sports glasses in many styles. Many players play in their everyday glasses, including bifocals and trifocals. Some can play with them just fine, but if you find that you're struggling to strike the ball on the sweet spot of your paddle, the problem may be your bifocals. See Chapter 10 for more on dealing with vision issues.

TIP

If you sweat a lot, you may need glasses that have extra ventilation and don't fit super snugly against your face to reduce fogging. You may also want to throw some anti-fog glasses cleaner and a cleaning cloth in your bag.

WARNING

We've seen some players wear eyeglass frames with the lenses popped out. Although this approach is probably better than nothing, it doesn't offer full protection for your delicate eyeballs, so we can't recommend it. Whatever glasses you get, they need to be comfortable so that you won't be tempted to play without them. We recommend that you invest a little more in a stylish, high-quality pair that you don't mind wearing (and that won't negatively affect your game). Please be proactive and protect your peepers, people!

Going Gaga for Gadgets and Accessories

As with most sports, pickleball enthusiasts tend to love their gadgets and gear. You can make pickleball a very inexpensive sport to play, or you can spend every available dime on more gear. It's totally up to you! (If you have a significant other, they may have an opinion on this as well, but that's between the two of you.)

Bag it up

You'll definitely want a bag of some sort to carry your gear to and from the courts. Players use all types of bags — totes, backpacks, sling bags, and tennis or racquetball bags. Of course, if you want to up your "cool factor," a pickleball-specific bag is both hip and functional. (We may have just ruined our credibility regarding the "cool factor" by using the word "hip.")

Here are some features you may want in a pickleball bag:

» **Multiple pockets of varying sizes:** Nobody wants to spend ten minutes digging through a cavernous bag to find their asthma inhaler. Most of us appreciate having multiple pockets so that we can find things easier. Then there's coauthor Mo, who is just confused by too many pockets and can never remember where she stashed anything.

» **A padded paddle compartment:** A padded compartment is the perfect way to keep your precious paddle(s) safe without needing separate paddle covers. You also get the satisfying feeling of slipping your paddle into its "holster" at the end of a hard play session.

» **A separate and vented shoe compartment:** You'll want one of these to keep your smelly shoes away from your less smelly stuff.

» **An insulated area to keep your cold stuff cold:** Nothing perks you up like warm, greasy salami on tournament day. If you're planning any long days or hot afternoons at the courts, an insulated area in your bag is a great feature.

» **A hook to hang your bag on the fence:** In our opinion, this is an absolute must. If your bag doesn't come with a hook but has some sort of top loop or handle, you can always add your own carabiner.

TIP

Get a bag that is just big enough for what you actually want to carry to the courts. If you get a giant bag, you will most likely fill it with things you don't really need. That means more wear and tear on your body every time you have to hoist that thing like a soldier in boot camp. A smaller bag also makes stuff easier to find. For tournament play, a larger bag can be very helpful, however. ("See, honey? I do need two bags!") You may need clothing changes, towels, food, an extra paddle, and room for all your medals.

Grasping at grips, gloves, and overgrips

The original factory grip on most paddles is just fine. It will get you going and stay nice and tacky — until it doesn't anymore. Friction from repetitive use, sweat, and dirt will cause your grip to become less tacky over time.

Instead of tossing your paddle, try one of these solutions:

» **Replace the original factory grip.** You can purchase either the same or a different grip for around $10. Some great videos online show exactly how to replace your old grip. If you purchase from a local tennis/pickleball shop, ask them to wrap it for you.

» **Try a contour grip.** One option to consider is to replace your grip with a contour grip. This is a style of grip that has raised ridges to fit your fingers into. Many players like the feel of the contour grip because it helps give them a more consistent hand position.

» **Add an overgrip.** The most popular and economical way of dealing with slippery grips is the addition of an overgrip. They are thin wraps that go over your regular grip. They absorb sweat and add tackiness. You can find videos online that show you how to apply an overgrip.

» **Wear a glove.** Many players choose to wear a glove to keep their hand from slipping. We find that wearing a glove may sacrifice some of the "feel" you need to finesse your shots. If you do wear a glove, make sure it fits well, tending toward being slightly tight. Shop for pickleball, racquetball, or golf gloves.

» **Try a grip-enhancing product.** Many products are on the market that help absorb sweat and improve tackiness. You can use a liquid or powder grip enhancer, such as those used by gymnasts and weight lifters. You can also try a tacky towel, much like what woodworkers use to remove sawdust from their projects.

Unpacking the world of portable nets

If you're playing on a court that doesn't have a permanent net installed, you'll need a portable net. These can range in price from $100 to over $2,000. At 215 pounds, the Douglas Premier net isn't really all that portable, but it's amazingly sturdy and better than many permanently installed nets. PickleNet makes several popular models that won't break the bank. For a lightweight net that assembles quickly, the SwiftNet 2.1 is considered by many to be the top choice.

When shopping for a portable net system, consider the following features:

» **Weight:** If you're carrying the net to the courts every time you play, you want a lightweight net. If the net will be left up all the time, you want a sturdier, heavier net that won't blow over with the slightest breeze.

>> **Dimensions:** If you plan to use the net for regular games on a standard-sized court, double-check that the net you're buying is regulation width (22 feet). Mini or half-court nets are available if you're just using them for practice sessions.

>> **Frame construction:** Almost all nets are made of powder-coated steel or aluminum. Most nets have horizontal crossbars along the bottom, but the shape and placement varies. Almost all regulation-sized nets have a solid vertical center rod that maintains the 34-inch net height in the center.

>> **Assembly time:** When shopping for a portable net, you see that nearly all of them claim to be quick and easy to set up. Generally, the fewer parts, the better. We find that the PickleNet and SwiftNet nets are relatively quick and don't require an engineering degree to assemble.

>> **Wheels:** If you're looking for a net that will be left inside a gym or other multiuse facility, get one with wheels on it. With luck, the nets can simply be moved out of the way when not in use. Wheels add weight (as well as cost and assembly time), so if you're setting up and taking down the nets frequently, don't get one with wheels.

>> **Replacement net availability:** Nets take more abuse than you may think. Between all the setup and takedown, balls pummeling the nets at high speeds, players running into them, and harsh outdoor elements, you will need a replacement net long before the frame wears out. A temporary net left permanently outdoors will be looking pretty sad after about a year. Find out whether the manufacturer of your net system sells replacement nets, and if so, how much they cost.

Investing in a ball machine

One of the tools that can help a player improve is a ball machine. A ball machine launches pickleballs over the net repeatedly, allowing you to practice certain shots over and over. It can be a fun and efficient way to work on your game, either with friends or by yourself.

The three most popular ball machine brands are Pickleball Tutor, Lobster, and Simon. Ball machine prices range anywhere from $700 to well over $2,000, depending on the brand, accessories, and features you choose.

Here are aspects to consider when buying a ball machine:

>> **Portability and weight:** Remember that this is probably going to be a solo activity, so it will be up to you to get it in and out of your car and transport it from the parking lot to the court. Some ball machines have wheels, but if you

have a long distance to go, you may want a separate hand cart or wagon to make it easier.

>> **Battery versus AC power:** Battery-powered machines are extremely convenient, but make sure the battery has enough capacity to last your desired length of session. AC-powered machines are great if you have a nearby outlet.

>> **Spin capabilities:** Some models give you the ability to add top-, back-, or side-spin to the balls it feeds.

>> **Number of speeds:** For a well-rounded game, you want a machine that can feed the ball at varying speeds.

>> **Remote control:** The ability to start or stop the machine from a distance prevents wasted feeds. It's also a nice safety feature if you need to suddenly stop the machine for any reason.

>> **Oscillation:** A non-oscillating machine feeds balls in the same direction until you physically move it. An oscillating model shoots balls to one side of the court and then the other, which is especially great if you're practicing with a friend or want to work on your footwork.

>> **Capacity:** The more balls the machine can hold, the longer you can practice without having to stop and pick them up.

WARNING

Ball machines are a great practice tool, but they have limitations. They aren't always as accurate as we'd like them to be when practicing a very specific shot. Don't expect to be fed the exact same ball every time. Also, they can get jammed easily. Ball machines can potentially be dangerous: Don't ever walk in front of a ball machine that is running.

Buying equipment locally and online

Now that you have a serious wish list going for pickleball gear, where do you buy it? Obviously, if you live in an area with few brick-and-mortar sporting goods stores, you'll probably need to shop online. The major online retailers are Pickleball Central, Total Pickleball, Pickleball Galaxy, Fromuth Pickleball, and Amazon. You can also purchase directly from the manufacturers' websites. Some online retailers will let you try paddles, or offer you a free return if you don't like the paddle you bought.

Large sporting-goods chains are starting to clue in to the pickleball craze, and we're seeing more equipment available there. However, these chains typically carry only one or two brands, so your selection will be limited. The staff is also unlikely to know enough about pickleball to guide you in any way.

PICKLEBALL RETAIL THERAPY: MORE FUN ACCESSORIES

There are dozens of other pickleball-related items that you may want to purchase to overstuff your pickleball closet, garage, or warehouse.

Here are some of our favorites:

- **Suction cup ball retrievers:** If your back goes out more often than you do, you may try adding a rubber suction cup ball retriever (such as the PickleUpper) to the handle of your paddle. This contraption allows you to pick up a ball without having to bend over as far.

- **Rolling ball collectors:** If you *really* don't want to bend over, and you have a lot of balls to pick up (such as when using a ball machine), try the Kollectaball. It looks like a Bingo hopper on a stick, and it "sucks up" pickleballs as you roll over them. Not only is it great for picking up a lot of balls quickly, it's really fun to use, which means you may be able to use the Tom Sawyer approach to convince others to pick up the balls for you.

- **Tube-style ball collectors:** You can also try a tube-style ball collector. Coauthor Mo has even made her own out of PVC pipe and zip ties, but she's exceptionally clever — just ask her. You can easily find these for purchase online or at your local paddle sports retailer. Franklin and Tourna make popular tube models.

- **Pickleball pouches:** For those of you who want to carry a few balls on you at all times but don't have pockets in your stylish pickleball clothes, you should check out the Ballszie or the Handy Hopper. These pouches strap around your waist with a lightweight belt and can hold up to a few dozen balls.

- **Start Rite Grip trainer:** If you're struggling to maintain a proper grip (that is, constantly sliding your hand all over your paddle in what we call the "Eastern Western Southern Northern Grip"), you may want to invest in a Start Rite Grip Trainer. It helps to lock your hand in place so that you can be all continental, all the time.

- **The Tourna Hot Glove:** To keep your paddle hand nice and warm in the winter, try the Tourna Hot Glove, which is a fleece mitt that fits completely over both your paddle hand and handle. Your hand will stay warm without losing any of the feel you're accustomed to.

(continued)

(continued)

Cooling towels, targets, cones, scoreboards, paddle covers, misting fans, water bottles, and sunscreen should fill up your available storage space nicely, but rest assured: There's always more stuff you can buy, but very little that you actually need in order to play pickleball.

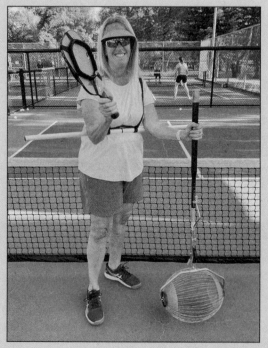

© John Wiley & Sons, Inc./Photo Credit: Mo Nard

Our favorite option for purchasing gear is to support local small businesses. You get the best-quality service and your dollars stay in your community. There are most likely players and dealers in your area who represent various brands and allow you to purchase paddles from them directly on the courts. Small tennis/paddle sports shops are a great place to shop, too, because they usually have demo paddles to check out. They are also fine places to try on and buy court shoes.

REMEMBER

You can spend as much or as little as you want on gear. Pickleball is a very affordable sport. If you have a decent paddle, a ball or two, good stable court shoes, and eye protection, you are ready to hit the courts!

Chapter **4**

Heading to the Courts

A s a beginning player, you are totally focused on getting the ball over the net; we get that. In this chapter, however, we broaden your view of the sport and help you understand the different kinds of courts to play on, the etiquette of pickleball, and some particularities (or maybe peculiarities) of this sport.

Depending on where you live, you might have dozens of different venues to choose from when you start to play. It can seem overwhelming at first to figure out where to play, what time, and with whom. On the other hand, your town may have only one or two established clubs, and you may feel intimidated about being the new guy or gal. As a new player, finding your niche can sometimes take a little time. The good news is that with the exploding popularity of the sport among people of all ages, genders, backgrounds, and athletic abilities, you're sure to find a tribe (and build some amazing new friendships along the way).

Through familiarizing yourself with pickleball etiquette and culture, you'll gain the confidence to visit new venues and become a pickleball chameleon, ready to mingle and fit in with all kinds of groups. (Or at least you'll know, "It's not me, it's them" if you aren't digging the vibe at certain courts.) The global pickleball community is full of wonderful, friendly people with an enthusiasm for sharing the game they love. Don't be scared to jump in with both feet!

It's All About That Court, 'Bout That Court

Now, armed with your paddle and ball, you want to find a court so that you can actually play. But you might find it helpful to understand the differences in courts — whether the court is indoor, outdoor, dedicated, multiuse, public, or private. The topic really is not that complicated, and we simplify it so that you can find the right court environment that works for you. We also happen to know plenty of pickleball players who will play on any kind of court, anytime — just to play!

Keep in mind that no matter the court, some elements of the game remain the same:

>> The court dimensions are always 20 feet wide by 44 feet long.

>> The net height is the same: 36 inches at the sidelines and 34 inches at the center.

>> The rules are the rules — they always stay the same.

See Chapter 2 for more information on court specifics.

Playing on outdoor courts versus indoor courts

There are three main (and fairly subtle) differences between outdoor and indoor courts: the environments; the balls used; and the court surface. Although playing on both kinds of courts involves a learning curve, making the transition back and forth between them becomes easy after you understand the different characteristics of each.

>> **The physical environment of the courts is different.** On outdoor courts, the sun, wind, haze, mist, dampness, shadows — you get it — can affect play. Even a gentle breeze can affect how and where the ball travels, despite your best intentions. With the wind behind you, for example, you barely have to hit the ball to send it sailing to your opponents, or worse, beyond their baseline. If it's blazing hot, you need sunglasses and a hat or visor, and you need to make sure you stay properly hydrated. Assess the weather factors each time you set out to play. (See Figure 4-1 for an example of an outdoor court.)

On the other hand, some people prefer playing on indoor courts because the experience is more consistent. The lighting is usually bright, and none of those pesky weather conditions is an issue. Depending on the acoustics of the indoor courts, playing indoors can be much louder than outdoor play. The biggest complaint about playing indoors is that gymnasium-type facilities have their floors lined for basketball, volleyball, badminton, and pickleball. That's a lot of lines! It can be quite difficult to call the lines when you're looking at a court like that. Finding and holding your position at the kitchen line with so many other lines nearby can also be a challenge. Just remember that it's the same game, so have fun! (Figure 4-2 shows a dedicated indoor court and Figure 4-3 shows a multiuse indoor court.)

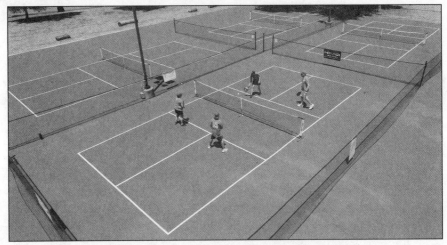

FIGURE 4-1:
Enjoying the pickleball life on an outdoor court.

WARNING

We recommend that you never, ever, ever play on wet courts; they are a hazard for slipping and falling. Yes, you can sing in the rain, but please, please don't play pickleball in it!

The best you can do is to be aware of the variations in playing pickleball outdoors and indoors. The availability of outdoor and indoor courts will vary too, of course, depending on where you live or travel. Always pack your paddle!

» **The pickleballs used outdoor versus indoor are different.** Outdoor balls, engineered to minimize wind disruption, are harder, heavier, and have 40 holes. (Don't make the mistake of one of the authors and get so excited about buying new balls that you order the pretty-colored but cheap ones online that barely bounce after three plays.) On the flip side, indoor balls are softer, lighter, and have 26 holes that are slightly larger than their outdoor cousins'. (See the section in Chapter 3 about counting the holes and other minutiae on balls, if you're that sort of person.)

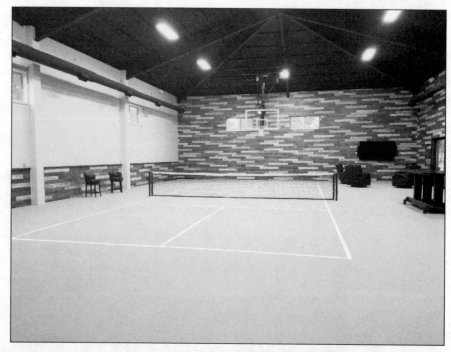

FIGURE 4-2:
An indoor court lets you play rain or shine!

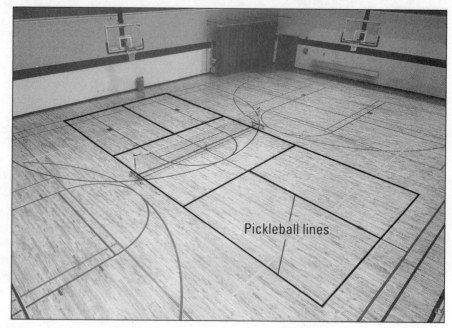

Pickleball lines

FIGURE 4-3:
A multiuse indoor court shows lines for different sports.

>> **The surfaces differ on outdoor and indoor courts.** An outdoor court has an asphalt or a concrete surface. The ball tends to bounce lower and move faster, which means that you have to react more quickly and bend your knees more to make good returns. On indoor courts, the surface is usually like a basketball court with a more flexible wooden surface that is kind to your knees. These same gentle floors can also be quite slippery, glossy, and reflective. You'll want a nice "sticky"-soled indoor court shoe to avoid slipping; see Chapter 3 for more details about shoes. Playing on an indoor court means slower-moving balls and longer rallies back and forth; also, the shots will travel exactly where you send them because of the lack of wind.

A rare find is an indoor facility that has an outdoor surface. Basically, this is an indoor area where the facility has installed asphalt tennis, Futsal (a type of soccer), or, better yet, dedicated pickleball courts. If you happen to find one of these gems, use an outdoor ball because it will perform better on the more abrasive surface.

As a budding pickleball player, you likely have plenty of options on where to play. You'll quickly discover whether you prefer playing pickleball on outdoor or indoor courts, or are fine with both. Read on, Grasshopper, to learn the differences between dedicated and multiuse courts, and public-versus-private courts.

Playing on dedicated versus multiuse courts

Dedicated courts are always the ideal place to play because you don't have to compete for time with other sports, (tennis and basketball, for example), and the lines are clearly marked and easy to see. After you have played on a dedicated pickleball court, it's hard to go back.

On multiuse courts, players can sometimes find all the different lines confusing. Many multiuse courts require you to bring your own net (see Chapter 3 for tips on buying one). Others utilize the existing tennis net, which you can lower using an adjustable strap in the center. Most parks provide these on multiuse courts, or you can purchase a net height adjustment strap from a pickleball equipment supplier.

The advantage to multiuse courts is accessibility. Many local Recreation and Parks departments choose to include multiuse courts in their facilities so that they can appeal to a wider audience playing different types of sports. Because the pickleball craze is relatively new, it's much quicker and cheaper for them to simply paint lines on existing tennis or basketball courts. You can go just about anywhere these days with your pickleball paddle and ball in hand and find a lined court to play on.

If not, it should be a relatively easy sell to ask your local park to paint pickleball lines on a seldom-used tennis court.

Joining in at public versus private venues

Because the popularity of the sport of pickleball is sweeping the nation, you need to learn the ins and outs of playing at both public and private courts. Fortunately, we have a bunch of combined experience with both. Connecting with other players, signing up for pickleball clinics, and taking a lesson or three from a certified coach are all great places to start. The internet will certainly open up a world of pickleball playing possibilities (say that three times fast) near you. We go into more depth on finding places to play later in the chapter.

Many community parks have pickleball courts, although they are most likely multiuse courts. Pickleball courts are a popular amenity for newly built communities because they don't take up a lot of space and offer family- (and senior-) friendly recreation for residents. Sometimes there is a reservation system, and sometimes it's just a matter of knowing that certain groups play at certain times. Check with your local Parks & Rec department to see whether groups exist for you to play with, or just go to a court and talk to the players who are there. You're likely to find nice folks who are eager to share the info you need to play in that area. Pickleball people are great!

TIP

Don't worry if you haven't found a group to play with yet. All you need is three more people who want to learn as you do. Many sports stores and facilities rent paddles for a limited time if you're just figuring out what kind of paddle you like, or want to see whether you like playing in the first place. (Trust us, you will like — no, love pickleball — and so will the friends you recruit to play with you. Warning: It's addictive!)

Private venues have memberships to play at gyms, sports clubs, country clubs, and other sports facilities. The costs of membership vary greatly, or nonmembers may have to pay a daily drop-in fee. The advantage of membership is knowing you have a place to play, other players are there wanting to play, and you can reserve a court, stop by a drop-in clinic, or join designated play times. Many private venues are used only for residents of particular communities. So, the next time you're ready to move, be sure to check out the pickleball situation. Some communities have dozens of dedicated pickleball courts just for their residents.

Building your own home pickleball court

Here's the inescapable truth: Most people who play pickleball end up being addicted to the sport. Fortunately, pickleball is fun, good exercise, and super social, so it's a healthful, safe addiction. If you eventually turn into a pickleball fanatic, you may be tempted to build your own court in your backyard — although it probably helps if you own a "back 40." If you are tempted to build an indoor court in your home, you are probably a gajillionaire and have people reading this section for you right now while fanning you with palm fronds.

If you really do want to build your own outdoor court, you have some options and definitely have some considerations. Imagine, the true pickleball lifestyle awaits you as you build your dream. (Cue the harp chords.) The amount of money you spend varies tremendously. You can do as little as tape down lines on cement and put up a portable net, or you can have it built professionally with specialty surfaces and coating as a more permanent structure.

But first, as Sergeant Joe Friday would say, "Just the facts, ma'am . . ."

>> **Pickleball court specifications:** 20 feet by 44 feet for both singles and doubles play

>> **Net height:** 36 inches at the sidelines; 34 inches in the middle

>> **Playing Area:** 30 feet by 60 feet when converting a tennis court, but 34 feet by 64 feet is preferable for tournament play and for a stand-alone court

Nets are sometimes strapped down in the center of the court to maintain regulation height and have supporting posts positioned just outside the perimeter of the court.

Deciding on DIY or hiring a builder

The first decision to make is whether to build a court from scratch or create a court on an existing surface. (Who needs that giant back driveway/patio anyway? Your brother-in-law has been parking his RV there for far too long.) Second, decide on your budget for the project. Read on to learn about more points to consider before you begin building your own court.

If you plan to build from scratch, consult with a professional, licensed contractor to build your private dream court. Costs start at about $30,000 (plus add-ons) but may be more or less depending on where you live. The general cost of building a court is between $11 and $22 per square foot. (This would total about $30,000 for a standard 30-x-60-foot pickleball court.) Figure 4-4 shows the dimensions of a standard pickleball court.

"Hey, it's cheaper than a pool and less maintenance!" is something an ardent pickleball player with his own backyard league tells us. USA Pickleball (www. USAPickleball.org) sells a manual for the construction and maintenance of courts. It would also be good to be pretty darn handy and have craftsperson-level friends waiting to help you.

TIP

If you're a pickleball purist, don't read this tip. Although a standard court is 30 feet by 60 feet, you can reduce the dimensions if you want to practice a lot but don't really have the room for full-on pickleball courts.

REMEMBER

Another factor to keep in mind is whether you actually have the needed space available for a private court, as well as adequate perimeter space for running around and returning deep serves. You're also likely to need room on the sidelines for other players to watch.

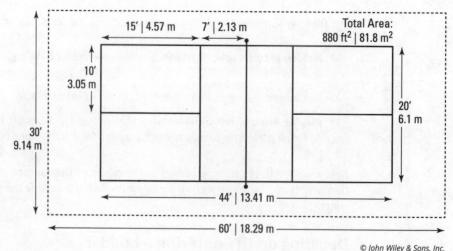

FIGURE 4-4:
Standard pickleball court dimensions.

© John Wiley & Sons, Inc.

In addition to knowing the proper dimensions, it's also important to figure out the correct directional orientation of the court because you want to avoid facing directly into the sun if possible. Almost all courts are oriented north/south because the sun rises in the east and sets in the west.

Choosing a court surface

The next consideration is the outdoor court surface material. The most common are concrete, asphalt, and snap-together plastic. Here are some options:

» **Concrete** is the best in terms of durability and value but it's hard on your joints.

» **Asphalt** is a more affordable route but can require additional maintenance. Plan on resurfacing every two to five years.

>> **Snap-together plastic**, a less common option, can be applied over concrete or asphalt and is an alternative surface if you don't want a permanent surface for a multiuse space. However, many players report that the ball does not bounce correctly on these types of surfaces. It's best to try any alternative surface before investing in it.

As mentioned earlier in the chapter, you can also repurpose an existing tennis court by taping or painting lines over the surface (see Figure 4-5). You can learn more about how to create a temporary court setup using a tennis court or other surface from USA Pickleball at https://www.usapickleball.org/what-is-pickleball/court-diagram/temporary-court-setup/.

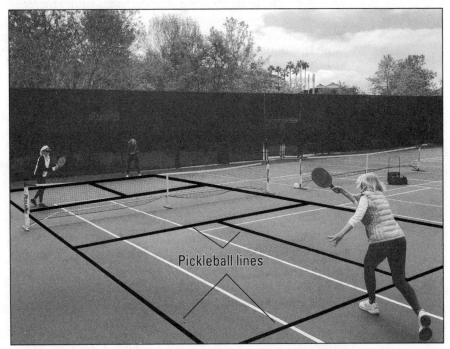

Pickleball lines

FIGURE 4-5:
Pickleball lines on a tennis court.

© John Wiley & Sons, Inc./Photo Credit: Mike Branon

Other options for courts are applied liquid coatings, poured-in-place surfaces, and cushioned surfaces. A contractor can go over the pros and cons of each option and the costs associated with them. Be cautious with cushioned surfaces because they can cause the ball to lose its bounce. Pickleball can be pretty tough to play if the ball doesn't bounce. (Figure 4-6 shows professionally built courts.)

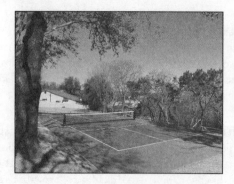 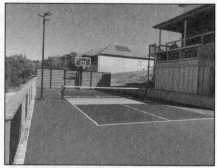

FIGURE 4-6: The dream: Professionally built, private pickleball courts.

Finally, perimeter fencing is a consideration, with wire fencing being the most common. You may also want lighting (and electricity), and in these areas, city codes and neighborhood Covenants, Conditions, and Restrictions (CC&R's) dictate. The fun part for you will be in design, color, court accessories, and amenities.

WARNING

We've already told you that playing pickleball can be addictive. In researching this book, we ran across dozens of people who have their own mini clubs and courts in their backyards. These "operators" are real characters who simply want to share the "Pickleball Love." Some of them have highly organized personal leagues with special uniforms, plus they teach and have tournaments, mascots, and even specialty cocktail recipes with the best happy hours in the neighborhood. We warned you!

Wanna Play? Finding Courts and Players Near You

Now that you know all the different kinds of courts and places to play (we are currently advocating for NASA to put a pickleball court on the moon), you have several options to find courts and players near you. The following websites and organizations are dedicated to helping players connect and play everywhere.

Referencing Places2Play

Places2Play is a helpful database created by USA Pickleball that helps you find courts and clubs near you. It's very easy to access online at www.places2play. org/. The map is also an app — just type in your location, and all the places to play pickleball in your community come right up. In the "Comment" section, details about each location, drop-in times, and so on appear. Although the tool is free to use, USA Pickleball encourages you to become a member.

TIP

One idea to keep in mind about Place2Play is that not every venue keeps their information current at all times. If a contact number or email is given, it's wise to reach out first before turning up somewhere new with your paddle in hand.

Using PlayTime Scheduler

PlayTime Scheduler (https://playtimescheduler.com) is another free online tool that can be extremely useful in finding courts and play sessions in your local area. It's a community-driven website through which players invite others to join them by posting sessions for a specific time, place, and skill level. You can RSVP by simply clicking a button to add your name to the list. After at least four players sign up, it's game on! PlayTime Scheduler makes it easy to see where your friends are playing on any given day, or to meet new players with similar skill levels and schedules. You can even sign up for email notifications so that you never miss a game!

Some players utilize the "invite only" feature to create private sessions for their friends, ladder leagues, or other groups. Keep in mind that PlayTime Scheduler is an invitation system, not a court-reservation system. Most public parks do not allow you to reserve courts, and private venues use different systems for reservations.

PlayTime Scheduler is a great resource when traveling because you can easily hop between different cities and check out the action on the local calendar. Although some cities are more active than others, the site is used on six continents across the world and is growing in popularity every day.

Reaching out to USA Pickleball Ambassadors

USA Pickleball has created an Ambassador program to promote its organization and the sport of pickleball. Ambassadors are volunteers who pledge to promote the sport in the local area that they represent. They work directly with communities, clubs, and other recreational facilities as advocates and guides to help build pickleball programs for all to enjoy. Ambassadors work together within their designated districts as well as across multistate regions to enhance the development of USA Pickleball and pickleball in general. To contact the Ambassador for your area, go to https://usapickleball.org/get-involved/usa-pickleball-ambassadors/. The program is a wonderful resource for quickly getting plugged into what's happening in your local community.

Searching social media

Tapping into social media to search for players and courts is another way to connect. Most local pickleball clubs have Facebook groups, making it easy to connect with other players in your area. There is a huge amount of enthusiasm from players on Facebook, Twitter, and Instagram, and you could easily spend all day scrolling through pickleball content of all kinds.

USA Pickleball (`https://www.usapickleball.org/member-news/are-you-a-social-media-butterfly/`) promotes events and tournaments through social media channels as well. When Nationals and other big tournaments are being played, it's a great way to find out what's happening in real time — both on the court and behind the scenes. Most upcoming tournaments are listed on PickleballTournaments.com. You will find no shortage of opportunities to compete if that becomes your thing.

Picking Up on Pickleball Etiquette

Anytime you try a new sport, you might notice a certain etiquette that players follow. These are the unwritten rules of the game that aren't set in stone in any rule book. In pickleball, proper etiquette is very important because it's such a social, inclusive game. If you find yourself on the court and aren't sure what to do, just ask a more experienced player. They will be happy to help, we promise! In this section, we give you some good guidelines to follow, both on the court and on the sidelines. For example, Figure 4-7 shows the customary paddle tapping between teams at the end of the game, with everyone saying, "Good game!" (Or something nice like that.)

In addition to understanding the etiquette, we shed some light on the quirks of pickleball culture, as well on how drop-in play works and the ins and outs of playing with strangers. Pickleball players are a pretty nice bunch!

Striving to be safe, courteous, and honest

When you're new at playing pickleball, chances are you're focused on the rules and mechanics of playing. Getting to know the etiquette of the sport, however, is equally important. Sometimes safety, honesty, and courtesy may seem like common sense, but it's still good to understand the "manners" when in a new social setting. Pickleball is definitely an inclusive, considerate sport, in which integrity is key.

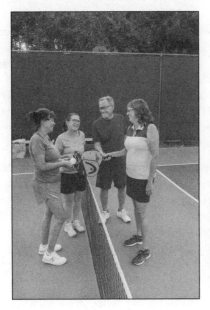

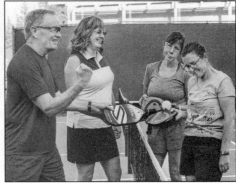

FIGURE 4-7: Tapping paddles at the end of the game, always! (left) Guess who won? (right)

© John Wiley & Sons, Inc./Photo Credit: Aniko Kiezel

Here are ten tips for good pickleball etiquette:

» **Wait until all four players are ready before you serve.** Sometimes random balls from other courts roll onto your court, or one person has some other distraction. Wait until everyone is focused to begin to play.

» **Call the score clearly.** Call the score loudly enough for everyone playing to hear it before serving the ball. It's easy enough to lose track of the score, but if you haven't been able to hear your opponent call it for three points, good luck!

» **Say "Nice shot."** Congratulate and encourage not only your partner but also your opponents when they make a great shot. Pickleball players like to encourage each other — remember that you're having cooperative fun. (You can still want to win, too!)

» **Be aware of the time you are using the court.** If many people are waiting to play, be aware and respectful. Don't stand there chatting for ten minutes. You can do that off the court. If you have played a bunch and people have been waiting, maybe sit out a game after you've played two or three. Different clubs and venues have their own rules, and they are usually posted by the courts. Use common courtesy and treat others the way you would want to be treated.

» **Don't walk through someone's game to get to another court.** Instead, wait for a break in the action and then quickly get to your court. Your foursome should all go together so that the players don't have to stop their game multiple times.

>> **Call "Ball on!" loudly when your ball ends up on another court.** You immediately and safely alert the players about a ball on that court so that they won't trip and fall. The play is stopped, the ball is politely retrieved, and the rally on that court is replayed. If your ball is not in any danger of injuring anyone on the other court (for example, it's up against the back fence) and the players haven't noticed that your ball is on their court, wait until they finish their point and then ask for your ball back. "Better safe than sorry" is the rule here, so it's always better to stop play than put anyone at risk.

>> **Don't coach other players unless they've asked you for it.** Pickleball players like to help each other, and nothing is wrong with that. If you want to share your wisdom with another player, ask them first; for example, "Would you like some advice about your backhand?" Don't be offended if they decline your advice. Often players would prefer to work with an actual coach, or they may not be in the mood to work on their strokes that day. Also, please don't delay games by doing an extended coaching session, especially if others are waiting for a court.

>> **If an opponent has restrictions, don't deliberately lob a ball so far behind them that they can't possibly get to it.** That's just not nice, and it's a cheap shot. Intention is what makes the difference. If you're playing with someone who is older or injured and unable to move quickly, don't take advantage of that when playing recreationally. Be kind. Now, if it's a tournament, that changes things a bit. That player entered the tournament and you are all there to win. So, players will play to that end.

>> **Walk to the net after every game and tap paddles with the other players.** It is customary after the game has been played for the players to approach the net and gently tap their paddles, saying things like "Good game!" and "That was fun!" (Some people prefer to tap their paddle handles instead because they don't want to scratch the face of the paddle, but either way is fine.)

>> **Lose and win graciously.** No one likes a sore loser or a gloating winner, and we want you to be liked! Pickleball is supposed to be fun, and nothing sucks the joy out of the room like players who take themselves way too seriously.

>> **Bonus tip: If you are a new player, we have good news for you.** Almost everyone makes a point to play with new players. "It's how we learned to get better," other players will tell you enthusiastically as they insist you join in. Patience, encouragement, and kindness are hallmarks of this game.

Understanding pickleball culture: OMG! (One more game!)

The very first time you play pickleball, you remember it. Almost universally, people are surprised by two prominent features of the sport. First, it's easy to play, even the very first time you try. Most people, despite their level of athleticism, can hit the ball and rally the first time they play. You can easily improve within a few weeks of playing regularly, or with a lesson or two.

Second, pickleball is an inviting, inclusive, and courteous sport. You don't need to be a big-time jock to enjoy it. It's not segmented by a player's size and strength, gender, or age. As we mention earlier in this chapter, public courts are readily available everywhere — in parks, schools, community centers, churches, and new housing developments. Courts are popping up at private clubs like crazy because of the sport's exploding popularity. People are even building their own courts in their backyards.

A big difference between pickleball and other sports is seeing *smiles everywhere!* It's impossible to walk past a pickleball court without hearing laughter. This holds true even at the most advanced competitive level. Friendships grow almost instantaneously. Kindness and positivity are hallmarks of the pickleball experience.

Coauthor Carl started playing about three years ago. Like most people, he had never even heard of pickleball then, and after one game, he was hooked. People are excited to welcome others into the sport. It's not unusual to see an experienced player happily going over the rules with a first-timer who is just learning to play.

Sure, pickleball has a funny name. It's a sport that was created in the 1960s. (See Chapter 1 for a brief history of pickleball.) Now it's one of the fastest growing sports in the country. USA Pickleball estimates that more than 4.8 million Americans played pickleball in 2021. That number will continue to grow exponentially as families and friends play together all over the world. Who knows — one day, pickleball may be in the Olympics.

The culture of pickleball has deep roots in fun and camaraderie. (See Figures 4-8 and 4-9 for a glimpse of the fun.) Here are some ways to familiarize yourself with this growing sport even further:

>> **Find your tribe:** If you want to play once a week just for laughs and a little exercise, you'll find your group. If you want to meet more regularly for a game or three, you'll find your people. Or if you want a more competitive environment, most likely you can find tournaments going on in your local area all year-round.

>> **Become star struck:** You know pickleball has gone mainstream when celebrities are out there playing, often on their own personal courts! Some of the pickleball converts are Reese Witherspoon, Kim Kardashian, George Clooney, Matthew Perry, Amanda Peet, Bill Gates, Rick Barry, Nick Foles, Larry David, Jamie Foxx, Owen Wilson, and more.

>> **Dive into media:** You can watch professional players on TV. ESPN, CBS, Fox Sports, and Tennis Channel have regular broadcasts. *Pickleball Magazine* is the official magazine for USA Pickleball, and there's also a high-end magazine called *InPickleball*.

>> **Travel the world:** You can find pickleball camps and resorts all over the world for intense instruction and enjoyment. Even major cruise lines now offer "pickleball cruises."

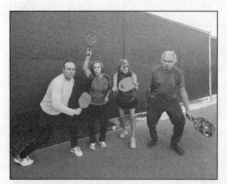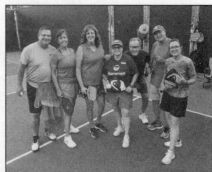

FIGURE 4-8: Pickleball = Fun.

© John Wiley & Sons, Inc./Photo Credit: Aniko Kiezel

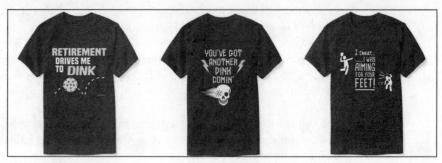

FIGURE 4-9: Having a healthy sense of humor is a huge part of pickleball culture.

© John Wiley & Sons, Inc./Photo Credit: Reine Steel

Even more reasons why you should play pickleball

Pickleball is much more than just a sport; it's a community. It's social. Chatting with your partners and competitors during a match is expected. Good sporting conduct and courtesy are key elements of the game and experience.

WHY PICKLEBALL IS GROWING SO FAST

- There's a low barrier to entry because courts are easy to access in most parts of the country. (Pickleball has a drop-in play culture that welcomes new players.)

- Little investment is required. All you need is a paddle, a pickleball, and preferably some court shoes.

- You can buy equipment easily online or at most sporting goods stores. Most tennis shops are selling just as much pickleball as tennis equipment these days.

- It's easy to begin to play. In very little time, you can be playing competitive games.

- The nets are lower than tennis and the court space to cover is about one-fourth the size of a tennis court. You don't have to already be in incredible shape to play pickleball.

- Pickleball is practically perfect for the baby boomers who now have free time to have some fun, as well as any other demographic who want more joy in their lives. The serve is underhand, which saves the shoulder a lot of stress. It mostly involves doubles, which means more social connection and less running. Because the court is small, it's easier to socialize while playing.

- The rules are simple compared to most sports. (People say pickleball scoring is weird, but who came up with "love, fifteen, thirty, deuce" anyway?)

- Drop-in fees and club memberships are relatively inexpensive or often free.

- Thousands of pickleball videos are available online to teach you every aspect of the game from the comfort of your home.

- You can find pickleball teachers and coaches out there to help you (including two of the authors of this book.) Lessons and clinics are reasonably priced, or sometimes even free.

By playing pickleball, you will likely improve your physical fitness and have a more positive mental state of mind all at the same time. We think the world will become a kinder, gentler place when pickleball takes over!

Civility, as we've mentioned, is a big part of the game. Players typically do their best to make honest line calls. It's not uncommon to see players calling a fault on themselves when they find that they were in the kitchen while volleying. For many players, winning or losing is secondary. It's a unique sport that way. Fun and friendship are at the core of the experience. Pickleball brings back recess for adults!

The more you dive into the pickleball universe, the more you will want to play with other like-minded individuals who want to enjoy themselves and get some exercise. In the next section, we steer you through the ins and outs of drop-in play.

Navigating drop-in play rotation

Pickleball is unlike tennis or golf because it encourages players to play in organized drop-in games, or *open play*. Open play allows strangers to meet and play together. Some open play sessions are organized by skill level, whereas others aren't, giving beginners a chance to learn from more experienced players. Pickleball truly is inclusive, which makes the play more fun. Even if you are an advanced player, we recommend mixing with other levels occasionally — it can be a lot more fun than you may think!

Venues that offer drop-in play typically use some kind of rotation rules or organization system to help manage court traffic. Some common methods include

» **Paddle line-ups and paddle racks:** Whether people simply hang paddles on a fence or use a specially designed paddle rack, most courts have a system for determining who's next in line.

» **Four on, four off:** In this common rotational system, a foursome finishes their game and all four players come off the court. The next four waiting in line then take the court.

» **Winners stay and split:** In this case, only the losing team rotates off the court, and two new players come on to replace them. The winning team splits up so that they each play with one of the oncoming players.

» **Winners stay together:** Often referred to as a Challenge Court format, winning teams stay on and continue to play together as long as they keep winning. After each game, the losing team exits and two new "challengers" come on to face the winners.

» **King/Queen of the court:** In this format, courts are designated from the lowest to highest level. As teams win their games, they move "up" to a higher court, sometimes splitting partners. The losing team moves "down" to a lower-level court, or back to the waiting area if they are already on the lowest court.

These are just a few of the most common court rotation methods. Each venue has its rules for rotating onto the courts. The rules are usually posted in writing, but if not, just ask the friendliest person you see. After you join in open play a few times, you'll see a friendly rhythm to it.

WARNING

When leaving or entering your court, make sure you don't cross the back of a game in play. You don't want to be a distraction for the other players or possibly injure yourself.

With drop-in play, communication is key. Don't be afraid to ask questions if you're unsure of how the rotation is going — pickleballers love to help new players. It's the nature of the game!

Playing nice: Being a good neighbor

You may find pickleball courts nestled into quiet neighborhoods. In that case, it's important to keep your noise level in mind (as when shouting "Wahoo!" at the top of your lungs when you score, for example) and not offend the nearby neighbors. Make note of the set hours of play that are posted and honor those guidelines. Think about it: The people living in homes near pickleball courts may not even play pickleball, and they get to hear *a lot* of dinking and wahoo-ing most days. Just as with any facility, remember to leave the courts clean and the gates closed when you leave. Please don't ever toss broken pickleballs onto the grass at your local park. They jam up the expensive lawn mowers very effectively. With just a few simple acts, you can help to make sure that neighbors welcome pickleball, not fight against it.

If you are considering building your own private court, how close you live to other neighbors will be a significant factor to consider. Sure, as pickleball players, we love the sound of a good "dink-dink-dink" rally. Your neighbors may not so much. So before you sink a bunch of money into building a court, our advice is to work with the neighbors on sound and traffic levels well in advance. Who knows? Maybe you will turn your neighbors into pickleball fans and players as well.

TIP

Consider installing soundproofing windscreen material to reduce the pickleball noise. Some manufacturers say their materials can reduce the noise up to 50 percent. (This will not apply to the loud whoops every time Uncle Larry wins a point.)

Chapter **5**

Transitioning from Other Sports: You Can Do This!

In today's world of sports, pickleball is unique because it's a relatively new sport that's exploding in popularity. Most people had never even heard of pickleball before five or ten years ago. Unlike some other sports, you won't find players who grew up attending pickleball camp every summer, or who went to college on a pickleball scholarship. The majority of players you'll encounter have been playing for fewer than several years.

This situation is exciting because it fills the pickleball community with all kinds of people, coming from widely diverse athletic backgrounds. Players are bringing their skills from all kinds of sports — from table tennis to taekwondo — and finding ways to make them work on the pickleball court. This great "melting pot" of individual talents and experience helps account for the rapid evolution of the game. By deciding to take up pickleball, you've caught the wave of something sensational, so go ahead and pat yourself on the back! Then read on to learn how you can incorporate your own unique skills and talents from your other athletic endeavors into your blossoming pickleball career. Or if you've never played competitive sports before, that's okay, too. Don't believe us? Skip to the last section of this chapter to find out why sometimes a blank slate is the best starting place of all.

Making the Leap from Other Racquet and Paddle Sports

If you've played any type of racquet or paddle sport in the past, you'll probably feel right at home on a pickleball court. Pickleball is often described as a combination of tennis, badminton, and table tennis. Some people view it as miniature tennis, or table tennis on steroids. Neither analogy is entirely accurate, but the similarities between these sports clearly exist.

As a beginner, your past experience in racquet or paddle sports can definitely give you a leg up, but you also need to be aware of some key differences. Simply trying to play tennis on a smaller court will get you only so far. Pickleball is its own game, and exploring the nuances is half the fun!

Tennis

Of course, when thinking about sports that are similar to pickleball, tennis is the first that comes to mind. No doubt, tennis players are flocking in droves to this sport and having a blast. Currently, the majority of top pickleball pros are former college or professional tennis players who are enjoying newfound passion and success in the pickleball world.

Pickleball incorporates many of the most fun aspects of tennis into a tinier package. You're still hitting groundstrokes, approach shots, volleys, lobs, and overheads, to name a few. Shot selection and execution remain your primary weapons. Many tennis players enjoy pickleball because it's more social than tennis. The court size makes player interaction easier during the game. Also, players often don't show up as a foursome; you can go out to the courts and play with whomever is there!

Along with a smaller court size that requires less running and fewer hard stops, one of the biggest motivators for tennis players to switch to pickleball is the underhand serve. The pickleball serve is much gentler on your back, neck, and shoulders than the overhead tennis serve. What a relief!

As you cross over from tennis to pickleball, here are some of the skills that will easily transfer:

>> **Shot accuracy:** Tennis players have trained to hit and develop accurate shots. You'll find that you're much better at placing your pickleball shots early on compared to other beginners. This previous training is especially helpful if you decide to take up singles.

» **Spin:** Topspin, slice, and sidespin are all tools you already have in your toolbox. Knowing how and when to execute different types of spin is considered an advanced skill in pickleball.

» **Footwork:** Your customary footwork on the tennis court may be your biggest advantage over those who haven't played tennis. You've already developed muscle memory for important footwork such as drop-stepping, side-to-side shuffling, split-stepping, and setting up to the ball.

» **Finishing shots:** Tennis players already know how to hit effective volleys and overhead smashes, and naturally go for angled winners. You've already been trained to look for the open court and to hit "slow side" (behind your opponent) as opposed to hitting right back at them (a common mistake among beginners).

» **Net play:** In both tennis and pickleball, when playing at the net, the goal is to elicit a pop-up from your opponent by hitting low or neutral balls that will force them to swing upward. In tennis, you're trading volleys, whereas in pickleball, you're trading dinks, but the concept is the same.

» **Switching and poaching:** Doubles tennis players already understand how to communicate and move fluidly with their partner. Concepts like "switch," "stay," and using hand signals are already familiar to you. Many beginning pickleball players feel that they must stay trapped on "their side" of the court and don't easily recognize poaching or switching opportunities.

Until you begin to understand the differences between the two sports, some of your deeply ingrained tennis habits may trip you up at first.

If you want to become a great pickleball player, watch out for the following issues:

» **Adjusting to paddle length, bounce, and net height:** The very first time you step on a pickleball court, don't be surprised if you "whiff" a few times! A pickleball paddle is much shorter than a tennis racquet, and the plastic ball doesn't bounce off the ground nearly as high. In addition, the net height relative to the court size is much taller.

» **Big backswings:** A tennis player is usually easy to spot because they tend to take large backswings. In pickleball, your strokes need to be much more compact. Minimize your backswing, but keep that long, pretty follow-through from tennis.

» **Not coming to the line:** If you were a baseline player in tennis, you may be tempted to continue playing in the same style. In pickleball, however, points are won at the kitchen line. You rarely win points with your groundstrokes against a team who has come to the line and closed off all your passing and angle opportunities. Staying back puts you at a huge disadvantage.

>> **Attempting to "chip and charge":** In tennis, this means to chip or slice your return of serve and charge forward by running toward the net. The method of properly transitioning to the line in pickleball looks very different. (See Chapter 11 for a detailed description of getting to the line.) Attempting to chip and charge in pickleball usually results in having the next ball blasted right past you!

>> **Driving the ball too often, and too high:** On a shorter pickleball court, your tennis-style drives will fly too high, allowing your opponent to easily slam them back at you. You need to learn to hit drop shots (or dropping drives) that curl over the net, forcing your opponent to swing up. The narrower court also means fewer passing opportunities, making drives less effective in general.

Badminton

The badminton birdie is recognized as the fastest-moving object in sports. The current world record was a smash clocked at 306 MPH! In comparison, pickleballs travel at a top speed of about 50 MPH. If you come from badminton, a pickleball will seem as though it's moving in slow motion.

Your badminton experience gives you some other definite advantages:

>> **Quick reflexes:** Badminton players are used to dealing with a very fast-moving shuttlecock and no kitchen to act as a buffer area. Your quick reflexes will transfer over beautifully, and you'll be known for having "fast hands" at the kitchen line.

>> **Familiar court size:** The badminton and pickleball court sizes are identical. You'll come to pickleball with good spatial awareness of where you should be standing to effectively cover the court, and where you need to aim to keep the ball in bounds.

>> **Snappy overheads:** In badminton, the power generated on an overhead with the wrist flick is significantly stronger than a full arm swing. As we describe in Chapter 9, a snappy, well-placed overhead in pickleball is a great way to put the ball away.

>> **Deception and pattern changes:** This important strategic tool in badminton applies to pickleball as well. To keep up with the high-speed rallies, your opponent must try to guess what shot you're about to hit, before you actually hit it. By deliberately projecting false information about your shot using your body, eyes, or paddle, or changing up your typical shot patterns mid-match, you can fool them into moving the wrong direction.

Clearly, a badminton racquet and shuttle are very different objects than a pickleball paddle and plastic ball. A pickleball is much heavier than a birdie, and there aren't any strings on your paddle to give it significant rebound.

Here are some other potential challenges to watch out for as you learn to play pickleball:

>> **Using too much wrist:** Because badminton is so wrist-heavy, you may not be used to swinging through your shot using your full kinetic chain (legs, hips, core, and arm). Adding a wrist flick on most pickleball shots leads to inaccuracy.

>> **Adjusting to spin and bounce:** When it comes to spin, the visual rotation of a ball reads differently than a birdie. You also have no bounce to worry about in badminton. A pickleball can sometimes skid strangely off a line or crack. When hitting a groundstroke in pickleball, you need to be extra ready to adjust your footwork at the last moment.

>> **Hitting behind you:** In badminton, because the racquet and shuttle are so light, power can still be generated even if the shuttle has wound up behind your body. In pickleball, it's crucial to always try to hit the ball out in front of you, with forward weight shift.

>> **Excessive lobs:** A reset shot in pickleball is a drop or a dink, but in badminton, it's a lob (known as a "clear"). Those are polar opposites! It may take some getting used to the idea that your best defense is a shallow drop rather than a high lob.

Racquetball

Racquetball is another one of the fastest-moving racquet sports. Quick reaction times, great footwork, and anticipation are essential. Doubles racquetball requires you to be in sync with your partner (and, to some degree, your opponents) as you move with each other around the court so as not to collide. The beautiful "dance" between perfectly in-tune racquetball partners looks similar to that of an experienced pickleball doubles team.

If you're coming to pickleball from racquetball, some of the other skills that assimilate nicely include:

>> **Backhand groundstrokes**: In racquetball, if you try to avoid hitting your backhand by running around it and hitting a forehand, you will literally run into a wall! Skilled racquetball players usually have a backhand that they believe in.

>> **Quick hands:** Racquetball serves have been clocked at close to 200 MPH. You'll never see a pickleball flying quite that fast! But you've developed fast reaction times and ball-tracking abilities, and as a result, you should be quite formidable during rapid volley exchanges.

>> **Baseline footwork:** If you don't get your feet to the ball on a racquetball court, you'll have to dive — ouch! When hitting a pickleball, great footwork will help you get the ball into your ideal strike zone. We rarely see racquetball players getting too "stuck in cement."

>> **Swinging through the ball:** In both racquetball and pickleball, trying to poke or jab at the ball is ineffective. Pushing forward through the ball, with a full follow-through, gives the best results.

Of course, there are many differences between racquetball and pickleball, from the paddle and ball to the layout of the court. When transitioning to pickleball, watch out for these potential pitfalls:

>> **Wild kitchen footwork:** Your fast-moving racquetball feet may help you in situations farther back in the court, but when dinking up at the kitchen, you need to calm those prancing hooves. When at the line, you want to remain stable and balanced, moving only when required.

>> **Hitting too hard:** You may be used to hitting every ball extremely hard and low. In pickleball, it turns out that hitting the ball very hard at the bottom of the net is a fault. (Somebody should really do something about that rule!) Most racquetball players need time to learn to slow down and hit the ball softer.

>> **Lack of topspin:** In racquetball, you don't use spin because the moment the ball hits the wall, the spin stops, rendering it useless. Topspin may be a brand-new skill for you.

Table tennis

If you gather a group of pickleball players together for a party, don't be surprised if they spend most of their time congregating around the table tennis table. Table tennis is one of the sport's closest cousins, and many people enjoy dabbling in both.

If you've played table tennis competitively, you come to pickleball with a huge advantage. You will be one of the few players with prior experience using a solid paddle to control a plastic ball, as opposed to a racquet with strings and a rubberized ball.

In addition to the advantages already noted, here are some others you find in coming to pickleball from table tennis:

>> **Ball tracking:** In table tennis, you have only 9 feet of table between you and your opponent, and the tiny ball is moving at over 60 MPH. When the action speeds up at the kitchen line in pickleball, you will bring a much faster reaction time than most players because of your heightened ability to track the ball.

>> **Fine-tuned movements:** Table tennis is highly explosive, yet it requires precise movements and paddle positioning to keep the ball under control. Quickly getting your paddle into the right position, with a correctly angled paddle face, will be second nature to you.

>> **Mastery of spin:** Table tennis players can spin a pickleball in ways that most players have never seen! Your incredible reflexes and paddle face awareness mean that you can select and apply spin at the last moment, without telegraphing your intentions.

Pickleball may feel like oversized table tennis at first. Although many of your skills will transfer easily after being amplified in scale, here are a few key differences to watch out for:

>> **Volleys:** This will definitely be a new skill for you because volleys are illegal in table tennis. You may feel tempted to step back and let the ball bounce instead of volleying. Preventing your opponent's ball from bouncing negates much of the nasty spin that you must deal with in table tennis.

>> **Paddle size and composition:** In table tennis, because of the rubber on the paddle, the ball comes off with great speed and spin with very little effort on the player's part. The composition of a pickleball paddle does not offer much in the way of energy or spin. The way you hold the paddle may also need some adjusting; a Penhold grip doesn't work well in pickleball.

>> **Court coverage:** You're accustomed to playing behind a table, not standing on the table. On a pickleball court, you'll need to learn where to stand and how to position your body in order to take shot options away from your opponents.

Transferring Skills from Non-Racquet Sports

Many new pickleball players express concern that they will struggle if they haven't played a racquet sport before. Rest assured that if you've participated in any kind of sport before, you'll find elements that transfer nicely to pickleball — perhaps in ways you didn't expect.

Whether you possess specific skills like footwork, ball tracking, and positioning, or more general ones like teamwork and mental focus, you have plenty to bring to the table. In this section, we look at some of the similarities and differences among the skills required in pickleball versus some popular non-racquet sports.

Volleyball

Volleyball isn't a racquet sport, but it is a net sport. Clearly, the net is much higher on a volleyball court than a pickleball court. However, keep in mind that when compared to the overall size of the court, a pickleball net is still a relatively tall obstacle. You need to carefully consider when it's appropriate to lift the ball up versus "spiking" it down.

Players of both indoor and beach volleyball will come to pickleball with an understanding of blocks, attacks, and deep serves.

Here are some other skills that transfer nicely between volleyball and pickleball:

>> **Court awareness:** Especially if you come from beach volleyball (which is played as doubles), you already have an understanding of how to position yourself relative to your partner for optimal court coverage. You're also used to reading your opponent's positioning and anticipating their next play, so you can get into the best position before the ball comes back.

>> **Bump, set, spike:** You can apply the classic volleyball offensive play to pickleball strategy as well. Think of your third-shot drop as the "bump" pass to your partner: You can imagine the setter on your side, close to the net where you want the ball to reach its apex before dropping over the other side of the net. The "set" in this case comes when your opponent accidentally pops the ball up. You need to wait for a good set before you "spike" the ball. On a pickleball court, we love nothing more than receiving a poorly executed lob to spike back over the net.

>> **Defensive digs:** Both sports use the term *dig* to mean defending a low ball, usually a hard attack aimed down at the ground. Your volleyball instincts will encourage you to go for more difficult digs. (Knee pads or not, we can't recommend diving on a pickleball court!)

As you're enjoying the opportunity to bump, set, and spike with a paddle and a plastic ball, you'll also need to spend time practicing some new skills:

>> **Patience.** As one player put it, "In volleyball, the mentality is kill or be killed. Pickleball is more of a cat-and-mouse game." Often, you best set your team up for success by prolonging the point until your opponent makes a mistake. Not every play involves an attack.

>> **Considering the bounce.** In volleyball, after the ball hits the ground, it's dead. In pickleball, your opponents have the option of letting it bounce. Spiking a pickleball incredibly hard, straight down, will just cause the ball to bounce up higher, giving your opponents more time to hit. A better attack would be more precisely aimed at the opponent's feet or angled off the court.

>> **Avoiding kitchen faults.** Attacking right at the net is a hard habit to break. With pickleball, you have to stay behind the kitchen line to legally volley, which can be an adjustment.

>> **Around the Post (ATP) shots.** Volleyball players are in the mindset of always keeping the ball inside the net antenna; hitting around the post is not allowed. When playing pickleball, you may need some time to recognize ATP opportunities and remember that they're legal. (See Chapter 14 to find out more about ATPs.)

Basketball

You can easily spot basketball players on the pickleball court because it's impossible *not* to see them; they are seemingly everywhere at one time! As a basketball player, you know how to occupy space, whether you're blocking an opponent's ability to pass or setting up a screen. In pickleball, this ability gives your opponents the impression of having very few open spaces to hit.

Here are some more skills that give basketball players an edge in pickleball:

>> **Lateral movement:** In basketball, quick lateral movement is essential. The defensive stance that makes you fast in basketball is very similar to the "at the line" ready position in pickleball: feet shoulder width apart; weight on the balls of your feet; knees slightly bent. When dinking, the ability to quickly slide laterally to get in front of the ball is important.

» **Anticipation:** Basketball players constantly read their opponent's body language and eyes to see where they are looking to pass the ball so that they can attempt a steal. In pickleball, you can also anticipate where the ball is going next by analyzing an opponent's eyes, paddle face, or body positioning. This will allow you to start moving into position to poach or hit an Erne (see Chapter 14) before your opponent strikes the ball. A deceptive "no look" shot is a sneaky play in pickleball, too.

» **Keeping your chin up:** When dribbling or passing, you can't stare at the ball the entire time or you won't be able to see what's happening on the floor. Basketball players learn to "feel" the ball and trust their muscle memory to know where the ball is in relation to their hand. We always recommend keeping your chin up when playing pickleball, too, rather than staring at the ball hitting the paddle.

» **Teamwork and communication:** In basketball, you rely on your teammates to help cover the court. When playing one-on-one defense, you expect help if the player you're guarding gets by you. When playing zone defense, the whole team moves together as a unit. Players must constantly communicate to work in sync as a team.

If you are coming from basketball, a few pickleball skills may feel new to you. Here are some issues to watch for:

» **Differences in footwork:** Basketball players may have a tendency to lunge or reach for the ball using large steps. In pickleball, you want to use big steps to cover the court quickly but use smaller adjustment steps as you get closer to the ball. Cross-stepping can also cause you trouble in pickleball. When at the kitchen line, if you need to pivot or move sideways, take a side step with your outer foot rather than cross over.

» **Digging balls at your feet:** Most of the passing and shooting action in basketball happens above the waist. Having to get low and deal with pickleballs constantly aimed at your feet may feel awkward at first.

» **Adjusting to lack of touch:** You're used to handling a basketball with your fingertips, which contain thousands of touch receptors. When you pick up a pickleball paddle, you lose this sense of intimacy between you and the ball. You have to develop the sense that this foreign object — your paddle — is an extension of your hand.

» **Shoulder and trunk rotation:** Basketball players do a lot of passing and shooting motions straight out from their chest or over their head. In contrast, many pickleball shots require more of a sidearm motion, with a full shoulder and torso rotation.

Baseball/Softball

Whether you grew up playing America's pastime or have only ever played catch in the backyard, throwing and hitting a ball lends some useful muscle memory that can help you develop solid pickleball strokes.

An overhead smash in pickleball is very similar to throwing a baseball. The pickleball serve is similar to an underhand softball pitch. Baseball and softball players instinctively reach out for balls coming toward them, a great habit that encourages playing in the "V" (as explained in the Chapter 6).

Here are some other baseball and softball skills you bring with you to the pickleball court:

>> **Bisecting angles:** When fielding a ground ball, a baseball player must quickly analyze its trajectory and determine what direction to run in order to meet up with the ball along its path. This determination is based on the velocity of the ball and the speed at which the player can run. This skill transfers directly to pickleball. If a ball is traveling toward you at an angle, you can't run straight toward it or it will pass you by. You must move at an angle that ensures you will intersect with the ball at the right moment.

>> **Bunting:** A great bunter is likely to be a great re-setter in pickleball. You already know how to absorb power off a ball by relaxing your body and slightly pulling back your bat (paddle) at just the right moment.

>> **Using your kinetic chain:** The term *kinetic chain* refers to different body parts working in sequence to create a desired movement. When swinging a bat, for example, the chain starts with your legs and then moves to your hips, torso, arms, and hands, transferring all the energy to the tip of your bat. This same kinetic chain works beautifully when hitting a pickleball serve or groundstroke.

>> **Reading pitches:** A baseball or softball batter has less than half a second to react to a pitch. In this moment, they must analyze speed, spin, and trajectory to determine their ideal swing path and timing. The ability to read a pickleball in this same fashion will be a huge advantage for you.

>> **Drop-stepping for overheads:** You've been trained that when a fly ball goes over your head, the safest and most efficient way to move is to drop-step with one foot and then run. This is a great habit for pickleball because it will prevent you from back-pedaling with both feet, which can lead to a nasty fall.

We've coached many baseball and softball players and found they have a few old habits that can trip them up. Be conscious of the following issues when playing pickleball:

>> **Windshield wiper backhands:** When a baseball or softball is hurtling toward your chest, you catch it with your palm facing outward. In pickleball, you actually need to turn your hand the other way around and hit a backhand. Flipping your paddle around the wrong way can be a hard habit to break and can lead to what's known as a *windshield wiper backhand.* Chapter 9 explains how to fix this problem.

>> **Setting up to the ball:** Baseball players are trained to get in front of a ball when receiving it and to catch it in the middle of their chest. In pickleball, this technique works great for blocking, but for groundstrokes and dinks, you need to line up more to the side. Aiming your belly button at the ball will leave you jammed up.

>> **Adjusting to constant play action:** During a typical baseball play, you're lucky to get to touch the ball once or twice; often, you won't touch it at all! You may even go several innings without being directly involved in a play. Pickleball is very different. You can expect to hit the ball many times, and in rapid succession, throughout each rally. No picking daisies in right field!

Soccer

Soccer is a team sport that appears to have little in common with pickleball. In soccer, you can use any body part except your hands, but in pickleball you can use only your paddle and the hand attached to it — the total opposite!

Keep in mind, however, that both games are played on a rectangular playing surface, with the goal being to create and defend open spaces. Your ability to recognize open passing lanes and prevent your opponent from finding holes in your own team's formation will give you a strategic edge.

Here are some other soccer skills that transfer over to pickleball:

>> **Understanding triangles:** Being familiar with triangle plays in soccer means you can clearly visualize the position of your teammates, opponents, and the ball, as well as the angles that connect them. Imagine that your pickleball opponent is about to strike the ball — that's one point on the triangle — and you and your partner are the other two points. You now have an idea of what angles are possible and how to defend them. As the ball comes to your side, reverse the triangle and look for the open angles where you can hit between your two opponents.

» **Keeping the ball in play:** In both pickleball and soccer, keeping the ball in play means keeping it in bounds. A soccer goalie's primary objective is to ensure that the ball doesn't get past them. You will rarely find players with more grit and determination to chase down every ball, lunge, dive, or do whatever else is needed to keep a point going.

» **Agile footwork:** It's no surprise that soccer players have great footwork. They are trained to change speed and direction quickly, make fine-tuned foot movements for various types of touches, and stay in balance at all times. Quickly moving to the ball and then decelerating into smaller, controlled steps is an important skill in both sports. Soccer players are also used to constantly moving even when they don't have the ball. They understand the value in using these moments to get into a good position.

» **Utilize touch and finesse:** Scoring a goal in soccer is not about kicking the ball as hard as you can. Often, a soft touch and creative shot-making are required to fool the defenders. "Placement over power" is a tenet of smart pickleball strategy as well. A short, backspin dink when your opponents are busy retreating to defend against a smash is a great point-ender. Think of it as being like a soft shot into the corner of the goal when the goalie has already leapt in the air.

We hope we've managed to convince you that soccer and pickleball have a few things in common after all. However, there still are some obvious differences to note:

» **Hand-eye coordination:** Unless you're a goalie, you've been trained never to use your hands — even an accidental touch is a foul. Although your foot-eye coordination is amazing, your hand-eye coordination may need some additional practice. Finally, your hands get a chance to play, too!

» **Physical contact:** Soccer is an aggressive contact sport. In pickleball, you're limited to channeling your aggression through your paddle. (Try to resist the urge to slide tackle your partner after they miss three backhand poaches in a row.)

» **Throwing motion:** Soccer rules dictate that with the exception of the goalie, a throw-in must be done straight overhead with both arms. This motion is nothing like swinging a paddle, which has more in common with throwing a baseball or football using a full shoulder rotation.

Martial arts

If you've practiced martial arts in the past, you are probably familiar with the importance of discipline, repetition, and mental focus. You've been trained to use your entire body as a weapon and do only what is necessary through efficiency of movement.

Though different martial arts styles vary in their philosophies and applications, here are some skills you can take from your prior experience to apply to pickleball:

» **Anticipation:** Martial artists have trained to pick up on minute visual cues to anticipate what their opponent will do next. Watching not only the ball but also your opponent's body, eyes, and paddle to guess what they will "throw at you" next is an important skill in pickleball.

» **Meeting force with force:** In some martial arts styles, an attack is met with equal or greater force. Certain plays in pickleball, such as counterattacking on an attack, can help destabilize your opponent.

» **Meeting force with softness:** In other martial arts styles, the goal is to meet force with softness and throw your opponent off-balance by redirecting their momentum. This tactic can be compared to a reset shot in pickleball, in which you absorb the power off the ball and change the pace unexpectedly.

» **Reduced flinch response:** When a ball is slammed right at you, having your eyes open and staying square to the ball gives you the greatest chance of handling it. Martial artists train repeatedly to defend against strikes to their face and body, meeting attacks without flinching or recoiling. Your confidence and bravery to "lean in" to a fast-moving pickleball will serve you well.

Your martial arts training clearly brings a lot to the table. However, here are some aspects of pickleball that may be different or new to you:

» **Working with a partner:** As a martial artist, your focus is primarily on yourself. In doubles, you need to strategize as a team and stick to the joint plan. Going for all the glory with a flashy kill shot may be seductive, when in fact the smarter play may be to just hit one more unattackable ball and set up your partner for the put-away.

» **The patience to strike last:** If you come from a martial arts style that treats striking first as the objective, you may have trouble navigating the patience required in pickleball. Knowing when to attack versus when to hit a neutral or defensive shot, or simply to wait for your opponent to make the first error, is an important skill. Patience, Grasshopper.

» **Attacking the open court:** You've been trained to directly attack the person or object threatening you. Your tendency when you begin playing pickleball may be to constantly hit the ball straight at your opponent. Learning to recognize and hit to the open areas of the court, rather than right back to your opponents, will take time.

Enjoying Pickleball As Your First Sport

When coauthor Mo was a young airman in the U.S. Air Force, she had to learn to shoot a gun. Many of her fellow airmen had grown up shooting and hunting, so she worried she wouldn't measure up. She watched and listened closely to the instructors. Much to her amazement, she earned the Expert Marksman ribbon. The firearms instructors explained that this was possible because she arrived with no bad habits to overcome.

If you are arriving to the game of pickleball as a clean slate, you have the opportunity to develop only good habits and build from a solid foundation. Pickleball, much like expert shooting, is all about precision and hitting targets. Consider taking lessons early on so that you can learn good fundamentals. Then keep practicing and building from there. You may just earn a ribbon that you can wear around and later brag about in a book! Or you can certainly become a skilled player (earning medals instead of ribbons).

No matter your athletic background, we encourage you to enjoy improving at your own pace. Don't fall into the trap of comparing yourself to others. Yes, a 5.0 tennis player may start out playing pickleball at a higher rating than you. That doesn't mean you won't eventually meet or surpass them. (See Chapter 15 for more thoughts on this topic.) Pickleball is all about enjoyment, so if cutthroat competition isn't your thing, there's no pressure to play in tournaments. If drilling a particular skill repeatedly sounds boring to you, don't drill! People have enough tedious chores in life without turning pickleball into another one.

While researching for this chapter, we interviewed athletes who had competed at elite levels in their various sports. For the final question, we asked what they enjoyed most about pickleball. Almost everyone mentioned the social aspect: meeting new friends; being part of a community; and sharing spirited competition. Many also spoke about how fun and rewarding it is to learn a new skill and then work hard to improve it. You don't have to be an elite athlete to find these same aspects of pickleball enjoyable. Whether or not you have ever picked up a paddle or racquet, or stepped onto a court or ball field before, the joy is in the journey!

2
Getting into the Swing of Things

IN THIS PART . . .

Understanding the body mechanics of playing pickleball

Finessing the first three shots

Dinking 101

Smashing, volleying, and so much more

Avoiding injury

Chapter **6**

Building Solid FUNdamentals

Before we can get into the finer points of dinking, dropping, and driving, you need to start with the fundamentals. Pickleball is a sport that is very easy to pick up; most people can successfully rally and play games their first time out on the court, without needing to take a bunch of lessons first. (As teaching pros, we would never discourage taking lessons, though!) It's incredibly easy to get off and running, but if your goal is to keep improving over time, you want to solidify good habits right from the start so that you have a solid foundation to build from. Undoing habits becomes more and more difficult later on down the road.

In this chapter, we start with the basics, beginning with how to hold your paddle. We tell you about a couple different grips and which one we recommend the most. Next, you find out the proper ready position, how to hit the ball accurately with a compact swing, and how to locate and move to your strike zone, plus more technical tips.

Getting a Grip

The way you hold your paddle is extremely important. It's extra challenging to hit nice shots if you're holding your paddle in a "creative" way. (That was the nicest way we could think to put it.) Would you want your tattoo artist to hold their tool using just their thumb and pinky? No! They need a good stable grip as they're applying that flaming pickleball tattoo to your arm, and so do you when you're playing pickleball. You have myriad grips to experiment with, but the two covered here are largely what you see used in pickleball. Just be sure that the grip you're using is working for you.

The versatile continental grip

The most commonly recommended grip in pickleball is the *continental grip*, with which you position your hand neutrally on your paddle. Hold your hand like you're giving your paddle a handshake — "pleased to meet you!" — and you see that your hand, between your thumb and index finger, makes a "V" shape. The bottom point of that "V" should be placed over the medial bevel of your paddle's handle. (Figure 6-1 shows a proper continental grip.)

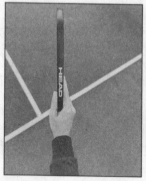 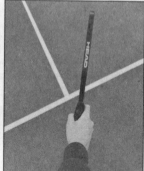 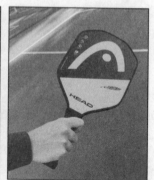

FIGURE 6-1: How to achieve a continental grip.

© John Wiley & Sons, Inc./Photo Credit: Aniko Kiezel

The easiest way to find this grip is to lightly pinch the top of your paddle between your thumb and the other four fingers of your hand. Then just slide your hand down the edge of the paddle, and when you get to the handle, give your paddle a nice, relaxed handshake.

Many videos are available online that will walk you through the steps of finding that perfect continental grip. They are particularly nice to watch while enjoying a continental breakfast.

TIP

To give yourself improved directionality and control, especially on your forehand shots, make sure you have enough space between your index and middle fingers. Note the space between the fingers in Figure 6-1.

Most coaches recommend the continental grip because it's a neutral grip that is good for hitting both forehands and backhands. Pickleball is a very fast-moving, dynamic sport, and you have only a teeny, tiny fraction of a second to change your grip as the ball comes right at you. The continental grip will "serve" you well.

The eastern forehand grip

The *eastern forehand grip* is achieved by rotating your hand so that the index knuckle (the second metacarpophalangeal joint) is on the flat surface of the grip. Many advanced players employ this grip. (See Figure 6-2.) *Note:* Don't worry, "metacarpophalangeal" will definitely be the longest word in this book.

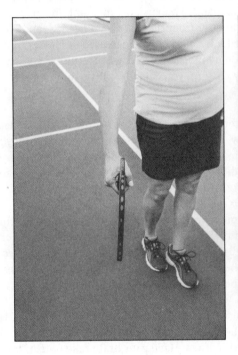
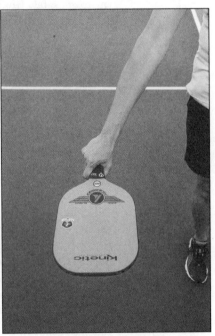

FIGURE 6-2:
The eastern forehand grip.

© John Wiley & Sons, Inc./Photo Credit: Aniko Kiezel

This grip can be useful for players who are trying to add more topspin and power to their forehand groundstrokes or serves. It puts the bulk of the hand a little bit more behind the paddle. This position puts more energy directly behind and under the paddle, giving the ball more forward rotation and creating a downward Magnus effect, which causes the ball to drop, hopefully within the boundaries of the court.

Fun physics fact: The *Magnus effect* is the force exerted on a rapidly spinning cylinder or sphere moving through air or a fluid in a direction at an angle to the axis of spin. This force is responsible for the swerving of balls when hit or thrown with spin. Another excellent use of the eastern forehand grip is hitting attack volleys, especially if you don't have great range of motion in your wrist.

WARNING

Please notice that this grip is *not* called the *eastern forehand–backhand* grip. Unlike the continental grip, it does not work for the backhand, so you will be faced with the added difficulty of switching your grip during the rally.

Getting the feel for proper grip pressure

Golf has an old adage about grip pressure: Hold the bird, but don't kill it. This wisdom applies in pickleball as well. If you have a death grip on your paddle and appear ready to hammer a nail into a wall, your grip is too tight. The ball will zing wildly off your paddle, perhaps scaring a passing flock of geese that was just trying to get safely from Canada to Mexico. If you maintain a more relaxed grip pressure, you can absorb energy from the ball when needed, and (counterintuitively) also be able to hit harder because of the increased wrist flexibility that will naturally result. This idea may indeed seem counterintuitive, but try it and you'll see that when you relax your grip, you can add a little more juice (also known as zip) to your shots.

WARNING

Holding your paddle too tightly is one of the primary causes of lateral epicondylitis, a.k.a. *tennis elbow*, which is a common injury among players. Try to get a "hold" on proper grip pressure early on in your pickleball career to avoid this painful — and very difficult to get over — condition. See Chapter 10 for more information on dealing with lateral epicondylitis.

Typically, as players move forward in the court toward the kitchen line, they get excited and tense and their grip pressure gets tighter and tighter. They are literally "white knuckling" the paddle. This is the time when you need to learn to relax the most. Your goal is to absorb power when blocking hard shots at the net, as well as to attack any high balls with accuracy and authority.

TIP

You can use a little trick to get a feel for a softer grip pressure. Hold your paddle as you normally do. Then release your pinky finger from the paddle as though you are enjoying a lovely cup of tea. Have your brain take note of how that grip pressure feels. It should feel kind of medium loose-ish (the technical term). Now, reapply your pinky so that it's gently resting on the paddle. Try to remember what that level of pressure felt like, and keep it as best you can throughout the game. Do not play with your "having tea" grip; just make note of that level of pressure on the grip. Is anyone else craving scones now?

Ready, Set, Go! Perfecting Your Ready Position

Ready position refers to the stance a player takes right before the action is about to begin. We cannot overemphasize the importance of the ready position, and readiness in general. By improving your readiness, you have more time to think about and execute your shots. The game starts to slow down, and you enjoy more chances to play the point on your terms instead of just reacting to what your opponent does. Everything builds from readiness!

Out of the blocks: Taking a stance

TIP

The most important part of your ready position is squaring your body to the ball. Many players square their body to the net and play that way no matter what is going on around them. If the ball is coming toward you, pivot so that your major joints (shoulders, hips, knees and ankles) are facing that direction. (See Figure 6-3.) This stance helps you to hit from a well-balanced position, with less reaching and fewer awkward movements. As the ball moves around the court, learn to track it with your body, not just your head.

Your ready position should change throughout any given point, depending on where you are in the court:

>> **Use a track stance when deep in the court.** If you're deep in the court, closer to the baseline, the ball you need to be ready for will be a lower one. (If you get a high ball while you're deep in the court, just let the ball go out.) A low ball headed your way requires your full attention and some solid footwork. Get your hands out in front of you, but not too high, because that position will slow you down when you have longer distances to cover. Hold your paddle at about navel, or even with the top of the net. Get a tiny bit lower in your stance, but don't squat. Stagger your feet, with your stronger leg *slightly* back. This is called a *track stance* and makes you faster by giving you a leg to push off from. (See Figure 6-4.) Competitive track athletes and swimmers always have one foot back when they are in the starting blocks. You should, too.

>> **Incrementally increase the height of your stance as you approach the net.** As you work your way from the baseline up to the kitchen line, through the *transition zone* (see Chapter 11 for more about moving through this zone), you get the opportunity to start looking for higher balls and possibly pounce on them. Incremental increases in the height of your posture — and your paddle — as you near the net help you to see, cope with, and possibly dominate those higher balls. If you're crouched too low as you move forward

in the court, you won't be able to see or hit these balls until they've dropped down lower, meaning you won't get to be as offensive as you could be. Stay in your track stance as you move through this zone so that you can quickly launch forward if you have the opportunity to hit a volley instead of a groundstroke. Your ability to accelerate in midcourt is essential.

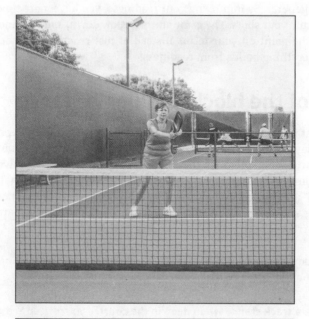

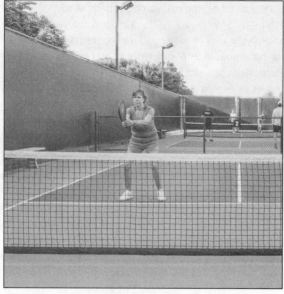

FIGURE 6-3:
A player squared to the ball (top) versus one squared to the net (bottom).

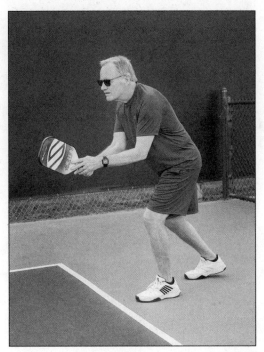

FIGURE 6-4:
The proper ready position at or near the baseline.

>> **At the kitchen line, stand mostly upright with your toes pointing forward.** After you arrive at the kitchen line, you want to be mostly upright. You should have your hands out in front, with the paddle in front of your sternum and your shoulders in line over your hips and ankles. Your knees should be slightly bent and your feet just wider than shoulder-width apart. Now, instead of that staggered track stance, both feet should be even with each other, about 1–3 inches from the kitchen line. Keep your weight slightly forward on the balls of your feet, but not up on your toes. Standing on your toes makes it too easy to fall forward into the kitchen. Try to envision wearing skis on your feet. You want your skis pointed forward, not turned inward (snowplow) or outward (splits). (See Figure 6-5 for the proper ready position at the kitchen.) You'll be quicker this way. As the ball moves around the court, shift your weight just slightly toward the leg closest to the ball so that you still have a leg to push off from if a sudden movement is necessary.

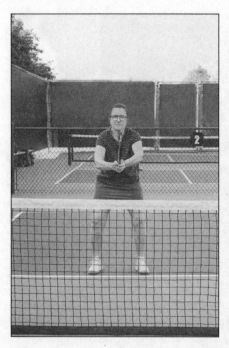 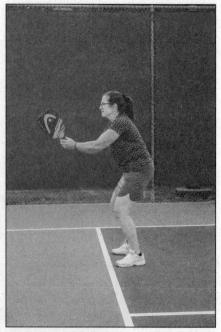

FIGURE 6-5:
A front and side view of the kitchen line ready position.

Keeping your chin and paddle up

As coaches, we never tell our students, "Watch the ball." Instead, we tell them, "Keep your chin up." When you keep your chin up throughout the rally, you find that you have fewer mis-hits, as well as more information on where to aim your next shot. For example, if you've dropped your head down to watch the ball bounce in front of you, you won't see that your sneaky opponent has moved to the middle to poach the next shot. (Figure 6-6 demonstrates the "chin up" position.) Lifting your chin up, you can see your paddle contact the ball and, in your peripheral vision, what your opponents and partner are doing. So you are indeed watching the ball, but also seeing the full situation that is unfolding in front of you.

Along with keeping your chin up, keep that paddle up, too. You spent good money on your paddle, so you should keep it in your sight at all times. (That guy on the next court with a cape and handlebar mustache does look a little shifty, and he's been eyeing your paddle all morning.) Keeping your paddle up means having less distance for it to travel when you receive a hard shot to your body; it also makes your reaction times faster. See Chapter 11 for more information on a technique called *paddle tracking*.

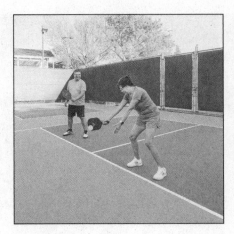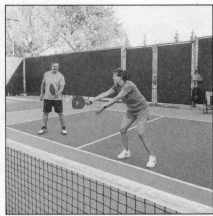

FIGURE 6-6: A player's line of sight when her chin is down (left photo) versus up (right photo).

© John Wiley & Sons, Inc./Photo Credit: Aniko Kiezel

Hold your paddle about chest height. (As noted previously, you should hold it slightly higher at the kitchen line than when you're at the baseline.) If you have trouble remembering how high, just think, "protect the heart." Your elbows should be slightly bent, leaving enough room for a small beach ball between your wrists and your chest. If your arms are fully extended with locked elbows or collapsed in toward your body, you have fewer options for adding or removing power on your shot. If you imagine a clock face, the tip of your paddle should be pointing to either 11 or 12 o'clock (for righties; see Figure 6-7) or 12 or 1 o'clock (for lefties). This position will allow you to quickly execute either a forehand or backhand.

TIP

By keeping your paddle and chin up, and squaring toward the ball, you present an imposing figure to your opponents. Nobody wants to hit the ball to a player who looks like they're ready to eat it for lunch; your opponent will be left scrambling to find a different target. Never let your guard down. By dropping your paddle down below your waist, you're sending a clear signal to your opponent that you're not ready. Your opponent will smile an evil grin and send a lob over your head or a body shot straight to your armpit. (Yes, we attack armpits in this sport. We never claimed it was a gentlepersons's game.)

Using your nondominant hand

You may have noticed that you're being encouraged to have your *hands* out in front, not just your paddle hand. Getting your nondominant hand out in front along with your paddle hand will help to keep you from dropping your paddle down toward your ankles. Your hands naturally want to be at the same height; if one hand drops, the other will eventually drop, too. Get in the habit of always having both hands raised out in front in your ready position. It will start to feel strange when they aren't, which will remind you to keep your paddle up.

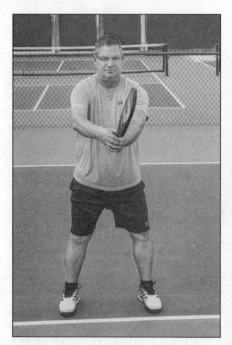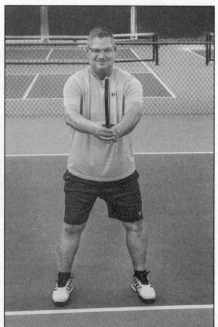

FIGURE 6-7:
An 11 o'clock (left) and 12 o'clock (right) paddle position.

Keeping your hands working together makes all the difference in keeping your body balanced. If your dominant hand is always way out in front and your other hand is draped lazily along your side as dead weight (something we lovingly refer to as *corpse arm*; see Figure 6-8), you are simply out of balance. Hitting out of balance negatively affects not only your current stroke but also your ability to recover for the next one. Tightrope walkers do not stick one arm out and leave the other hanging down. They want to avoid missteps at all costs, and so do you. Figure 6-9 shows properly balanced positioning.

It's up to you exactly where to place your nondominant hand. Unless you are planning to hit a two-handed backhand, it doesn't necessarily need to be on the handle. In fact, it doesn't need to be touching the paddle at all, though that usually feels more comfortable.

Don't worry, you don't need to keep your nondominant hand out in front of you while hitting every single shot, but it is an important part of the ready position. You may also find that having both hands out in front helps you engage your torso when swinging through the ball, as opposed to poking or jabbing at the ball solely with your arm. If you have two arms, make them both work for you.

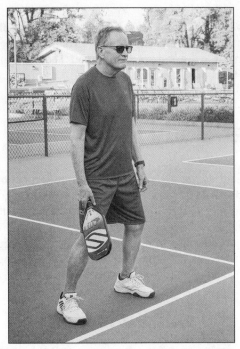

FIGURE 6-8:
A player who has dropped his paddle because of the dreaded corpse arm.

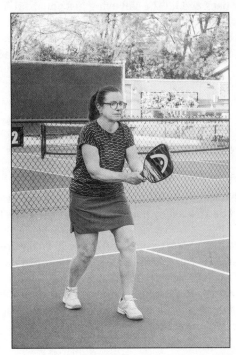

FIGURE 6-9:
A player in balance with both arms up.

If you're reaching way out in front for a ball, such as when volleying a shallow pop-up from the kitchen line, you can actually extend your reach by stretching your nondominant hand and arm back behind you. See the section on swinging volleys in Chapter 9 for more on this technique.

Using Good Upper-Body Mechanics

Playing pickleball requires the use of all your currently functioning body parts. Your upper body and lower body must be a team that works together. If you plan to hit every ball using only your arm, you should also plan to visit your doctor and physical therapist regularly. Your arm needs the support of the rest of your body, not only to avoid injury but also to produce consistent, high-quality strokes. In this section, we first look at how the various parts of your upper body can get involved; then we talk about what your lower body brings to the team.

Contacting the ball out in front

As you're beginning to play, one of the most important things to focus on is hitting the ball out in front of you. If you allow the ball to get even a little bit past you, you have to reach back and hit the ball using just your arm. Your shots will be less accurate, less powerful, and impose a lot of strain on your wrist and elbow. When you contact the ball out in front of you, you can actually see the ball hit your paddle, and your legs and torso can rotate through your swing, adding power and consistency.

Visualize a large "V" in front of your body. To do this, hold your arms out in front of you, each at exactly a 62.5° angle from your torso. (We may have just made that number up in an attempt to hawk our next product, the Pickleball Protractor. Approximate measurements are actually fine.) Figure 6-10 shows the all-important "V."

Your new mantra is "No ball gets past the 'V'!" When you can deal with every ball within this area, you'll be amazed by how much easier the game becomes.

Think of this "V"-shaped area as your *workspace*. If you were typing at your computer, whittling at your workbench, or performing open-heart surgery, you probably wouldn't set up your workspace off to the side — or worse, behind you. You would keep your hands, tools, and patient right in front of you. Pickleball is no different: You do your best work when you keep your hands, paddle, and the ball all within a comfortable workspace.

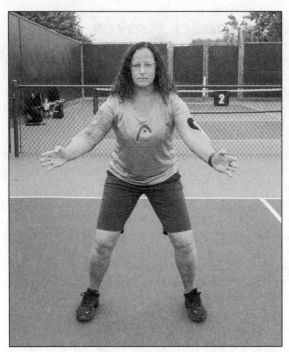

FIGURE 6-10:
An example of a player's "V," or ideal contact area.

REMEMBER

Earlier in this chapter, we talk about the importance of squaring to the ball when in ready position, as opposed to just facing the net at all times. If your upper body is already square to the ball as it comes toward you, your "V" naturally opens up square to the ball, as if you were trying to catch it, or give it a big hug.

When you contact the ball in front, you can see the ball, your paddle, and your opponents at the same time. If you wait until the ball is even with your body, you're too late. Either you will strike the ball blindly, or you will be forced to turn your head and lose track of what's happening on the other side of the court.

A ball struck too far behind you also means you'll also have to use your wrist and elbow to make the shot work. When you use your smaller joints, you lose consistency and accuracy. Your shots that hinge from your larger joints (shoulders, back, and hips) are more reproducible. Using your larger joints is also safer, meaning that it won't help line your doctor's pocketbook, thereby leaving more money for you to buy pickleball books. Isn't that the goal?

TIP

All this may sound simple enough, but contacting the ball late is an extremely common issue. Most players are not aware that they're striking the ball too far behind them. Ask a friend to record a short video of you playing, and then watch it in slow-mo to see exactly where your contact points were. You may be surprised by what you see!

Creating compact strokes

Pickleball is played on a small court, typically crowded with four players and divided by a net. This situation requires players to hit their targets, lest the ball go out of bounds, into the net, or straight to their opponent. Pickleball is a game of pinpoint accuracy! Placing the ball exactly where you want will win you many, many more points than just blasting away with all your might.

Consider the game of darts. A competitor who is trying to hit the bullseye doesn't take a big windup way behind their head and then throw the dart as hard as they can, like a cricket bowler. It just doesn't work (and would turn darts into a very bloody pastime). The more advanced dart thrower uses a very short, compact motion to achieve perfect accuracy. The same holds true in pickleball. A compact swing gives you more accuracy, allowing you to collect more medals and fame.

When talking about the compact stroke, we really mean that the backswing is compact. (See Figure 6-11 for a proper backswing.) For your groundstrokes, take your paddle back just past your hip. On other shots, the backswing is even shorter — and in some cases nonexistent. It all depends on the amount of power you need to generate and the amount of time you have to prepare to hit the ball. (Chapter 9 goes into the compactness of various types of volleys in more detail.)

TIP

It is much more common to take too big of a backswing on the forehand side than on the backhand because it's hard to reach way back behind your body on the backhand side. If you find that your backhand is more accurate than your forehand, an oversized backswing may be the explanation. Two-handed backhands tend to have the perfect amount of backswing, making them a very formidable shot.

REMEMBER

Don't forget that your primary goal is to always contact the ball within your "V." If your backswing is too large, and therefore takes too long to allow you to hit the ball before it passes your "V," you need to shorten it. You sacrifice a tiny bit of power, but accuracy and placement are more important. When hitting a soft shot, such as a drop shot or dink, think of the word *push* as you guide the ball forward with a slower stroke. When hitting a hard shot, such as a drive, think of the word *hit* and swing a little faster with more "oomph."

So you've taken your short backswing and are all set to contact the ball out in front. The ball enters your workspace — gulp — and it's now time to hit it! Swing forward, leading just a bit with your wrist until you reach the point of contact. The moment your paddle touches the ball, your paddle face should be "flat" (perpendicular to the ground) and facing toward your target. Strike the ball and continue swinging forward, guiding the ball over the net. As your paddle passes in front of your body, relax your elbow and wrist a little as you're following through, forward and upward. Figure 6-12 shows the flat paddle face at contact.

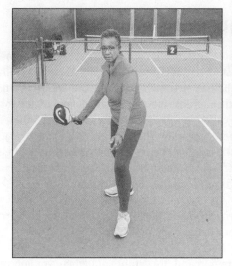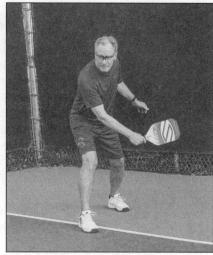

FIGURE 6-11:
A compact backswing on forehand (left) and backhand (right).

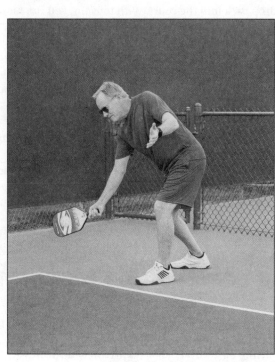

FIGURE 6-12:
A player with a "flat" paddle face at contact.

Achieving topspin

Many players claim that they don't use spin, aren't ready for spin, or don't understand it. They are almost always already using spin and don't realize it! Spin refers to the rotation of the ball as it travels through the air. Here on planet Earth, a pickleball never floats through the air completely devoid of any rotation. If the ball rotates forward, that's called *topspin*. If it rotates backward, that's called *backspin*. (Where do they get these names?) There is also *sidespin*, when the ball rotates horizontally (think of a basketball being spun on someone's finger) and *cork spin*, which is basically any off-axis (diagonal) spin. See Chapter 14 for a more in-depth look at using different types of spin.

TIP

Learn from our experience. Do not type "sidespin" into your search engine unless you're ready to see a lot of pole dancing content.

Topspin is the most common and important spin whenever you're playing a game over a low net, such as tennis or pickleball. Topspin causes the ball to arc over the net and then drop back into the court. With topspin, you can hit a nice, crisp serve or groundstroke and it will still land in bounds on your opponent's side, assuming that you haven't drastically over-hit.

The good news is that even if you are new to racquet and paddle sports, you can start using topspin in your game right away. To achieve topspin, just hit the ball out in front of you (in your "V") with a flat paddle face and an upward follow-through. This will magically (or seemingly so, to those not super big on physics) cause the ball to rotate over on itself. That's topspin! You did it!

Focusing on these fundamental upper body mechanics — contacting the ball out in front with a short backswing, flat paddle face, and pretty follow-through — not only gives you a solid start but also serves you well throughout your pickleball career.

Understanding Lower-Body Mechanics

The lower half of your body is another key component to playing good pickleball. When your upper body and lower body fail to work as a team, you'll be constantly off-balance. Hitting an accurate shot is extremely difficult when your two halves are going in different directions! You also need to use the muscles in your legs and waist to hit with any real power, and you need those feet to get you to the ball. We've noticed that when we're tired, our lower body doesn't always show up for us, or we're so focused on what we're doing with our paddle that we forget our feet are even there. Your legs and feet came to play, too, so wake them up and get ready to move!

Finding your strike zone

Your *strike zone* refers to the ideal place where you want your paddle to contact the ball. For either your forehand or your backhand, this magical zone is out in front of you, toward whatever side you're hitting on. This means that when you hit a forehand, that ball is out in front of your dominant side. For a backhand, it's still out in front, but on your nondominant side.

Pickleball is a fast-moving sport, and you typically don't have time to do a *unit turn* (also known as a *closed stance*), which is when you turn your body fully to the side before hitting the ball. A unit turn can allow your body to wind up and unleash a wicked shot, but it takes a few seconds that you often don't have in pickleball. When you aren't able to turn, you're left in a more *open stance*. That's okay; no need to worry. The closed and open stances are both fine, and you can generate plenty of power from either.

When hitting from a closed stance, your strike zone is about even with your forwardmost leg. When hitting with an open stance, your strike zone is out in front of both legs and off to either the forehand or backhand side. Figure 6-13 shows the strike zone in both closed and open stances.

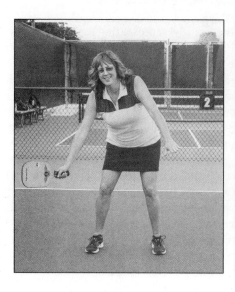 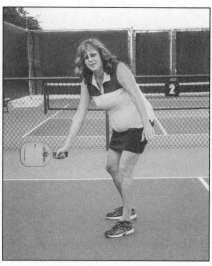

FIGURE 6-13:
The strike zone in both open (left) and closed (right) stances.

© John Wiley & Sons, Inc./Photo Credit: Aniko Kiezel

TIP

We encourage you to create a 3D visualization of your strike zone to give it more spatial meaning. You may imagine it as a glowing orb, a cloud of pixie dust, or a neon cube. Your strike zone is constantly attached to you as you move around the court, so make sure it's something you enjoy having around!

When you start to discover your strike zone and hit within it, your game greatly improves. Sadly, despite your strike zone's being made of magic pixie dust, those stubborn pickleballs do not just magically float straight into it. It's up to you to move your strike zone *to* the ball. For that, you need footwork.

Footing the bill: Effective footwork

Footwork essentially means getting your booty to the ball. Any questions?

When you see that the ball is heading toward you, call the ball ("Mine!"), present your paddle out in front of you within your strike zone, use big steps to quickly get to the general vicinity of the ball, and then take small steps to dial in.

REMEMBER

The whole sequence we just described builds from being super ready and tracking the ball as it moves around the court. (See the section "Ready, Set, Go! Perfecting Your Ready Position," earlier in this chapter, to find out about the ready position.) If you're staying focused and are eager to blast out of the starting blocks the moment your opponent hits the ball, you will get there much faster than your buddy who is casually standing and listening to onlookers talk about what a bold choice you made with those white spandex shorts.

TIP

You may have noticed that we advise presenting the paddle out in front before you zip over to the ball. This is a fantastic trick that helps you to figure out exactly where your strike zone is before you dial in that footwork. Your paddle becomes the target — all you need to do is aim yourself so that the ball collides with it. This technique also eliminates an unnecessary backswing when you arrive at the ball; the backswing takes longer to execute and can cause your weight to shift backward as you're hitting. Remember, if your lower body is going backward at the same time that your upper body is going forward, you won't have a good result.

As you start moving to the ball, keep your weight forward on the balls of your feet, but not on your toes. Take large steps to cover the court quickly, followed by tiny steps to adjust your position. You can think of it like using binoculars or a microscope: The big knob gets you close, and the little knob refines. Stay confident. If your internal monologue is saying, "I can get there," you're much more likely to get there.

Gettin' shifty: Watching for weight shift

You've arrived. The ball is in your strike zone. You have taken your compact backswing. You're moving your paddle forward, hitting through the ball. As all this is happening, your weight should be shifting forward.

Ideally, your shots are hinging from your shoulder and your waist. When you use your major joints and muscle groups, including your legs, your weight naturally shifts forward as you swing. You should feel your pelvis open up toward your target as you complete each shot with a pretty follow-through. This forward weight shift adds a great deal of power and accuracy to your shot because your torso and legs are getting in on the action. You will know whether your weight has shifted forward if you notice that your back heel has lifted up slightly. Figure 6-14 shows a forward weight shift as the player completes the follow-through. If you're in a completely open stance (both feet facing the net) don't dismay — you can still use good forward weight shift with just your upper body. Lean in slightly and push forward through your shot.

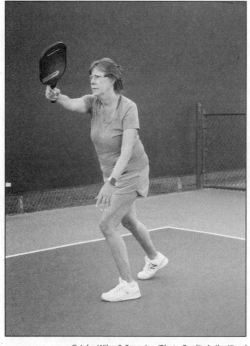

FIGURE 6-14:
A completed follow-through with a forward weight shift.

A forward weight shift also sets you up to move in behind the shot. You always want to try to move *forward* in the court. Moving forward puts pressure on your opponents, cuts off their possible angles, and gets you closer to the net. The player who is closer to the net is the player who can hit down on the ball, or at least cut the ball off earlier, taking time away from their opponents. You and your partner should be like a tsunami wave pressing toward your opponents. Imagine what this looks like from the other side of the net, as opposed to a team who is stuck in mud, or moving backward in retreat.

Chapter 7

Starting the Point: The First Three Shots

Before you get into the fun of dinking and banging, you need to know the fundamentals of starting play in pickleball: the serve, the return, and the all-important third shot. This chapter covers all three of these initial shots, plus their mechanics, goals, and targets. We guide you through the rules of serving and explain how the Two-Bounce Rule affects the nature of these first three shots.

Each point starts with a serve. Although the rules ensure that your serve is unlikely to overpower the receiver for an "ace," you want to learn to serve accurately and strategically so that you can start each point in your team's favor.

We often say that the serve return is the most underrated shot in pickleball. A strong return can help force a weak third shot from your opponents. A weak return can lead to your opponents taking the offensive early on in the point. These points typically don't end well for your team! Later in the chapter, we take you through the basic mechanics behind forehand and backhand groundstrokes, as well as the goals and targets for the serve return.

The third shot determines whether the serving team can move forward to join the battle up at the kitchen (non-volley zone, or NVZ) line, or if they will have to stay back and try, try again. Your best options for a third shot are either the iconic "third-shot drop" or a well-placed **drive.** You find out how and when to hit each of these shots so that you can get **to** rallying, and most of all, having pickleball fun!

Serving It Up

At the very beginning, you start a pickleball point with a serve. The rules of pickleball are designed with the idea that **the serve** puts the ball into play. (Although tennis is known for powerful "ace" **serves,** in pickleball, aces are rare.) For your team to start off with an advantage, it's more important to focus on *the quality* of your serve, rather than pure power. You **want** to put your best foot forward and serve up the ball right!

Keeping it legal

We touch on basic serving rules in Chapter 2, but this section goes into more depth on those rules. Before you solidify **any bad habits,** you need to thoroughly understand all the requirements of a legal serve. Here are some rules to keep in mind:

>> **Strike the ball below the waist.** Figure 7-1 shows you the difference between legal and illegal contact points. Because you're playing a sport that involves getting the ball over a **net,** this low-contact point means that you have no way to hit downward on the ball, as you can with an overhand tennis serve.

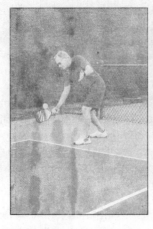 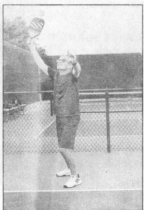 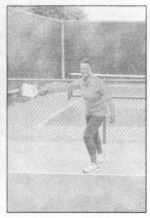

FIGURE 7-1:
Legal (left) and
two different
illegal (right)
contact points on
a serve.

© John Wiley & Sons, Inc./Photo Credit: Aniko Kiezel

>> **Serve the ball using a low-to-high underhand motion.** This seemingly small detail is a major part of why people of a wide variety of ages and physical abilities can take up the sport in the first place. Many older athletes find that their shoulders don't enjoy coming up and over anymore, as when throwing a baseball. (Coauthor Mo has a shoulder that is essentially dangling by the threads of her tired shoulder ligaments, but she can still hit a pickleball serve pretty darn hard.) Thankfully, the pickleball gods smiled upon the world and gave us a serve that we can all do a lot more comfortably.

>> **The highest part of the paddle cannot be higher than your wrist.** Figure 7-2 shows examples of an illegal "cocked wrist" serve compared to a legal one. You shouldn't spend too much time worrying about this rule, because serving this way would be very awkward unless you're attempting to add a heavy slice or spin to the ball.

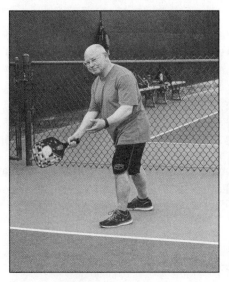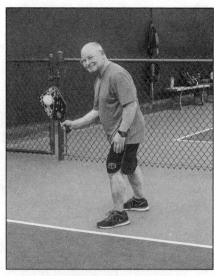

FIGURE 7-2:
A legal serve (left) versus an illegal cocked-wrist serve (right).

© John Wiley & Sons, Inc./Photo Credit: Aniko Kiezel

>> **You may strike the ball out of the air, before it bounces, or you may drop the ball and let it bounce before striking it.** The first option is often referred to as the traditional serve, because for many years this was the only legal way to serve. Introduced in 2021, the drop serve now allows you to hit the ball off a bounce, but be aware that the ball cannot have any energy added to it. Simply put, you may not toss or bounce the ball with any force; you must simply drop it and let gravity do its thing.

» **Strike the ball while standing behind the baseline.** You should be standing behind the service box on the correct side of the court. (See Chapter 4 for specifics about the layout of a pickleball court.)

» **Always call all three numbers of the score before serving.** You have ten seconds after the score is called to unleash your beautiful beast of a serve on your opponents. If someone questions the score, you may correct yourself and call the score again. (See Chapter 2 for details about keeping score.)

» **You must hit the ball crosscourt so that it lands in the service box that's diagonal from you, on your opponents' side of the court.** If the ball lands on the baseline, sideline, or centerline, the serve is considered in. If the ball lands on the kitchen (NVZ) line, it's a fault.

» **If the serve goes in the net and doesn't make it to the other side of the court, it's a fault.** If the serve touches the top of the net and lands in, the ball is live and must be played. If the serve touches the top of the net and does not land in, it's a fault.

» **You get only one fault on your service attempt.** If you miss your serve, it's your partner's turn to serve or it's a sideout, depending on whether you were the first or second server (or considered the "2" because it was the first serve of the game).

Preparing to serve: This is your moment!

Serving is your big moment to show everyone on the court what you've got. It's also the only shot in pickleball that lets you work entirely on your own terms. Rushing through the serve is one of the most common causes of service faults. Take your time to do it right and make sure you've completed the following steps before you serve it up:

1. **Let the previous point go.**

   If you lost the previous point, take a moment to think about what you could have done differently. Then forgive yourself and let it go. A brand-new point means new opportunities to succeed where you previously may have faltered.

   TIP

   Before serving, a quick check-in with your partner through eye contact, a paddle tap, and some encouraging words ("We got this!") can quickly erase any past regrets while lifting your team up at the same time.

2. **Create your own serving routine and stick to it.**

   You may try bouncing the ball five times, drying your sweat on your shirt, twirling your paddle in your hand, or whatever repetitive action helps you refocus for the next rally.

3. **Note where your opponents are standing and then choose a target.**

   Is the receiver standing way off to one side, perhaps to avoid using their forehand or backhand? Are they standing inside the baseline, or several feet back? These are all clues as to where you may want to aim your serve. Be sure to select your target before you begin your service motion!

REMEMBER

   The receiver's partner, who is standing up at the kitchen line, may try to intimidate you by hugging the centerline. Don't let this tactic influence you into serving out wide if that wasn't your plan. If your serve just so happens to end up hitting this player, it's your point!

4. **Call the score and let it settle.**

   Sometimes the other players on the court don't agree with the score you've just called. It's best to get the matter of the score sorted out before beginning the next point. Also, many players tend to serve while calling the score simultaneously, which typically results in less than optimum results. Not only is this illegal — the rules say you must call the entire score before beginning your service motion — but it's also needless multitasking! It's the same reason we stopped chewing gum while juggling on our unicycles.

Mastering Serving Mechanics

In pickleball, no two players' serves are exactly alike. The truth is you can hit a good serve in a thousand different ways. Fortunately, all you need is one. Above all else, keep it simple. Start with solid serving mechanics that will be easy on your body and lead to consistent, replicable results.

When it's your turn to serve, follow these steps:

1. **Point your front foot toward your target.**

   Your front foot is the opposite foot from your paddle hand and should generally point to the middle of the service box to which you are aiming. Your back foot may also point the same direction, or open slightly to form a "V" shape. Your stance should feel comfortable and totally in balance. (Figure 7-3 shows the best ways to stand when serving.)

WARNING

   Avoid lining up completely sideways to your target, with both feet parallel to the baseline. This position will force your back to unnaturally twist in order to direct the ball crosscourt. Besides, we'd rather you spend your hard-earned money on pickleball books than weekly visits to the chiropractor.

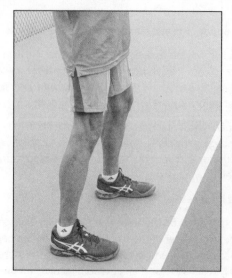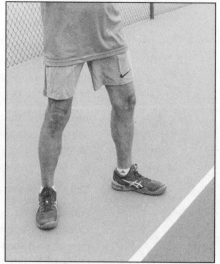

FIGURE 7-3: Recommended ways to stand when serving.

2. **Present the ball out in front.**

   Whether you are using the traditional (out of the air) serve or the drop (off the bounce) serve, be sure to present the ball far enough out in front of you. You don't want to get jammed up as you swing, or contact the ball where you can't see it. Your non-paddle hand also has a very important job to do on the serve; it must "tee" up the ball in the perfect position every time, ideally along the natural swing path of your paddle. If you toss or drop the ball in a different place each time, you will be forced to chase after the ball with your paddle, leading to inconsistency and frustration.

   TIP

   If you're having difficulty with the rule about contacting the ball below your waist, focus on presenting the ball at a lower height. It helps to bend slightly at the waist and use a dead drop rather than an upward toss.

3. **Abbreviate, or eliminate, the backswing before you make contact with the ball.**

   When you're first learning to serve, a shorter backswing can resolve timing issues and help ensure that you make solid contact with the ball in your paddle's sweet spot. Think "short-to-long" — short backswing, long follow-through toward your target. (See Figure 7-4 for an example of an abbreviated backswing).

4. **Hinge from your shoulder and waist, and follow through upward.**

   Swing forward through the ball on your serve, continuing with an upward follow-through. The paddle should wind up near your ear, or just above your head, over your opposite shoulder.

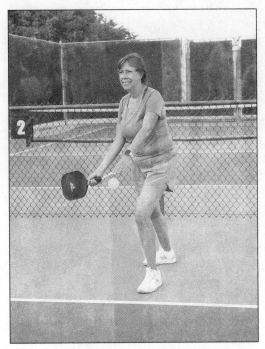

FIGURE 7-4:
Abbreviated backswing on the serve.

5. **Strike the ball with the paddle at an angle of 45 degrees. (See Figure 7-5.)**

Avoid dropping your paddle head vertically so that it's perpendicular to the court. Hitting the ball at an angle allows you to generate much more topspin. The full vertical paddle drop also tends to be inaccurate and inconsistent because even the tiniest variant in the paddle face direction causes the ball to fly out. We want your serves to go *in!*

WARNING

Some pickleball instructors teach a full paddle drop, or what we call "the bowling serve," to beginners. Although this variation guarantees a legal serve, it's not a great technique to build on.

6. **Transfer your weight from your back foot to the front foot.**

Your back heel should pop up a bit, indicating that your weight has indeed shifted from the back foot to the front. (See Figure 7-6.)

TIP

If you struggle with this stance, put your paddle down for a few minutes and practice tossing some balls underhand over the net. You will find that your weight naturally shifts forward in the direction you're tossing the ball. Then pick up your paddle and do the exact same weight shift as you serve.

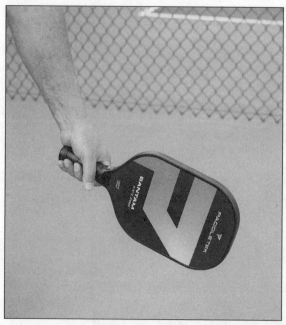

FIGURE 7-5:
The recommended angle at which to hold the paddle when serving.

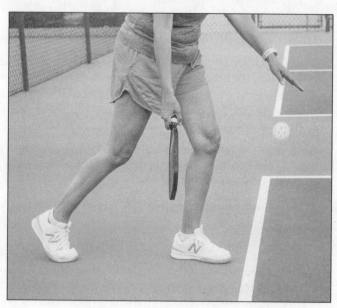

FIGURE 7-6:
A proper weight shift with heel lift.

7. **End with your hips pointed toward your target.**

Your pelvis should open and end up facing your target. (We feel kind of funny commenting on what you should be doing with your pelvis, but correct positioning in pickleball does matter. #yourpelvisisyourbusiness)

TIP

If your serves are going too far to the left or right, check where your hips are pointed after you hit the ball. Adjust your stance accordingly so that next time, your hips will end up square to the middle of the service box.

MAKING THE SERVE YOUR OWN

After you're getting at least 85 percent of your serves in, it's time to start experimenting with adding your own variations and personal flair. We encourage you to make your serve your own; it's your fingerprint. You can try any of these variations as you continue to develop your personal serving style:

- **Try pointing your lead foot toward your target and your rear foot to the side.** This creates more of an "L" shaped stance. You may find that this stance allows your hips to rotate faster through your swing, generating more power.

- **Take a step toward your target as you're striking the ball.** Many players find that this step leads to a more natural and complete weight transfer.

- **Use a larger, more looping backswing to generate more power and topspin.** Just be sure you're not contacting the ball late because of the added time it takes for your longer backswing.

- **Experiment with using both the traditional serve and the drop serve.** It's perfectly legal to switch between the traditional serve and the drop serve throughout the match. It's fun to keep your opponents guessing by adding more variety to your serving toolbox.

- **Add sidespin, either through the toss or by changing your swing path.** We go into more detail on how to achieve spin in Chapter 14.

- **Try a backhand serve.** If you're having trouble with your forehand serve, or simply want to mix things up, try serving from your backhand side. Line up with your front foot pointed at the far net post. Present the ball out in front so that the paddle will connect with it on a natural swing path. Backhand serves can be useful for disguising from your opponent where the ball may go, but they generally lack power.

Settling on serving targets

When you serve, your three primary goals should be (in this order):

>> **Get it in.** Remember, you get only one chance to serve, and your team can win points only when you are serving. You don't want to give up your opportunity to score points with big, risky serves that end up being faults more often than not. Although it's fine to occasionally "go big" with your serve, you should be getting at least 85 percent of them in before you get too fancy.

>> **Hit it deep.** Basic pickleball strategy calls for keeping your opponents back as long as you can. A deep serve helps prevent them from hitting an offensive shot and quickly moving in toward the kitchen line. As a beginner or intermediate player, aim your serves for the back third of the service box.

>> **Direct it toward your opponent's weaker side.** In most cases, an opponent's weaker side is their backhand side. As you become more accurate with your serves, you can also pay attention to whether your opponent prefers a high-bouncing or low-bouncing serve, and how they handle different types of spin.

The more you practice with these goals in mind, the better off you'll be! A deep serve to the opponent's backhand side is an excellent go-to serve in many situations. However, we still recommend that you ultimately keep a few different serves in your toolbox. Figure 7-7 illustrates a few of our favorite serving targets. These serves are not only fun to practice but also extremely satisfying to unleash on your opponents at unexpected times.

Try these different serves to determine which serves to use:

>> A hard, deep serve aimed to either the right, left, or middle of the service box.

>> A soft, short serve that will cause a back-footed or slow player to hit outstretched and on the run.

>> A deep, high-bouncing lob serve that pushes your opponent back into the fence.

>> A sneaky, short-angled serve that often leaves the court before your opponent has time to say "Doogie Howser!" (Pickleball players employ *very* creative cuss words.)

Serve and step back (more than just a dance move)

Earlier in this chapter, we discuss the importance of establishing a service routine. However, your routine is not over as soon as you have struck the ball. You still have one more dance move in this cha-cha, one that we like to call "Serve and step back."

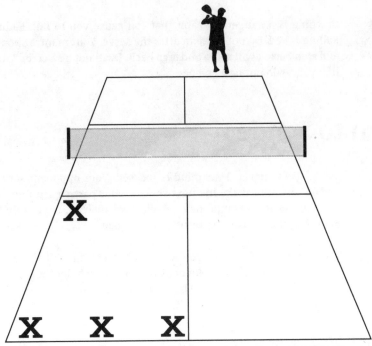

© John Wiley & Sons, Inc.

FIGURE 7-7:
A variety of
targets to aim for
when serving.

After you have served the ball, your momentum (and your brain's desire to "fol-low the ball") has a tendency to pull you forward into the court. You may find yourself standing several feet inside the baseline as you wait for the ball to come back. In pickleball, this is known as *creeping*. Don't be a creeper! This advice goes for the server's partner as well. As part of your service routine, make a habit of stepping (or staying) back behind the baseline after you've completed your service motion.

REMEMBER

Because of that pesky Two-Bounce Rule, you must always let the serve return bounce before you can hit it (see Chapter 2). If you have crept forward toward the net and your clever opponent notices this and hits a deep return to you, coping with your next shot will be difficult. You will be dealing with a ball bouncing right at your feet or, even worse, several feet behind you. By staying farther back after your serve, you will be able to contact the ball in front of you with a forward weight shift, rather than have to try to back pedal and hit a ball that is already past you.

Although it's true that occasionally you will get a short return that requires you to run forward on the court, you're still better off staying back in case of a deep return. It is easier (and safer) to run forward than to run backward. Remember to use your "track stance" from Chapter 6 so that you have a leg to push off from in case you do need to run for the ball.

Creeping is a dangerous habit that can cause you to fall. Falling is bad. Repeat: Falling is bad. Do not creep in after the serve. Your mantra should be, "I will serve and step back. I will serve and step back. I will not be a creep." In pickleball and in life, please do not be a creeper.

Return to Sender

The players are set. Your mind is focused. Your opponent serves the ball to you. It's up to you to make the next shot — your partner isn't even allowed to touch the ball. What do you do next? Panic? No! Instead, try calmly returning the ball back over the net with a pretty groundstroke.

A groundstroke is a shot you hit after the ball has hit the ground — hence the name. Owing to the Two-Bounce Rule, you have to let the serve bounce before you can hit your return. So stand back deep in the court and be ready for either a forehand or backhand groundstroke.

Finessing the forehand groundstroke

A forehand is any shot hit on your dominant (paddle hand) side. If you're a right-handed player and the ball is headed toward your right side, that's a forehand. If you're a left-handed player, a forehand will be struck from the left side of your body. Either way, you want to follow these steps to hit a solid forehand groundstroke:

1. **Present the paddle out in front.**

    As soon as you see the ball coming to your forehand side, "flop" your paddle out in front of you toward your dominant side. This is a fun way of saying "present the paddle out in front of your body." It should feel as if you are going to catch the ball with an open palm. Do not take a large backswing by bringing your paddle way back behind you; doing so is unnecessary and can lead to striking the ball too late.

2. **Move your feet to the ball.**

    Because your paddle is already in position, you know exactly where you want the ball to be when you meet up with it. It takes some practice to accurately predict the trajectory and bounce of each serve, but doing so gets easier with time. Be sure to stay light on your feet so that you can make tiny adjustments at the last second, if needed.

3. **Contact the ball out in front.**

Figure 7-8 illustrates what we like to call your "strike zone." Much like a batter in baseball, your best shots will come from hitting a ball within your strike zone. Unfortunately, unlike in baseball, you can't just stand still in the batter's box and hope the pitcher throws a strike. It's up to you to move your strike zone to the ball. That's right — you must use your feet!

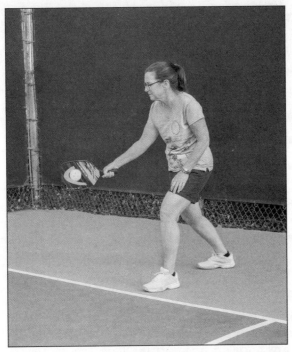

FIGURE 7-8:
An example of an ideal forehand strike zone.

4. **Hit through the ball with a forward weight shift.**

It helps to imagine that you're hitting through a line of three pickleballs, not just one. Push forward through the ball, guiding it forward, rather than carving or chipping at it. As you swing, your weight should transfer in the direction you're aiming the ball.

5. **Follow through upward.**

After you have finished the forward part of the swing, your paddle should come up and over your opposite shoulder, out in front of your ear. This is an excellent time to have your photo taken, because a great follow-through just looks cool!

Fear not the backhand groundstroke

We often hear players declaring that they "don't have a backhand." Or, more subtly, we see them running around the ball (usually way off the court) so that they can avoid hitting a backhand. The backhand can seem intimidating if you don't have experience playing racquet sports. Fear not, friends! With proper paddle preparation and a relaxed follow-through, you, too, can hit a beautiful backhand.

TIP

If you can throw a flying disc, you can hit a backhand. The motion is very similar. The good news is that even if you can't throw a disc, you can still hit a backhand!

Some of what follows will sound quite familiar (you're catching on!). If you're a right-handed player and the ball is headed toward your left side, it's time to hit a backhand. Once again, the opposite is true for left handers.

Follow these six steps and you'll prove to everyone (most of all, yourself) that you actually do own a backhand:

1. **Present the paddle out in front.**

   As soon as you see the ball coming to your backhand side, "flop" that paddle out there in front of you, this time toward your nondominant side. This is your compact, winning backswing that will reduce the chance of errors. Figure 7-9 shows the correct paddle presentation for a backhand groundstroke. It can help to use your non-paddle hand for support, regardless of whether you're planning to hit a two-handed backhand.

2. **Move your feet to the ball.**

   Use big steps to get to the general vicinity of the ball and then little steps to dial in to exactly where you want to have your paddle meet the ball. It's similar to using a microscope or binoculars: Use the big knob first, and then use the little knob for fine-tuning. Again, you want to steer your path so that the ball ends up landing right on your paddle at the point where you and the ball collide.

3. **Make contact with the ball out in front.**

   Figure 7-9 shows the ideal strike zone on your backhand side. It should be slightly on your nondominant side rather than in front of your belly button — give yourself space to hit.

4. **Hit *through* the ball with a forward weight shift.**

   It can be helpful to imagine guiding the ball forward over the net, rather than slapping or stabbing at it. As you hit, shift your weight in the same direction you want the ball to go.

5. **Follow through upward.**

   You should feel a slight stretch in your upper back and the sensation of your chest opening up. If you freeze your follow-through, you'll resemble the Statue of Liberty with your torch (paddle) held high in the air. Try to relax as you swing; many backhand issues come from being too tight and controlled, resulting in little to no follow-through.

6. **Sign autographs for all of the people who gather around to admire your stunning backhand.**

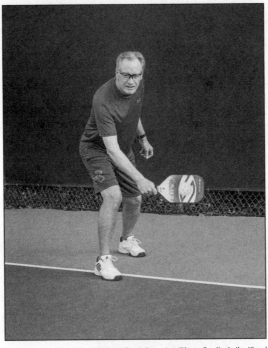

FIGURE 7-9: The ideal backhand strike zone.

Realizing your return of serve goals

Too many players hit their returns without much thought. In truth, the serve return is crucial to building a successful point for your team.

Your primary goal for your return should be to force a weak third shot from your opponents. In other words, don't give them a ball that will be easy to deal with! A short, high-bouncing return invites them to tee off with a blistering third-shot drive. Your team is now instantly on defense and will struggle to get back into the rally. A short return also makes it much easier for your opponent to hit a successful third-shot drop because they can come forward to the ball, hitting comfortably in their strike zone. For these reasons, we recommend hitting your returns deep.

THE PROS AND CONS OF TWO-HANDED BACKHANDS

Traditionally, most pickleball players use a one-handed backhand because of the lightness of the paddle. However, the two-handed backhand (meaning that both hands remain on the paddle handle for the entire swing) is gaining popularity among many pro and recreational players. If you're considering adopting a two-hander, you'll want to understand the pros and cons first.

Pros:

- **Increased power:** Increased torso rotation means more force behind your shots, as opposed to the force generated just by using your arm and hinging from the shoulder.

- **Improved consistency:** Hinging from your waist is very stable and can offer control and accuracy because of the added use of your torso.

- **Built-in muscle memory:** You may already feel comfortable with this hitting style if you come from tennis, baseball/softball, or golf.

Cons:

- **Limited reach:** The two-hander limits your reach pretty significantly, especially when the ball is down around or behind your nondominant foot. You need quicker footwork to get the ball in your strike zone.

- **Awkward learning curve:** If you're not used to this shot, it can feel unnatural because you are driving the paddle with your nondominant hand.

- **Special paddle requirement**: Unless you have small hands, they may not both fit comfortably on a standard-length handle. As the two-hander becomes more popular, manufacturers have started making models with longer handles. However, because of the restrictions in overall length, you will typically sacrifice some paddle face length for the extra handle length.

Your second goal for returning serve is to put your team in a winning position. Before the point began, your partner wisely took an offensive position up at the kitchen line. You'll want to join them there so that your team will be the ones hitting down on the ball. After you've hit your gorgeous return, hustle up to the line like a disco dancer from the 1970s. Don't run so fast up to the kitchen that you can't gently stop, though. Hard, jarring stops are terrible for your joints; they can also leave you off-balance for the next shot.

TIP

There's no shot like the present! Make sure you do only one thing at a time: Hit your return first, and then move up to the line second. There's no sense hitting your return into the net because you're so worried about getting into position for the next shot. Running through your shot almost always leads to regret.

As you line up before the serve, you should already have a target in mind — and that's one less thing to worry about as you're trying to hit! Here are a few solid choices for a target:

>> **Deep to the middle.** For beginner and intermediate players especially, it's usually a great idea to hit your returns deep and to the middle of the court (referred to as the "T," the spot where the centerline and baseline meet.) This forces the other team to quickly figure out who will hit the ball. You're also keeping them back away from the net longer. The longer you can keep your opponents back, the better off you are.

>> **Deep to your opponent's weaker side.** If you have noticed that one of your opponents doesn't have a stunning backhand like yours, try hitting to their backhand side. If their forehand shots are all going in the net today, hit to their forehand. Odds are, a return hit deep to an opponent's backhand corner is your best bet.

>> **Short drop shot into the kitchen.** If you've been consistently hitting deep returns the entire game, try occasionally hitting a drop shot into the kitchen that your opponents aren't expecting. A drop shot can be particularly effective if you sense that your opponent is getting tired toward the end of a match. Be cautious about using this shot with more spry players because you are essentially inviting them up to the net with you — which is something to avoid. Try it once and see how it goes!

The preceding three targets are enough to win you many points. We get into more in-depth return strategies in Chapter 11 so that you can return serve like a master pickleball player (which entitles you to a special license plate frame and keychain).

Hitting the All-Important Third Shot

After the serve (the first shot) has been made and returned (the second shot), the serving team hits (you can probably tell where this is going) the third shot. In pickleball circles, you hear much talk, debate, and pontification about the notorious "third shot." We're sure that in the Old West, the third shot discussions started many a gun fight.

Why all the buzz about the third shot? The explanation lies with the Two-Bounce Rule, which dictates that both players on the serving team must stay back to let the return bounce before they can hit it. (Unlike in tennis, employing a "serve and volley" tactic in pickleball is illegal.) By the time the return of serve comes back, both players on the receiving team have likely ended up at the kitchen line. They have formed a seemingly impenetrable wall. The serving team, now with a severe positioning disadvantage, must hit their third shot in such a way that they, too, can get up to the kitchen line. Any third shot that is *attackable* (meaning a ball that can be struck with a downward motion) will lead to the point being over very quickly. Although it's not easy (and some would whine "not fa-a-a-a-ir") for the serving team to have to overcome this inherent disadvantage, it's not impossible, either. You have two distinct options when hitting a third shot, so read on about how and when to use each one.

Drop it like it's hot

A *drop shot* is a low-energy ball hit shallowly into your opponent's court. A successful drop shot (or *drop,* for those in the know) is one that your opponent cannot attack because they can't swing downward (high to low), but rather must swing upward (low to high) in order to lift the ball up and over the net.

When you see your opponent swinging low to high, you're not currently in danger of having the ball blasted at your toes. You can safely move forward toward the kitchen line, at least two or three big steps. Yay — progress! Keep in mind that moving all the way to the line often takes more than one drop shot. Stay patient and hit as many drops as it takes to get all the way to the kitchen line.

REMEMBER

The team that gets to play closer to the net is more likely to win the rally because they get to hit down on a higher number of balls. Be that team! Don't give up and try to play every rally from midcourt. The odds will not be in your favor.

Now that we've convinced you of the need to have this shot in your repertoire, you need to know how to hit it. Start with the same good forehand and backhand groundstroke mechanics discussed earlier in this chapter. Nobody wants to learn dozens of different strokes, so just use your basic strokes with a few small differences, depending on your goals. Using the same mechanics for your various shots can also help to disguise your shot, keeping your opponents from easily predicting what you're about to do. (Three of the four coauthors are very sneaky, and we're not about to divulge which one isn't.) When hitting a drop shot, think of the phrase "slow push." Your goal is to guide the ball a few feet over the net, with very little energy behind it, so that it starts to die (drop) as soon as the ball crosses over into your opponents' court (see Figure 7-10). Be careful not to hit the ball too high in the air, or it will bounce up high after it hits the ground, becoming an easily attackable (for your opponent) ball.

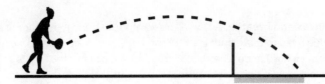

FIGURE 7-10:
The optimal
trajectory of a
drop shot.

© John Wiley & Sons, Inc.

Here are some of the keys to successfully hitting drops:

>> **Use a more relaxed, supple wrist and a lighter grip pressure.** Your goal is to absorb some of the power and take it off the ball, not add to it. Let the paddle be a little looser in your hand, but not so loose that you drop it!

>> **Give yourself plenty of room behind the ball.** It's absolutely crucial on drops to contact the ball out in front of you, with a forward weight shift.

>> **Gently push or guide the ball forward.** Be careful not to "scoop" under the ball too much, lifting it high into the air. Imagine a window or picture frame hovering just over the net. (The size of your window can depend on your current skill level.) As you swing, think of gently pushing the ball through the window. This visualization technique helps to ensure that your ball travels lower over the net.

>> **Swing slowly!** Whenever you're trying to hit a soft shot, like a drop, think instead of the word "slow." The word "soft" tells you the desired outcome, but not how to achieve it. The speed of your swing dictates the pace of the ball. For drop shots, it's even slower than you think, so hit that "slow-mo" button on your internal remote control!

>> **Think dink!** The third-shot drop is hit very much like a dink. The only differences are a forward step into the ball and a longer follow-through. You still push the ball softly over the net with your paddle low and out in front of you. If you try to hit or jab at the ball, you won't be able to properly control the shot.

>> **Be mindful of bounce height.** Even if you hit a beautiful rainbow of a drop that lands in the kitchen, a smart opponent will just step back and let it bounce. With too much energy behind it, a ball can easily bounce up to your opponent's attackable height. If you find your drops bouncing too high, swing slower and concentrate on hitting them lower over the net (through the imaginary window).

>> **Consider adding backspin or topspin.** Backspin helps to keep the ball from bouncing too high. Topspin helps the ball curl over the net with a lower trajectory. (Check out Chapter 14, where we put our own spin on the subject of spin.)

>> **Relax and breathe.** Anytime you want to slow down the pace of a pickleball, you need to relax, both in mind and body. We realize (all too well) that relaxing can be hard to do when you're frustrated. Don't put the fate of the world on the shoulders of your drop shot. Take a moment to put it in perspective. Take a time out, joke with your partner, or just pause and smile for a moment. Relax. You can do this!

THIRD-SHOT DROP TARGETS

Mo and Reine's favorite way to win a point in pickleball is to hit a drop shot so well that the opponent hits the ball directly into the net. We call this the Drop of Doom, or D.O.D. for short. Here are some excellent targets (see the following figure) that can turn an ordinary drop shot into a glorious Drop of Doom!

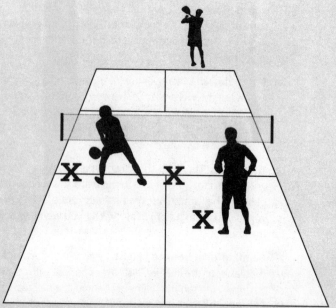

© John Wiley & Sons, Inc.

• **Aim for the feet.** Many players assume that a good drop shot must land well inside the kitchen. This isn't necessarily true. A drop that lands in the middle of the kitchen is often easier for your opponent to deal with than one that lands right at their feet ("Dance, pardner!"). If both opponents are up at the kitchen, aim your drops near the kitchen line. If one or both opponents are deeper in the court, aim at (or just behind) the current location of their feet.

- **Hit to the player who is back.** It's often a smart idea to hit your drop toward the player who just hit the return of serve. In addition to having more court in front of them, they are probably still busy recovering from their last shot, or are already on the move. In contrast, their partner is standing super ready at the kitchen line, so you have only a few feet in front of them to expertly place your drop. (Confession: Even the experts have trouble expertly placing their drops.)

- **Go crosscourt.** Whenever you're hoping that your ball will lose steam before it reaches your opponent, the longer distance of a crosscourt shot is more forgiving. In addition, the ball will be traveling over the lowest part of the net. Another advantage is that it puts the ball in front of your partner, who is certainly anxious to get involved and will be waiting for a chance to pounce on a poaching opportunity. (More on poaching in Chapter 14.)

Driving it home

Now that you've mastered the drop shot, we want to tell you about another option for your third shot: the third-shot drive. A *drive* is a shot that you hit with a lot of force in an effort to pass your opponents completely or put them off-balance with a hard shot coming straight toward their body.

TIP

The time to hit the drive is typically when your opponents have hit a short, high-bouncing return. A return like that makes these authors drool! Test your opponents early in a match to see whether they can handle a drive hit right at them. If they smack it back for a winner, it may be time to abandon the drive and instead execute the drop. If they miss the shot or let out a squeal, go ahead and keep driving the ball whenever you get a short return.

To execute the drive, start with the same groundstroke fundamentals covered earlier in this chapter, in "Return to Sender." A drive is the same shot but with a little more "oomph" and a few extra considerations.

Here are four tips for executing an effective drive:

>> **Get your feet set.** Hitting an accurate drive is very difficult if you are running through your shot. A drive is not a shot to attempt when you're reaching or off-balance.

>> **Take a slightly bigger backswing.** A longer backswing helps your paddle get up to a higher speed, but don't overdo it. You still want to keep your strokes compact to ensure accuracy and consistency.

- >> **Swing with 60 percent of your full force.** Using too much force causes you to lose accuracy, just as driving your car 100 miles per hour makes it quite a bit more difficult to stay on the road.

- >> **Utilize topspin.** Contact the ball out in front and follow through forward and slightly upward to achieve topspin. The drive will likely sail out if no topspin is helping the ball to arc downward into the court.

The most common error when hitting the drive is hitting it too hard, sending it well beyond the confines of the court and scaring small children and pets who were just trying to enjoy a relaxing day at the park. Focus on placement as well as power, and you won't need to hit your drives with every muscle fiber of your being.

Here are some suggested targets for your drives:

- >> **Hit directly at your opponent.** Although some people feel that this is not good sporting conduct, body shots are undeniably a part of the game. Hitting a ball directly at your opponent (preferably one standing up at the kitchen line), especially if they don't have great reaction time, often wins the point for you, or at least sets it up in your favor. See Chapter 12 for a description of a specific play called the "Shake 'N' Bake," which takes this concept to the next level.

- >> **Drive it down the middle.** It can be challenging for your opponents to deal with a ball driven down the middle, forcing a very quick decision about who will take the shot. If one of your opponents is currently on the move, or you see a big hole between your opponents, take advantage of this and aim to split the difference. (You'll often see your opponents looking dumbfounded after a shot like this, because they didn't communicate and the ball sailed right between them!)

- >> **Send it down the sideline.** Many intermediate players focus so much on playing in the middle of the court that they leave the sides wide open. Occasionally sending a drive down the line will force your opponents to start covering the sides of the court (we call it "keeping them honest"), thereby opening up more of the middle.

Chapter 8

Dinking: The Game within a Game

S ome recreational players spend their entire pickleball lives happily knocking the ball back and forth, having a great time, but never once hitting a particular shot called a dink. A *dink* is a soft shot hit from around the kitchen line, which lands in or around your opponent's kitchen. Much like the fabled third-shot drops you discover in Chapter 7, dinks are an iconic part of the game. You see countless pickleball company names and t-shirts referencing the word *dink*. Dinks are cherished in this sport for good reason. This seemingly wimpy shot is actually a powerful weapon in the right hands, and it's an essential element of winning pickleball strategy. Pickleball just wouldn't be the same without it!

Although hitting every ball as hard as you can may be incredibly fun (and therapeutic), the fact that coauthor Mo spent her first few months of playing without also knowing the joy of dinking makes her sad. Nobody likes a sad Mo. If you're playing pickleball, we encourage you to play *all* the phases of the pickleball point for maximum enjoyment (and maximum victories). We delve more into the four phases of a pickleball point in Chapter 11, but dinking is a big one.

Here's why dinking in pickleball is so important: Whenever all four players are up at the kitchen line, each one of them is looking for a high ball to attack and finish the point. By hitting soft, low-bouncing, unattackable dinks to your opponents, you are ensuring that they won't have that opportunity. When both teams realize this strategy, it can result in long rallies in which dozens of dinks are traded back and forth. The suspense builds until eventually one player makes an error, such as hitting their dink a little too high, resulting in an attackable pop-up for their opponent to happily smash.

This beautifully nuanced, back-and-forth dance, often causing spectators to hold their breath or "oooh" and "ahhh" with delight, is one of the things that makes pickleball so special. We get goosebumps just thinking about it! Embrace dinking and the game becomes more fun to play.

In this chapter, you find out how to dink with the best of them. We explain why dinking is like a chess match, and how you can become an Evil Dinking Genius who controls their opponent like a puppet on a string. We demonstrate the importance of keeping calm, and how to hit accurate dinks toward point-winning targets. Nothing wimpy about that — more like diabolical! You also discover how to defend against other great dinkers by using efficient footwork and protecting your hoop. (What? Hoops weren't mentioned in the chapter on required equipment! Read on to find out what we mean.)

Dinking Footwork: Calm Feet, Calm Mind

Pickleball is not considered a form of meditation, but maybe it should be. The more you can calm your mind and body, the more stable your footwork will become and the more precise your shots will be. This effect holds true throughout the point but is especially crucial when dinking.

Dinking is like a game within a game, in that it can sometimes involve a long, strategically played battle of wits. Your goal is to not only make sure your dinks are unattackable but also to be offensive in dictating how the rally progresses. Much like in a chess match, you need to be able to plan a few shots ahead and move your opponents around with intention. You also need physical and mental stamina, because dinking rallies can sometimes last for 10, 20, or even more shots. Engaging in long rallies requires concentration, knowledge, practice, and a calm — but alert — presence at the kitchen line.

When you arrive at the kitchen line during a point, remember to breathe. Players commonly feel excited or tense the closer they get to the net, and to their opponents. Give your paddle handle a little squeeze, and then release back to a lighter grip pressure. Doing so brings your mind's awareness back to your hand, which you need for the nuanced touch shots you're about to make.

Keep your back straight, chin up, and paddle out in front, with a slight bend in the knees. Think to yourself, "Time to settle in." You may be there awhile — hopefully as long as it takes for you to win the point. Be comfortable with this possibility, not fearful of it. Your calm, confident presence at the line will allow you to make more accurate shots while simultaneously stirring fear in your opponents' hearts.

Taming the tap dancing

One of the things that often breaks down a player's dinking is too much tap danc-ing. No, not the literal steel-toed type — we are referring to constantly shuffling or moving your feet. Dinking is hard enough when standing still, so imagine try-ing to finesse your dinks while simultaneously performing *Riverdance* (and get-ting more and more out of breath). If you find yourself dinking against a player who moves excessively, you are in luck. Your stable-footed self is about to best your overly fidgety opponent.

Here are some tips to keep in mind when practicing proper dinking footwork:

>> **Establish a home position.** Whenever you're playing up at the kitchen line, you want to develop a home position about 1–3 inches behind the line. By always standing in the same place, you'll have greater consistency when you play and practice, and you won't need to look down constantly to check where your feet are in relation to the kitchen line. You should be centered in front of the service box or just slightly more to the outside (see more about court positioning in Chapter 11).

>> **Be ready to move in any direction.** Don't lock your knees or have your weight back on your heels. Your feet should be about shoulder-width apart, toes pointing forward, weight just slightly forward on the balls of your feet. Bend your knees slightly, but don't crouch down or bend over at the waist. This posture is very similar to preparing to do squats, so if you're looking to tone your posterior, we think dinking is way more fun than hitting the gym!

>> **Leave your home position only when necessary.** Now that you're in your home position, your goal is to move your feet only when your opponent forces you to. You will be surprised how little you really have to move. Own your space. If you do need to move, make it a small step toward one side or the other. You should be able to cover just about any ball with one or two steps.

>> **If you do leave your position, immediately return to it.** Whenever you are forced to take a step, consider your last shot unfinished until you get back into home position. To dominate the line, you must remain vigilant about return-ing to your home position quickly after every shot.

>> **Pivot and square your hips and shoulders to the ball.** In Chapter 6, we explain proper ready position and "playing in the "V." You can avoid unnecessary movement at the line by always squaring your body to the ball as it moves around the court. You can do this by pivoting your feet and squaring your shoulders and hips to the ball. You don't need to chase after your last shot with your feet — just pivot! This technique makes it so that you can hit out in front of you, rather than reach behind your body or stretch way out to the side. We can't stress enough what a difference this will make to your game.

>> **Leave an anchor foot if you have to go into the kitchen.** Sometimes you'll receive a dink from your opponents that lands very shallowly in the kitchen, requiring you to step in and hit. Remember that as long as the ball bounces before you touch it, stepping in to hit is perfectly legal. If you do need to step into the kitchen at any time, try to leave an anchor foot behind in its home position. That way, you can step in and out of the kitchen without having to look down at your feet all the time. Just leave that one foot behind the line and return your other foot back beside it after your shot. Of course, if you do have to go all the way into the kitchen with both feet in order to get a ball, don't hesitate to do it, but be sure to hustle right back out. Remember, it's okay to be in the kitchen, but don't linger in there. No loitering!

Avoiding the cross step

When moving side to side at the kitchen line, it can be tempting to take a cross step. A *cross step* is when one foot has to cross in front of the other. (See Figure 8-1.) If you have to cross one foot in front of the other, the odds are that you have now turned your back to the court. This is, shall we say, not ideal; it's hard to see what's going on when you're facing the wrong way! In extreme cases, your feet may even get a bit tangled up, taking you completely out of the point for the next shot or two and leaving your partner with a lot of court to cover all by their lonesome.

Cross steps are common in other sports, so you may have some muscle memory to unlearn here. In pickleball, you don't have enough time or space to cross-step without negatively impacting both your current shot and your readiness for the next one.

REMEMBER

Cross-stepping completely closes your stance and sends your weight shift in a sideways direction. Remember, you always want *forward* weight shift in pickleball. More specifically, your weight should be shifting in the direction you're attempting to send the ball. It's difficult to hit an effective shot when your lower body is going in a different direction than your upper body.

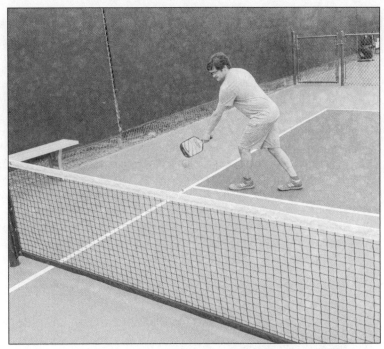

FIGURE 8-1:
A player doing the dreaded cross step at the kitchen line.

The trick to avoiding the cross step is to try to take the ball earlier, which means cutting it off before it gets past you. Readiness and focus are key. If you're square to the ball with your paddle out in front, you will gain a few extra milliseconds, allowing you to track and hit the ball earlier on its flight path. This may mean taking the ball out of the air rather than letting it bounce, which can feel a bit awkward, but it's frequently the best option. See "Protecting your hoop," later in this chapter.

TIP

If you can hit a dink just behind your opponent's foot on the backhand side, you may get your opponent to take a cross step. Take it as a mini victory! Your opponent has essentially turned their back to the court and opened a hole to hit through. Do not, repeat, do not let your opponent do this to you.

If your opponent does hit a fantastic dink that forces you to cross-step, don't panic and give up on the point. Cross-stepping will happen sometimes — just try not to make it a habit. Simply do your best to return an unattackable dink (aiming crosscourt is safest), untangle yourself, and get back to your home position as quickly as possible.

Dinking Strokes for Dinking Folks

To become the Evil Dinking Genius you aspire to be, your dinks need to be very accurately placed, so you need to learn and then practice the stroke techniques that create great dinks.

Imagine that you're at the kitchen line and a low ball is coming your way. If you've pivoted your feet toward the ball, you can most likely take it with a forehand, but regardless of whether it's a forehand or backhand, the same principles apply. Have both hands out in front of you, almost as if you were going to catch the ball. (See Figure 8-2.) Open your paddle face by tilting it slightly toward the sky and drop the paddle down in front of you so that you can lift the ball slowly. Contact the ball well out in front and guide the ball toward your target with a pushing motion.

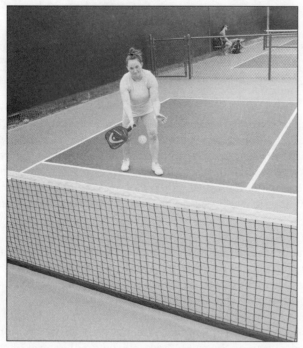

FIGURE 8-2:
A player ready to "catch" the ball.

The action should come mostly from your shoulder, not your elbow or wrist. As we explain in detail in Chapter 6, using your larger joints and muscles leads to more consistency. When small joints like your wrist get involved, shots become inaccurate. Many newer players attempt to flick or spin the ball using their wrist while dinking, which adds two new variables — timing and paddle-face angle — to a skill they haven't yet mastered. When you're learning to dink, keep it simple. Use a slightly open paddle face and a supple wrist, and hinge from your shoulder. The wrist is not invited to the dinking party! (See Figure 8-3 for the proper paddle and wrist positioning.)

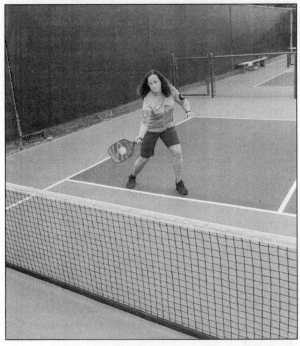

FIGURE 8-3:
A player dinking with a flat paddle face and supple wrist.

Extending the follow-through: Make it pretty!

The follow-through on your dinks should be long and pretty. Pose like you're a figure on top of a trophy or the cover of a pickleball magazine. Sure, it sounds weird, but whenever we tell players to make it pretty, their follow-through suddenly shows up. Don't question the magic.

Your oh-so-logical (soon to be Evil Dinking Genius) brain may try to tell you that because you're hitting softly, you should limit your swing by poking or jabbing at the ball with very little follow-through. In fact, the opposite is true. When hitting softly, you definitely don't want to wind up and take a huge swing, but make sure you are eliminating the correct part of the swing — the backswing. You don't need any backswing to generate power when hitting a soft shot, but you do need the follow-through in order to accurately place the ball.

A long follow-through gives the ball more time on your paddle, and therefore more guidance to its intended target. Whenever the ball comes to you, it's your turn to dictate where the ball goes next. Think of the duration of your stroke as being like a conversation with the ball. It's much less instructive to jab at the ball and yell "GIT!" than to say, "Ball, please go over there, to the back right corner of the kitchen, thank you kindly." Okay, we realize you can't talk to a pickleball; your paddle is how you communicate during those few moments it's in contact with the ball. Extend the conversation between your paddle and the ball by using a full follow-through, and it will be more likely to go where you tell it. (*Note:* We have seen players sometimes talk to, even plead with, their paddle. It happens, especially for a certain coauthor.)

TIP

Another benefit of a long, pretty follow-through is that you'll happen to finish the stroke with your paddle out in front of you — and voilà, you're already in a good ready position for the next shot! Holding your nondominant hand up during your entire dinking stroke is a great way to remind yourself to extend that follow-through so that your hands naturally meet out in front again at the end. (Figure 8-4 demonstrates this position.)

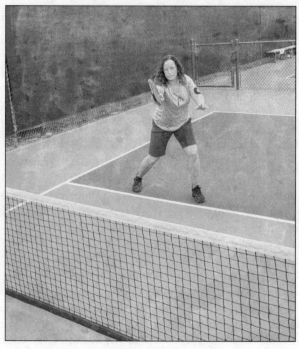

FIGURE 8-4:
An extended dink follow-through, guiding the ball toward its target.

© John Wiley & Sons, Inc./Photo Credit: Aniko Kiezel

Slowing your roll

Another common cause of dinking errors is swinging too fast. (This is also one of the six "scientifically" proven reasons for pop-ups that we outline in Chapter 14.) Remember that the energy behind a ball is dictated by the speed of your swing. When you send a dink with too much energy behind it, it will either sail high in the air or bounce up too high, giving your opponent an easy ball to hit down on, as an attack.

It won't take long to understand that your dinks need to be hit softly, or else they will be punished. Here are some keys to keeping your dinks unattackable:

>> **Think "slow" not "soft."** Instead of thinking in terms of hitting the ball "hard" or "soft," swap those two words for "fast" and "slow." These words actually provide your body with instructions on what to do, instead of focusing on the end result. Swing slowly when you want to hit softly, and fast when you want to hit hard.

>> **Hit the "slow-mo" button — it's slower than you think!** If you're a naturally speedy person, go search through the couch cushions right now and find your remote control, because it's time to hit the "slow-mo" button. You're probably swinging at least 50 percent faster than you should be. Next time you practice dinking, challenge yourself to swing as slowly as possible, and watch the results.

>> **Guide the ball forward over the net.** The good news is that swinging *too* slowly is almost impossible, as long as you contact the ball out in front and have a nice, extended follow-through (as described in the preceding "Extending the follow-through: Make it pretty!" section). Really focus on pushing the ball *forward* over the net, rather than scooping up under it. You may even feel a nice little stretch in the back of your shoulder. Breathe, swing slowly, and guide those dinks all the way home.

>> **Think "When it's low, go slow."** (Or "When it's lowly, go slowly" if you're picky on the grammar thing but like the catchy rhyme.) Be cautious of swinging fast anytime the ball is below the level of the net. Most of the time, this results in a hard shot straight into the net or a pop-up that zings right up to your opponent's paddle for an easy put-away. If your opponent is successfully sending you nice low dinks, that is not the time to try to speed things up. When it's low, go slow! See Chapter 11 for more on how to select the right shot in a given situation.

Protecting your hoop

When coauthor Mo started playing pickleball, she soon realized that when people hit the ball at her feet, she often hit a pop-up or some other weak shot. Worst-case scenario, she'd miss the shot altogether. She often felt like her opponents were trying to untie her shoelaces with the ball. (Now she always double-knots.) This situation was extremely frustrating, but when she learned about protecting her feet, a big light bulb went on over her head. (It looked weird and made it impossible to get in the car, so she had it removed.) But this new concept stuck with her and made a huge impact on her game. So how do you protect your feet? The key is to cut off the ball in the air before it gets close to them.

Follow these steps to put this technique of cutting off the ball into your game:

1. **First, determine what you can reach.**

   Standing at the kitchen line, use your outstretched arm and paddle to draw a semicircle in front of your feet and body. Be sure to include the areas to the right and left of you, as well as in front of your toes. (See Figure 8-5.)

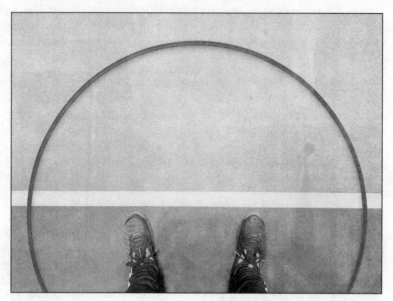

FIGURE 8-5: Imagine drawing a semicircle around your feet.

© John Wiley & Sons, Inc./Photo Credit: Aniko Kiezel

2. **Create a visualization of this semicircle in your mind.**

   You're envisioning a semicircle painted on the ground, or even more fun, a rainbow-colored plastic hoop that follows you throughout the court! Everyone's hoop is a different size because of differences in height, arm length, and flexibility. Understanding what you can reach is one of the most important things you can know about yourself on the pickleball court.

3. **Block any ball that comes toward your hoop.**

From this point forward, one of your primary goals is to prevent any ball from entering this zone. It's time to channel your inner hockey goalie! If a ball flying toward you looks like it's going to land in your hoop, block it from doing so by reaching out and taking it out of the air as a volley. This idea applies throughout the court, except when the Two-Bounce Rule applies (serve returns and third shots cannot legally be volleys). At the kitchen line, you'll be relying solely on your reach. In other places in the court, you may have time to also take a step forward as you reach.

This hoop trick is especially important when dinking. The more you let dinks bounce within your hallowed hoop, the more errors you will make attempting to dig them out of your shoes. You're hitting from an awkward position and swinging low to high, so it's no wonder your odds of popping the ball up just skyrocketed!

When you dink a ball that hasn't yet bounced, you're hitting what's known as a *dink volley.* Take the ball well out in front of you, as early as possible and at the highest possible point. Doing so takes reaction time away from your opponents and minimizes the amount of low-to-high arc on your swing path. You'll also be avoiding the temptation to back away from the line, giving up your offensive position and exposing your feet. Lean in, hold your ground, and keep that forward pressure.

As a budding Evil Dinking Genius, you've probably figured out by now that aiming your dinks toward your opponent's hoop is a great idea (assuming there's no obvious open court to hit to instead). Early on, you'll be playing lots of players who, for some unexplained reason, have not read this book and don't know how to protect their feet the way you do. You will be pleasantly surprised by how many points you'll win with this crazy hoop knowledge. Be sure to note your opponent's ability to reach. Are they seven feet tall? Their hoop is more like the St. Louis Arch. That's a player you may want to make move around more because their extended reach will make jamming them at their feet very difficult — *if* they are aware of their hoop.

Dink volleys may feel a little strange at first if you're used to backing up and letting every dink bounce in front of you. You will definitely have to take the time to practice taking balls out of the air. You'll need to be very conscious about leaning in and keeping your feet in place instead of backing away. With a bit of determination, you can change your dinking habits. Be sure to contact the ball well out in front of you, and guide it to its target with your long, pretty follow-through. It takes some repetition to learn how big your hoop is and to perfect your dink volleys. Carve out some time to practice this new skill, perhaps by letting other things in your life go. Do you *really* need to brush your teeth *every* day? (Whoops, coauthor Reine just remembered that her dentist plays pickleball and may read this. Sorry, Dr. Hana!)

Think before You Dink

Dinking is more than just mindlessly tapping the ball back and forth softly over the net. Significant strategy is involved, allowing you to be offensive at the same time as you're being defensive. Dinking is your chance to move your opponents around and force them to make errors. If you have honed your dinks in true Evil Dinking Genius fashion, you're ready to sneak up on your opponents like a ninja and slay the dragon. (We happen to be fans of both mixed doubles and mixed metaphors.)

Offensive dinking: Making a hole and hitting through it

In a nutshell, basic pickleball strategy could be described as "Make a hole and hit through it." This strategy is especially important to keep in mind when dinking.

To make a hole, you'll need to coerce your opponent out of their home position by moving them from side to side and back and forth. Ideally, you'll be the one maintaining your position while you gradually work your opponent out of theirs. It's like pushing someone around who is trying to play the game of Twister. If you can get them off-balance, they will most likely make a mistake and give you a ball that is attackable. You'll know you've reached true Evil Dinking Genius status if you can do so without their even realizing it! (Maniacal laughter while dinking is optional, but it's probably best not to do it out loud.)

Another offensive goal when dinking is to get your opponent to back away from the kitchen line, which makes them less able to hit down on the ball and opens additional angles and court real estate for you. Most important, it exposes their feet to being attacked. Most players have a very difficult time dealing with balls hit directly at their feet. When you can maintain your position 1–3 inches from the line, the net does some of the work of protecting your feet. Even getting backed off just a few steps will make your feet extremely vulnerable, like wading barefoot through a kiddie pool full of piranhas.

Here are some proven dinking targets and strategies that will win you points:

>> **Dink to your opponent's feet or behind their feet.** When you send a ball toward your opponents' feet, their tendency will be to back away from it so that they have more room to hit. If they aren't diligent about getting back up to the line afterward, aiming at their feet will gradually back them farther and farther away, putting them on defense. If they choose instead to hold their ground and let it bounce at their feet, they will be forced to hit from a very awkward position while swinging low to high — which sounds like the perfect recipe for a pop-up!

>> **Make them reach or change direction.** As your opponent backs away from the line, they open up more court for you to hit into. Start sending them dinks that cause them to reach, such as way out in front of them or off to one side. If you catch them leaning or shifting their weight to one side or the other, send a dink in the opposite direction. Don't give them a ball that is easy to deal with by sending it directly to them. Remember, you're playing pickleball, not catch. Your goal is to give your opponent trouble.

>> **Pull them out wide.** Use angled dinks to pull one of your opponents out wide and create a hole. Your opponent may be less likely to notice just how out of position they have become if you gradually move them a little farther over with each strategic dink.

>> **Mix it up and keep them guessing.** Your dink targets should continually change throughout the rally. Never let your opponent get into a rhythm. Hit two shots to the target behind their left foot, followed by a dink to the middle, and then back to their backhand side, and then shallow to the backhand, and then deep behind their right foot, and so on. (We go over some more specific dinking patterns in Chapter 12).

TIP

Many beginners think that dinks are shots that land in the kitchen. This is not necessarily true. Sure, many dinks will land in the kitchen, but many won't. You often want to push the opponent back off the line by dinking at their feet, which are located outside of the kitchen. Hitting the targets behind their feet requires you to dink even deeper. These more offensive dinks will be much harder for your opponent to deal with than ones that land in front of them inside the kitchen. (If you don't believe us, have a friend dink to you at a variety of depths, and see which dinks are easier for you to return.) See Figure 8-6 for some suggested targets.

Defensive dinking: When things are not going well

So far, we've focused on offensive dinking targets. If you happen to be facing another great dinker, you may find that things aren't going as well as you'd hoped and you are no longer in control of the point. You may be feeling your own puppet strings being yanked! Anytime you find you are hitting off-balance, or have been moved out of position with no time to return, it's time to dink more defensively.

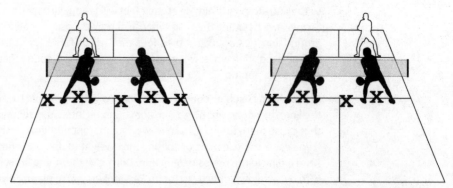

FIGURE 8-6: Offensive dinking targets for even-side (left) and odd-side (right) dinkers against right-handed opponents.

© John Wiley & Sons, Inc.

Here are some strategies to get you back on the offensive:

» **Reset the clock with a safe, shallow dink.** Defensive dinking is mostly about buying time. A shallow dink to the middle of the court is nearly impossible for your opponents to attack. Although it's unlikely to force an error and win you the point, it will force them to hit another shot and grant you a few extra seconds to safely get back into position. If you're lucky, you'll then have a chance to get back to your offensive plan.

» **Go crosscourt when pulled out wide.** If an angled dink pulls you out wide, but not wide enough to hit around the post (see Chapter 14), your best bet is to dink the ball back across the court. Compared to hitting straight ahead, hitting a crosscourt shot gives you 40 percent more distance, which translates to 40 percent more time to recover. If you completely leave the court and hit to the opponent right in front of you, all they have to do is block it back into the empty space you've left behind. A crosscourt dink also puts the ball in front of your partner, who has a better chance of being ready for the next shot should your opponent choose to hit it back straight ahead or toward the middle.

» **Avoid straight-ahead dinks down the sidelines.** For the even-side opponent who is right-handed (or odd-side opponent who is left-handed), straight-ahead dinks give them an easy forehand shot that they can place just about anywhere. Often, they rocket it sharply across the court toward your partner, sending them way out wide. If your dink floats a little too high, you're also inviting your opponent to hit an Erne. (We explain the Erne in Chapter 14.) Be wary of these dinking targets.

Patience, patience, patience

Many people get antsy during dinking rallies and feel they just want to get the point over with. That is not a good frame of mind for dinking. You should always assume you will be hitting 20 or more dinks and be comfortable with it.

There is a saying, "Patience wins points in pickleball." Some people are naturally more patient than others. Ultimately, patience in pickleball comes from confidence. We highly suggest you go out and drill and develop confidence in your dinking abilities. If you're confident that you can hit ten dinks in a row without an unforced error, whereas your opponent can hit only five, then even dinking conservatively becomes a valuable tool in your toolbox. You don't need to use spin or crazy angles to win the point if you can reliably outlast your opponents in every dinking rally.

Comfortably settling into a dinking rally doesn't mean you shouldn't be ready for someone to suddenly speed things up. There may be a higher ball that someone decides to attack — and that person may even be you. Everyone on the court needs to be ready in case the dinking rally turns into a rapid-fire volley situation (as it often does). Rapid volleys are great fun, but try not to initiate one unless it's the right ball at the right time. Are your opponents in good position, or do you see a hole to hit through? Are your opponents leaning forward or dropping their paddles down? Is one of them off-balance? If so, it may be a good time to attack with a body shot or an offensive lob. Otherwise, wait for the next ball . . . and the next . . . and the next.

Patience is the superpower of the Evil Dinking Genius.

You'll often see long crosscourt dinking rallies in which only one player on each team is actively involved. During these rallies, the inactive partners sometimes get bored or impatient. If they get bored, they tend to lower their paddle and lose their good ready position. Be ready to attack toward that player if you get a chance. "Surprise!" When players get impatient, they may try to poach and leave their position, or attack a ball that isn't quite high enough. If you ever do this, expect some serious eyeball daggers from your partner who just put in all that work hitting 37 dinks, only to have you jump in front of them and hit the ball into the net. Yikes!

Be patient, wait for your moment, but don't hesitate to attack when the moment is right. The more experience you gain on the court, the more you'll learn to recognize that special moment. You may even get a funny, tingly feeling all over. Of course, even the most advanced players get it wrong sometimes. It's all part of the joy of dinking!

Chapter 9

The Big Thrill: Volleys, Smashes, and Lobs

When coauthor Mo started playing pickleball, she just wanted to hit every ball really hard and low. (She was a former racquetball champion.) She soon found that in pickleball, the pesky net was not her friend. She was beating other players, but only to a certain level. She blasted holes through the net, which you should know does not win you any points. She then discovered a whole catalog of shots that she could develop to make the game her own. She could lift the ball, push it, smack it down, cut it off in mid-air, lob it over her opponents' heads, and, every once in a while, throw in a trick shot just for fun. The game is all about fun, so why not? This discovery of new shots caused a big jump in her skill level. She suddenly had this big smile whenever she stepped on the court. You don't want to see your opponent smiling like that!

It may seem difficult to learn all these different shots, but the journey is enjoyable, and adding these shots to your pickleball toolbox will help you to become a more well-rounded player who can adapt to any playing style. (See Figure 9-1.)

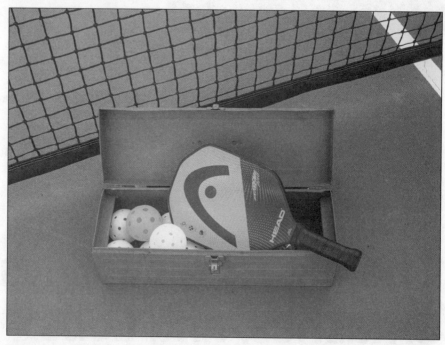

FIGURE 9-1:
Add some fun
shots to your
imaginary
toolbox!

Vying with Vicious Volleys

To *volley* means to hit a ball before it touches the ground. Volleys are extremely important in pickleball because they give you a greater chance of hitting down on the ball. Hitting down on the ball is very satisfying! You take precious time away from your opponents by not waiting for the ball to bounce before you send it back over. Taking time away from your opponents is a smart strategy; you want everything to slow down for you and to speed up for your opponents. (Cue the wicked laugh.) Another advantage of volleys is that you don't have to worry about the ball taking an unpredictable bounce, owing to spin applied by your opponents or a stray leaf or crack on the court. Those are three big plusses! For all these reasons, it's smart to try to volley the ball whenever you can. You have a variety of different volleys to hit depending on the situation. Read on to find out about the most common ones.

Punch volleys

The *punch volley* is the "high five" of volleys, consisting of a very compact swing path. It's a fantastic way to attack the ball when the time is right. Quickness, efficiency, and accuracy are the main strengths of this shot.

Whether you're hitting a forehand or a backhand, the mechanics are the same. From your perfect, upright ready position (described in Chapter 6), strike the ball out in front of you and punch it toward your target. No backswing is involved; a backswing only slows you down and creates more opportunity for errors. The power comes from the rapid acceleration of your paddle head. You should hear a satisfying "pop" or "snap" off your paddle when you hit a good punch volley. When you finish your stroke, the paddle face should be pointed toward your target on the other side of the net. If it points down toward the ground, there's a good chance the ball just went into the net. That is not so satisfying.

The punch volley is a great option when you're in good court position and are in a volley battle with a player whose reaction times you know you can beat. You're being aggressive by reaching forward on either your forehand or backhand side and repeatedly punching that ball right where you want it to go — preferably to your opponent's feet, angled off, or to an open area of the court. (Figure 9-2 shows forehand and backhand punch volleys.)

TIP

If you do decide to hit the ball right back to your opponent, another great target is along the dominant side of their body, especially their armpit or hip. You know your life has taken a strange turn when you find yourself talking about attacking someone's dominant armpit. That's okay; just keep hammering at your opponent with your annoyingly efficient and accurate volleys!

You can also use punch volleys to keep your opponents back in the court. Your goal is to send the ball back over the net as quickly as possible, before your opponents have time to take any steps and advance toward the kitchen line. Punch the ball back deep in the court, either at or behind their feet. Picture a row of cheerleaders chanting, "*Keep* 'em back. *Keep* 'em back. *Waaay* back!" There's no need to get fancy when the humble, no-fuss punch volley is so incredibly effective. Yay, team!

The most common errors to watch out for when hitting punch volleys are

>> **Allowing the paddle to become unstable:** If your grip or wrist is too loose, the paddle may wobble or collapse as you hit. Although we don't want you to ever grip too tightly (which can cause injuries), be sure to hold on tightly enough to keep your paddle face pointed toward your target for the duration of the stroke.

>> **Opening the paddle face:** If you're attempting to hit down on the ball, your paddle face should be slightly closed, meaning slightly angled downward. Attempting to hit a punch volley with an open paddle face (meaning angled upward) will result in the ball flying up, either popping up for your opponent to smash or sailing out of bounds.

>> **Aiming with your wrist or elbow:** If you're attempting to hit the ball straight ahead, your paddle face should be parallel to your chest and the net. You "punch" the ball by moving your paddle quickly forward. If you want to angle the shot to the right or left, avoid twisting your elbow or cocking your wrist. Instead, keep your paddle face parallel to your chest and rotate your torso in the direction you want to hit. You'll build consistency and accuracy by using the same motion every time, and by using your larger joints instead of smaller ones.

>> **Hitting while off-balance:** It's difficult to hit an effective attack — including punch volleys — while off-balance. Try to keep your head and upper body centered over your feet at all times — "nose over toes." Keeping centered may require a bit of extra footwork to get you closer to the ball instead of reaching for it.

>> **Taking too big of a swing:** No backswing is needed on this shot, and it requires only a short follow-through. You're more likely to "whiff" the ball completely, or contact the ball too late, if you spend precious time taking a big backswing. Be sure to follow through forward, toward your target, rather than down toward the ground.

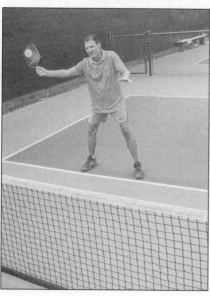

FIGURE 9-2: Photos of forehand (left) and backhand (right) punch volleys.

© John Wiley & Sons, Inc./Photo Credit: Aniko Kiezel

>> **Punching a ball that is too low.** Sometimes a ball coming your way may be dropping faster than you think. You set up to hit your perfect punch volley and then find yourself bending your knees, squatting lower and lower until your paddle is below the net. This is not the time to try to punch the ball; instead, try to dink it back over with a slow, gentle lifting motion. We've heard this described as lifting a chick into the nest, but we think people who use chicken metaphors have been cooped up too long.

Swinging volleys

Unlike a punch volley, a *swinging volley* utilizes a more significant backswing and follow-through. It's very much the volley equivalent of a groundstroke drive (explained in Chapter 7).

You'll want to primarily use swinging volleys as a midcourt (transition zone) shot. You're in the process of transitioning forward toward the kitchen when your opponent makes the mistake of sending you a high, floating ball. You take a compact backswing and an aggressive step forward, and then you swing through the ball, finishing with your weight and paddle face toward your target.

TIP

Your nondominant arm can play a role in executing killer swing volleys. Try using it as an opposing counterweight as you swing by throwing your elbow behind your body as you push forward with the paddle arm. This action helps to increase the speed of your torso rotation and therefore the speed of your paddle. It also looks really cool, which of course is the most important thing of all.

Two-handed backhand swinging volleys are becoming much more common in modern pickleball. Some players love the extra power and stability that two hands can give them. Because of limited reach, you need to be extra conscientious about moving your feet so that the ball is right in your strike zone. Make sure you are in good balance before you attempt this shot; otherwise, the accelerated rotation on the follow-through can easily cause you to stumble and be off-balance for your next shot.

Watch out for these common pitfalls when hitting both forehand and backhand swing volleys:

>> **Trying to hit too hard:** You don't need to break the ball in half, but instead place it exactly where you want it, with authority. Although the swinging volley has more of a backswing than a punch volley does, you still don't need a big windup because you're already getting a lot of power from your forward momentum and core rotation. Trying to also "muscle it" over with your arm

will more than likely cause the ball to go out. We recommend using only about 60 percent of your full power when driving or attacking the ball.

» **Following through toward the ground:** If you finish your shot with your paddle face far below the height of the net, you'll cause the ball to go very hard into the net. Not exactly your desired outcome!

» **Running through your shot:** Just take that one big aggressive step into the ball — don't sprint right past it. (See Figure 9-3.) You will likely miss your ideal contact point and end up putting too much momentum behind the ball, causing it to fly wildly over the back fence.

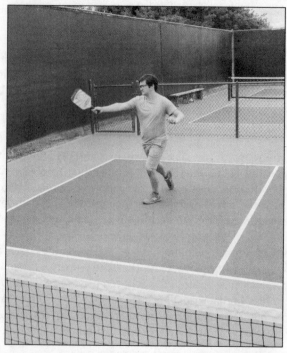

FIGURE 9-3:
An example of a forehand swinging volley with a big forward step.

© John Wiley & Sons, Inc./Photo Credit: Aniko Kiezel

Block volleys

Unlike the previous two volleys that we have discussed, which are primarily used for attacks, a *block volley* is considered more of a neutral or defensive shot. When an opponent hits a hard shot toward your body, your primary goal is to survive the attack and keep the ball in play. Ideally, you'll want to take some energy off the ball as well so that you can slow the rally back down to a manageable speed. Taking speed off the ball is often easier said than done, so if you can block the ball back without popping it up, consider it a success!

TIP

For a block volley, if you're using the ready position that we recommend in Chapter 6, your paddle is held out in front of you, about chest high. For blocking, many players find it helpful to keep their paddle slightly defaulted to the backhand side — 11 o'clock for righties, and 1 o'clock for lefties. When a hard shot comes right at you, you need to quickly make a decision: Forehand or backhand? You don't exactly have time to make a list of pros and cons, mull it over, and sleep on it. Fortunately, we can tell you in advance that most of your block volleys will be backhands.

Here's a visualization that can help: Imagine that you're standing in front of a standard-sized door frame. Any ball that comes through the doorway (in other words, right at your body) will be a backhand. Think of your paddle as your superhero shield, there to protect you from the deadly laser beams that your supervillain nemesis is zapping at you through the doorway. Hold your paddle just as you would a shield, with your knuckles facing out. To raise or lower your shield, simply bend your knees. When a ball comes toward you that is outside the door frame on your dominant side, it's time to switch to forehand. Take these balls as early as possible, well out in front of you.

When hitting a block volley, be sure to turn your paddle face so that it's nice and flat (perpendicular to the ground) or just very *slightly* open. (Figure 9-4 demonstrates open, flat, and closed paddle face positions.) Loosen your grip a little to help absorb some of the energy on the ball so that it's less likely to pop up. Hold the paddle out in front of your body with your elbows slightly bent, and let the ball strike your paddle. You can aim your block volleys by rotating your torso; don't attempt to aim by twisting your elbow into funny positions. Your paddle is essentially acting as a backboard, deflecting the ball back in whatever direction your paddle face is angled.

A player's struggle with the block volley is usually attributable to one of these issues:

>> **Fear of getting hurt:** If you're afraid of getting nailed with the ball, you may try to turn or back away from an attack instead of blocking it. Doing so actually increases your chances of getting hit because you're no longer watching the ball and have probably dropped out of your strong ready position. You're better off holding your ground and raising your paddle in front of you for

protection — shields up! Be confident and believe that nothing can get past you and your superhero shield. Remember, as long as you have your eyes protected, a pickleball can't do much to hurt you beyond a small cut or bruise. So be brave, lean in, and show your mettle.

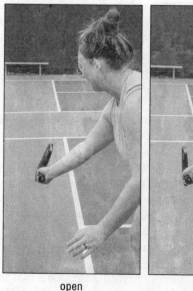 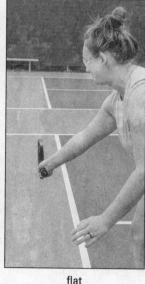 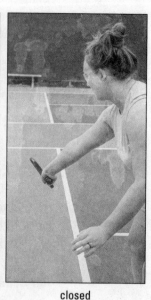

open   flat   closed

FIGURE 9-4: Open (left), flat (middle) and closed (right) paddle positions.

© John Wiley & Sons, Inc./Photo Credit: Aniko Kiezel

>> **Overgripping the paddle:** A looser grip helps you absorb some of the energy on the ball that your opponent has sent your way, which in turn helps keep your return shot lower and less attackable. If you panic and squeeze your paddle handle too hard, all that energy reflects back, causing the ball to fly off your paddle in an uncontrolled manner.

>> **Using too open of a paddle face:** If your paddle face is too open, meaning pointed toward the sky, the ball bounces off your paddle and flies right up into the air — a nice, juicy pop-up for your opponent to smash back! Remember, the ball goes wherever the paddle face is pointed. Coauthor Reine will tell you "Paddle face is everything!" (She has a bit of an obsession.)

>> **Swinging at the ball instead of just blocking:** Remember, you're getting attacked, so your goal is to be a backboard and keep the ball in play. Now is not the time to try to fire back by taking a big swing at the ball. Try for a

defensive or neutral shot — something low and slow that your opponent can't attack. If you have time, go for an open spot on the court. Make your opponent hit one more ball, and wait for your moment to go on the offensive again.

>> **Trying to "catch" the ball with an open palm:** If you were playing catch with someone and they threw a ball right at your belly button, your instincts would be to open your hand and try to catch it with your palm facing out. Unfortunately, this technique doesn't work well when you're holding a paddle (see Figure 9-5) because it's guaranteed to send the ball back high in the air. Instead of hitting with your palm facing out (a forehand), stick with the backhand block. Bend your knees if you need to connect with a ball that's dropping as it comes toward you. (See Figure 9-6 for an example of a backhand block volley.)

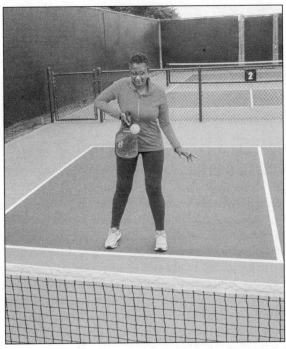

FIGURE 9-5:
A player trying to do a forehand "catch" at her belly button with a paddle.

© John Wiley & Sons, Inc./Photo Credit: Aniko Kiezel

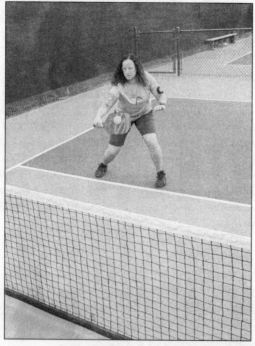

FIGURE 9-6:
An example
of a backhand
block volley.

BANISHING THE WINDSHIELD WIPER BACKHAND

Players often struggle when they're up at the kitchen line and the ball comes right at them on their nondominant side. Ideally, they should hit this shot as a backhand volley. Some players instead wave their paddle in front of them like a windshield wiper and hit it with the forehand side of their paddle. You'll know you're doing this if the palm of your hand is facing the ball, as opposed to the back of your hand (hence the term "backhand"). Most likely, this move is caused by muscle memory in your brain telling your hand that it needs to open and catch the ball. It may take a little time to retrain your brain to remember that you're holding a paddle, not a baseball mitt!

You may see some players pull this shot off with decent results, but as we've said, it's not ideal. It's very difficult to get your paddle face pointed in the right direction when making that awkward twisting motion. From your default ready position, it takes twice as long to flip the paddle all the way around as it would to tilt to the backhand. Not only is it less consistent than a regular backhand volley, but it also places excess strain on your elbow, wrist, and shoulder. Nobody needs more strain in their lives! Straining is for pasta, not pickleball.

If you are ever playing against a player who uses this shot, hit toward their nondominant side, down by their hips or knees. If they are really addicted to their windshield wiper backhand, they will struggle when you hit below their windshield. (The following figure shows an example of the windshield wiper backhand.) The ball will typically go into the net because the player can't get any kind of lift on it from that hunched-over position.

A great way to break the windshield wiper habit is to place the fingers of your nondominant hand on the back of your paddle face. As the ball comes toward you, your nondominant fingers will help you resist the temptation to flip your paddle over. (You can't hit with that side of the paddle when your fingers are still on it!) Just push your paddle forward, away from the hand that is supporting the back, and hit a simple backhand block or punch volley. The windshield wiper backhand can be one of the most difficult habits to break if you've been doing it for a long time, but with practice and determination, you can do it!

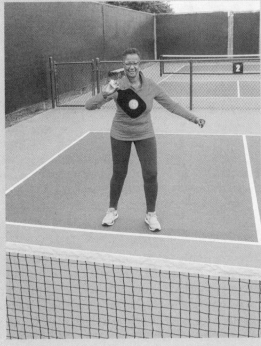

Drop volleys

A *drop volley* is a sneaky little shot that converts a hard shot from your opponent into a soft, typically back-spinning dink or drop shot. Drop volleys will win you more points than friends. It's typically used when your opponents are deep in the court and you're confident that they won't be quick enough to retrieve a ball returned short. (See Figure 9-7.)

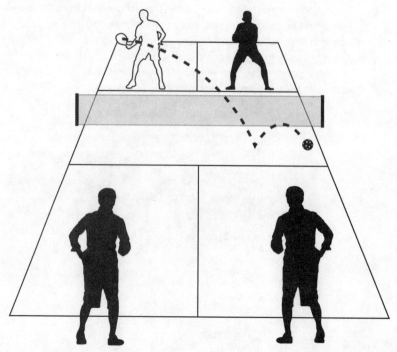

FIGURE 9-7:
Diagram of a player hitting a drop volley against deep opponents.

The drop volley is very similar to the block volley. The key difference is that you take most of the energy off the ball so that it will drop like a dying pigeon into your opponent's kitchen. ("Honey! It's squab for dinner!") Drop volleys are often hit with a significant amount of backspin, causing the ball to bounce back toward the net after it hits the ground and making it even more difficult for your opponent to reach. This shot also takes a lot of touch, practice, and a slightly evil heart (which in this case we encourage).

Follow these steps to hit a great drop volley that will leave your opponents cursing your name ("Dammit, Darla!"):

1. **Relax!**

   When you're tense, your body acts as a backboard reflecting all the power back over the net. Relax your neck and shoulders, bend your knees slightly, and think calm thoughts. Remember to breathe. If you have time between rallies, go take a yoga class and get a massage. Your partner and opponents may not appreciate waiting around, but you can explain that it will only help your team's chances of winning.

2. **Loosen your grip.**

   When you grip your paddle too tightly, your entire arm becomes an extension of the mass of your paddle. It's like swinging a sledgehammer versus a ball peen. As we learned in high school physics class, momentum equals mass times velocity. All that extra mass won't help to reduce the momentum on the ball. Loosening your grip and having a more relaxed wrist will help you absorb energy as the ball strikes your paddle. On a scale of one to ten, your grip pressure on this shot should be about a three.

3. **Keep your elbow in.**

   Rather than sticking it straight out horizontally, hold your elbow at more of a 45-degree angle to your torso so that you resist the urge to tense your shoulders and punch through the ball.

4. **Open your paddle face a bit.**

   On most shots, we like to avoid using an open paddle face because it often causes the ball to pop up in the air. In this case, because you aren't imparting any additional energy to the ball, you need a slightly more open face to make sure the ball goes over the net.

5. **Bring the paddle slightly backward at the moment of contact.**

   Imagine that someone just tossed you a water balloon and you don't want to get wet. You would try to catch it as softly as possible, absorbing some of the energy by bringing your arms in toward your body. Think of your paddle, and body, as being a pillow absorbing the ball into it.

6. **Use a very short and slow follow-through.**

   In most cases, if you move your paddle only backward, the ball won't have enough forward energy to go over the net; that is, you still need to push forward just a bit. Remember, when you want to hit softly, you swing slowly. Your forward follow-through on this shot should take up only a couple of inches.

7. **Add backspin or sidespin for maximum effect.**

   If you're comfortable hitting with spin, the drop volley is the perfect time to use some. On your forward follow-through, add a downward or sideways brushing or chopping motion, causing the ball to rotate backward or sideways on its axis. When the ball hits the ground, it will spin farther away from your scrambling opponent. HA!

The struggles that players can have with the drop volley are usually touch related. This shot requires a great deal of sensitivity and feel. You need to practice taking just enough energy off the ball so that it drops into the kitchen, but not so much that it goes into the net. Practice, practice, practice!

TIP

If your drop volleys are landing deeper than you would like, try going crosscourt. When hitting straight across, you get 14 feet of kitchen to work with. If you go crosscourt, you get about 20 feet — and that's 40 percent more kitchen. Your crosscourt drop will have a much higher likelihood of landing in the kitchen than a straight-ahead one will.

Crushing It with Overhead Smashes

Your poor opponent has just made the mistake of hitting a high pop-up or a not-quite-high enough lob (otherwise known as a *flob*, short for "failed lob"). This is the moment you've been waiting for! It's time to smash the ball down — *hard*. You start to drool, sprint toward the ball, unfurl a giant windup, take a flying leap, and then swing with all your might. You hit the ball harder than you ever thought possible — straight into the net. Sheepishly, you wipe up your drool and slink back to your position for the next point while purposely avoiding eye contact with your partner.

Stop! Time to wake up! Thank goodness, it was all just a nightmare.

Try that same scene again: The ball is sailing high and you've called the ball — "Mine!" You take a compact backswing, keeping your paddle in your peripheral vision. You are moving your feet to the ball so that you can set up in balance underneath it (see Figure 9-8) and strike it in your perfect strike zone, up high and out in front. You're reaching or pointing toward the ball with your nondominant hand, almost as though you're going to catch it. As the ball enters your strike zone, you bring your paddle forward and contact the ball out in front, following through toward your target. You've hit a crisp, accurate attack to an open area of the court. Your opponents didn't stand a chance! The crowd goes wild, your partner hoists you on their shoulders, and your phone immediately starts ringing with corporate sponsorship deals. ("How did they get my number?")

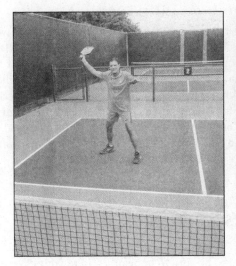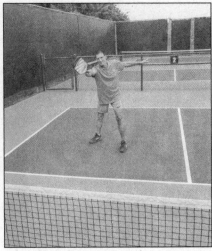

FIGURE 9-8:
The proper
overhead
preparation
(left) and
follow-through
(right).

We hope you noticed a few key differences between these two scenarios. When hitting an overhead smash, balance and accuracy are much more important than mustering as much power as is humanly possible. When you take a giant windup and swing, more often than not you end up contacting the ball either too late or too early, and outside your strike zone. This scenario causes the ball to fly over the back fence or hard into the net. Even worse, you may "whiff" the ball completely. Keeping your paddle where you can see it prevents this embarrassing moment from happening to you.

REMEMBER

The momentum from a huge swing can also cause you to hit off-balance, and wind up off-balance for your next shot. So can an unnecessary leap or jump while hitting an overhead smash. (Save the scissor kicks for your next synchronized swimming routine.) Remember, attacking when off-balance usually does not end well. Keep your nose over your toes at all times for best results.

When you're practicing your smashes, focus first on getting your feet under you and striking the ball out in front. Add more speed or snap to your swing after you begin to master the fundamentals, but not to the point that you're sacrificing accuracy. Never hit the ball like you're trying to crush it, thinking, "Now I can cancel my court-ordered anger management classes!" It is much more satisfying to win the point than it is to hit a hole through the net at 150 MPH.

TIP

Be mindful that many players who have strong defensive skills will be able to hit your amazing smashes back at you. (Yes, it's very obnoxious!) Be sure not to get caught stopping to admire your last shot; always be ready for it to come back to you. Against skilled players, it can sometimes take three or four smashes to successfully finish the point. If you feel that your smashes are ineffective, try angling them off the court more. This technique will often end with your opponent running into the fence in an effort to get your astonishing overhead. When the rally is over and you can see "grill marks" left on your opponents from being pressed up against the fence, you know you dominated the last point.

Loving Those Lobs

Another important tool to be sure to hone and add to your ever-expanding pickleball toolbox is the lob. A *lob* is a ball that is hit up, and hopefully over, your opponent's head, causing them to have to run to a spot deep in the court to retrieve it.

Lobs can be both offensive and defensive. We recommend focusing more on offensive lobs because they don't tend to be very effective for defense. In Hail Mary–type situations, a defensive lob can sometimes buy your team some time. However, these are often hit from a less than ideal position (such as reaching, or on a full sprint, or even over the shoulder). Consequently, most defensive lobs are executed poorly and are therefore ineffective. When in trouble, a soft crosscourt drop shot or dink is often a safer choice than attempting a lob.

The most common time for an offensive lob is during a dinking rally, which gives the lobber a chance to move their opponents out of position, away from the kitchen, forcing them to have to earn their way back up to the line again. Especially when well-disguised, the lob is a great surprise attack when your opponents have been lulled into thinking they were done chasing balls and would only be dinking for the rest of the rally.

For most beginner or intermediate players, the lob is considered a low-percentage shot. You must hit the lob just high enough to be out of your victim's reach but not so high that it takes a big bounce, giving them plenty of time to get there and hit. Tough to do with only 22 feet of court. However, with the right mechanics and a little practice, you, too, can become a skilled lobber.

Here's how it's done: You're dinking along patiently when suddenly your Evil Dinking Genius mind notices that your opponents don't look ready. They may be bent too far forward at the waist, have lowered their paddle, or possibly even yawned. It's time to lob!

Your lob stroke should look almost exactly like your dink stroke because it's important to disguise your lobs. (Refer to Chapter 8 to learn the mechanics behind great dinking.) When you get a slightly shallow dink that you can reach under, lift it skyward with a long, pretty follow-through. (See Figure 9-9 for details on a lob setup and follow-through.) Use your knees to create added lift while your paddle moves upward through the ball.

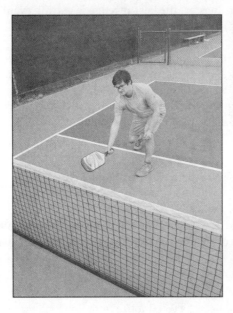 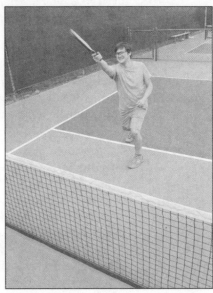

FIGURE 9-9: The point of contact of a lob being hit from a dink that has bounced in the kitchen (left) and a proper lob follow-through (right).

© John Wiley & Sons, Inc./Photo Credit: Aniko Kiezel

TIP

Be sure to hit your lobs with intention. Most players just think "LOB!" and hit the ball straight into the air, without much thought of where it may land. You can do better. Hit lobs to targets that you've selected and practiced. For example, if you've noticed during the course of the game that your opponents are not good at sorting out who takes the ball, try a lob deep to the middle. If one of your opponents has an obvious weakness, such as a poor backhand, exploit that weakness by lobbing to that corner. When possible, lob over the backhand shoulder of your opponent. Most players can't put away a backhand overhead as well as they would a forehand.

People who lob excessively (a.k.a "lobsters") are typically unpopular players. It can suck the fun out of a friendly match when you have to spend the entire time running back chasing lobs instead of happily dinking and volleying. We jokingly like to say, "Lobbers live alone" or "Lobsters, lose my number." You may be winning points, but don't be shellfish if you notice your fellow players are getting crabby and seeing red. All kidding aside, lobs are an important shot to master, especially for serious competitors looking to win tournaments. After all, when you encounter a vicious lobster, the best revenge is getting even! (We prefer ours dipped in garlic butter.)

WARNING

Many people consider it poor sporting conduct to lob over players who have limited mobility. We will leave these moral judgments up to you. However, when playing recreationally, we encourage you to be kind and put fun first. In tournaments, it's appropriate to play to win, knowing that all participants signed up expecting their opponents to play to their best ability.

Playing to the Crowd with Trick Shots

Trick shots are not part of standard pickleball instruction and often occur due to poor paddle position, but they're fun. Nothing is wrong with having fun!

Here are a few trick shots you can learn to dazzle the crowd:

>> **The Tweener:** This shot is hit when you're retrieving a lob that was hit over your head and deep in the court. Turn around and run directly at the ball. Try to time it so that the ball is about to bounce for the second time right under you. Still facing the back of the court, swing your paddle and strike the ball between your legs, taking care not to knock yourself in the tender bits.

>> **The Between-the-Legs shot:** This is not a lob retrieval but rather a fun Hail Mary shot that you use when your opponent has hit the ball to a spot directly between your legs, and you have missed the opportunity to hit it in front of you. Still facing forward, reach around behind you and hit through your legs, hopefully while video is being taken.

>> **The Behind-the-Back shot:** This shot is another hope-and-prayer shot that you hit when the ball is going by you on your nondominant side. You "simply" reach around behind your back with your paddle and strike the ball right next to your nondominant side. Often, if you can manage to get the ball over the net, the shock experienced by your opponents makes this a rally ender. If so, pause for compliments and applause, and then casually continue on with the game. (Figure 9-10 shows examples of these trick shots.)

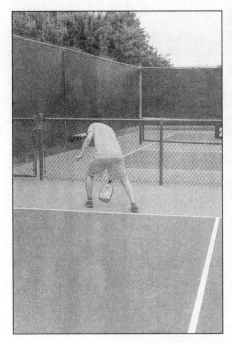 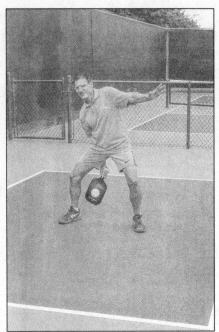

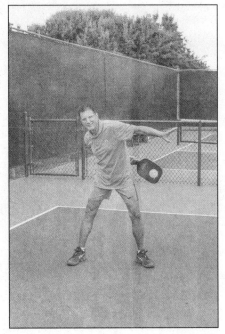

FIGURE 9-10:
A tweener (left),
between-the-legs
(right), and
behind-the-back
shot (bottom).

Chapter **10**

Achy, Breaky: Preventing Injuries and Managing Physical Limitations

Players often joke that the first few minutes of pickleball begin at the net, where both teams discuss all their recent aches and nagging injuries. Fortunately, pickleball is a kinder, gentler sport for joints, which is one of the main reasons everyone shows up in the first place. You can make some smart moves to prepare before a game in order to minimize your pain and maximize your enjoyment. Warming up properly, learning to move safely, and preventing common injuries are good places to start, as we describe in this chapter. We also address mobility issues and how best to play when you have them. As we say throughout this book, pickleball is a sport for everyone — including many people who use wheelchairs. There's an opportunity for fun for all!

Warming Up Properly

Most recreational players arrive at the courts, start casually dinking for a few minutes while visiting, and then suddenly announce that they're ready to play. We refer to this as the "dink and chat" warm-up, and although it's enjoyable, it doesn't do you much good as preparation for play. In this section, we describe a much more complete routine that warms up both your game and your body, helping you to play better and avoid injuries.

Warming up your body

When you arrive at the courts, first do some slow joint rotations from fingertips to toes. Rotations should be done both clockwise and counterclockwise. Rotations coat those joints with extra synovial fluid, making your joints function more smoothly.

Next, move on to some kind of a dynamic warm-up, like taking a brisk walk or jogging around the courts. Get your blood pumping! Your warm-up should literally warm your body temperature up by a couple of degrees. Warm up before you start stretching. You need your muscles to be a little warm before you try to stretch them.

Next it's time to stretch your muscles, but not your tendons and ligaments. You can actually injure your joints, especially your knees, by stretching the joint instead of the muscles around it. Breathe out as you apply stretch to a muscle. (Pro tip: Don't forget to breathe in again.) Try to stretch only one muscle at a time and on one side of the body at a time. Do *static stretching* first, which means to stretch a muscle near its limit, hold it for several seconds, and then relax. Next, do some *dynamic stretching*, which involves moving the various parts of your body and gradually increasing the reach, speed of movement, or both. After you've stretched, try some pickleball-specific moves. Do some *shadow strokes*, which means swinging without the actual ball. Move around the court like you're moving to an imaginary ball. Don't worry about looking silly. Gold medals never look silly, and wouldn't you rather wear one of those than multiple knee, elbow, and shoulder braces?

TIP

Try to stay warmed up despite long breaks between matches. You'll find that if you just plop down in a chair for 15 minutes while waiting, you'll be quite stiff when you get up. Try to keep moving if possible. While waiting, consider using a massage roller device to help move the metabolic waste out of your muscles, increase blood flow, and pamper those muscles. The roller not only helps with your performance but also feels amazing.

Be sure to also cool down after you play. A good way to cool down after you've been really exerting yourself is to basically reverse the order of activities you did in your warm-up. Do some of those pickleball-specific moves in a gentler way, followed by some dynamic and static stretching, and finish off with some light aerobic activity (which might just involve hauling your giant pickleball bag and chair back to the car).

WARNING

We're pickleball experts, not doctors (though coauthor Carl has often dreamed of playing one on TV). Our advice should not be construed as a substitute for qualified professional advice. It's a good idea to work with a physical therapist or certified personal trainer to develop a personalized warm-up and stretching routine tailored just for you. They can work with any physical limitations you may have, and show you how to properly prepare to play safely. Make sure that this person is familiar with the game of pickleball. Perhaps even buy them a book about it. (Hint, hint.)

Warming up your game

After your body is warmed up and ready to go, it's time to get your game itself warmed up. Practice all the shots you'll be using throughout the match.

Start with dinking. If you can, dink straight across as well as crosscourt. Be sure to hit both backhand and forehand dinks, and aim for a variety of depths and angles. One of the issues with "dink and chat" is that you might be too focused on your conversation and end up just mindlessly batting the ball back and forth. You're far better off hitting with intention throughout your warm-up — you should be dinking to win, just as you would in a game.

Next, have your partner stay put at the kitchen line while you take one step back after every few dinks. Magically, your dinks transform into drop shots as you retreat farther in the court. Keep hitting drop shots from all depths of the court, including the baseline. Be sure to hit forehand and backhand drop shots as well as drop volleys. Start working your way back up to the kitchen line by hitting drops all the way in. Then it's your partner's turn to do the same exercise and get their drop shots fully warmed up.

REMEMBER

Don't go too easy on your partner when it's your turn to feed. Your opponents won't gently feed the ball to you in the actual game (they are the *worst!*). Help your partner practice hitting drops off the type of balls they're likely to encounter in real game play. Give them a variety of speeds, make them move, and hit toward their feet. Make warm-up challenging!

Next, both partners should go back and hit some baseline shots to each other, again using forehands and backhands. Include some hard drives. Both of you should then come up to the kitchen line and do some rapid-fire volleys at each other. This routine warms up your volleys as well as your reflexes and reaction speeds (especially useful for those early-morning sessions and 8:00 a.m. tournament start times). Hit some overheads. Be sure to serve from both the right and left side of the court. Take note of the wind and work on adapting to it throughout your warm-up. Hit a lob or two, or any other shots you typically use in your game. Use the time to find your groove.

If for some reason you're in a situation that allows only a minute or two for warm-up (which happens in tournaments more frequently than you'd hope), concentrate on whatever shot you struggle with most. If your serve has been letting you down, hit mostly serves. If you're feeling confident in all your shots because you just read a great book about pickleball, focus your abbreviated warm-up time mostly on drop shots. These shots are the most critical to the game, tend to be more streaky ("I wonder if I brought my drop shot with me today?"), and are particularly affected by weather conditions. Drop shots are your key to getting to the net, where the game is won, so get them ready!

Moving Safely and Efficiently

Pickleball shoes are expensive. Joint replacement surgeries are even more expensive. You can save on both of these items by learning to move safely and efficiently through the court. Here are some suggestions:

>> **Move gently, with quiet feet**. Sneak around the pickleball court like a quiet ninja, waiting to pounce when it's least expected. Use big steps to get to the vicinity of the ball, and smaller steps to fine-tune your position so that you can contact the ball in your ideal strike zone (see Chapter 6 for details on your strike zone). If your shoes make loud squeaking sounds like a litter of puppies as you run, slide, and skid around the court, you should really work on using more careful movement.

>> **Slow down.** If you're running as fast as you can around a small pickleball court, you're also having to execute very hard stops and directional changes. Players who run hard to the kitchen line and then slam on the brakes are well-loved by their orthopedic surgeons ("Hey kids, looks like another trip to Disney World this year!"). That hard running and stopping is traumatic to your joints, especially when you consider how many times you do it per game. The sudden deceleration sends shockwaves up through your lower body and spine. Instead, walk toward the kitchen with big, dynamic steps with your weight slightly forward toward the balls of your feet. If you need to suddenly move to the left or right to get the ball, you can do so without having to make a hard stop or 90-degree turn at full speed.

>> **Stay aware of your court position.** You can minimize excessive or awkward movement by always being in a good position. (See Chapter 11 for our best tips on positioning.) Move to the ball as required, but remember to return to good positioning immediately after you hit. Getting stuck in cement — too often caused by stopping to admire your last shot — forces you to run harder to reach the next ball. If you're not in the process of hitting the ball, you

should be busy getting yourself into a better position. You always have an active role to play in helping your team win the point.

>> **Stand and walk fairly upright.** Bending forward at the waist is not only bad for your back but also puts your weight in your heels, which is not ideal when trying to react to the ball in a timely fashion. Stay tall and keep your chin up and sternum pointed toward the ball when it's in your opponent's court. Your back will thank you.

>> **Speed walk (but don't run) to the line after your return of serve.** The one time when we really want you to hustle up to the line is after you've just returned a serve. Briskly move to the kitchen line to join your partner already waiting there for you. Ideally, you want to get there before the ball comes back to your side of the court so that you can take it as a dink or a volley, rather than awkwardly dealing with it coming toward your feet in the transition zone. You should be able to accomplish this goal with a speedy walk. If not, try hitting your return deeper and with more loft so that it takes longer to come back.

>> **Never run backward!** If the ball lands deep in the court, whatever you do, do not run backward! Running backward often results in a fall. Turn around and run toward the ball, or better yet, just yell, "Yours!" Maybe your partner will get it. (This tactic has proven ineffective in singles.) If during a point you want to just move a few feet back, lean your weight forward and shuffle backward. It's almost impossible to fall back if your weight is forward. It's physics, or gravity, or something.

>> **Stay in balance.** Many players remember that they need to keep their paddle up, but they drop their nondominant arm down by their side. We call this corpse arm. Dropping your nondominant arm puts your shoulders and upper body out of balance. Try to stay in balance over your feet (nose over toes), with both arms up and out in front, and square to the ball at all times. Your movements will be much safer and more efficient when you're in balance. (Refer to Figure 6-9 in Chapter 6.)

Preventing Common Injuries

According to the USA Pickleball Association, 60 percent of core pickleball players are 55 or older. Whether we like it or not, aging bodies are more prone to injury. Many pickleball players are lifelong athletes still dealing with the effects of old injuries from previous sporting endeavors. Even if you happen to still be a young, lithe whippersnapper (get off my lawn!), you can take many actions to help prevent common injuries while enjoying your new favorite sport. Exercising regularly keeps your body and mind in shape, so we would never want you to avoid playing pickleball due to fear of injury.

Here are some "best practices" to help you play safely:

>> **Always wear eye protection.** Glasses, goggles or sunglasses are all fine. Pickleballs can cause serious and permanent damage to your eyeballs.

>> **Wear pickleball or court shoes.** These are designed to support you during your lateral movements on the court. Running shoes or shoes with knobby tread can cause you to trip or roll an ankle. See Chapter 3 for more information on proper eye and shoe wear.

>> **Warm up and streeeetch.** You should ideally stretch every day, but especially before you play. Always. You can access a plethora of online videos to learn the best stretches for playing pickleball. At the bare minimum, stretch out those shoulders, forearms, calves, back, and neck.

>> **Hydrate well.** Good hydration is an important part of your health in your daily life, and even more important when you are exercising. Even if you don't think you are perspiring or overheated, make sure to drink up when you have the chance! Consider adding an electrolyte product to your water. Quality electrolyte products like Jigsaw Health's Electrolyte Supreme, Liquid IV, Hydrant, and Pedialyte can all help you to compete better and longer.

>> **Protect yourself from the sun.** Our mothers always nagged us about wearing sunscreen, and although we hate to admit it, they were right. We've seen severe sunburns on pickleballers who were too excited about playing to notice that they've been roasting in the sun for hours.

>> **Sit out a game if you feel tired.** Listening to your body and sitting out to rest will invigorate you for that next game. There's also no shame in just calling it a day if you're not feeling your best.

>> **Know your limitations.** You don't need to push your body to the limit on every shot. Sometimes it's fine to just say, "Nice shot!" instead of lunging, diving, or body-slamming the fence. Relax; you'll get the next point! Pickleball is supposed to be fun, and nothing ruins the fun for you (and everyone else) as quickly as an injury.

>> **Maybe resist the urge for "one more game."** In pickleball, the acronym OMG stands for "one more game." Pickleball is so enjoyable that it can be hard to fight the temptation to keep playing even when you're already totally knackered. Too often, you announce you're ready to go home but your friends convince you to stay just a bit longer. ("Come on! We need a fourth!") Experience proves that "one more game" is almost always one game too many!

In the event you suffer an injury, fear not. Although we will always refer you to the medical experts, here are some common injuries and suggestions for dealing with them:

>> **Shoulders:** This pesky pickleball pain should not be ignored, or you could end up needing surgery. Exercises for strengthening back and shoulder muscles can help. Avoid overswinging at the ball. Be sure to read Chapter 9 for our advice on compact, efficient volleys and smashes.

>> **Knees:** Too much pivoting, shuffling, or squatting while playing can cause muscle, ligament, and tendon injuries in your knees. (Often, the pain is from a flare-up of an old injury.) It's not unusual to see a lot of players on the courts wearing knee braces and wraps. These wraps can help prevent you from overextending your knees past a safe range of motion. Try to move under control on the balls of your feet, not run at full speed, and stay square to the ball to minimize twisting. Hard stops or sudden changes of direction are very dangerous for compromised knees.

>> **Hands and wrists:** When you first start playing pickleball, these smaller joints and muscles may not be used to some of the unique movements and grip strength required. Hand and wrist muscles will strengthen over time from playing. You can help speed things along by doing exercises with small dumbbells, or silicone bands designed for hand strengthening.

>> **Hamstrings, calves, and other muscles:** Warming up, stretching, and staying hydrated with electrolytes are keys to avoiding muscle strain injuries. Compression sleeves can help with increasing blood flow and gently limiting movement of the targeted muscles. Some players find that kinesiology tape also helps; look for videos online explaining exactly how to apply it to different body parts. A massage roller device (or even a pickleball in a pinch!) helps roll out any knots or tension.

>> **Back:** If you're over the age of 30, you may already be in a standoff with your back every morning. "Don't you dare threaten to go out on me again! I'm just trying to put my socks on!" Compared to being sedentary, playing pickleball can actually improve your back health by helping you stay strong and flexible. However, it's extremely important to listen to your back when it starts giving you those warning tinges. Don't overdo it on the days your back is ornery. Consider doing yoga or other core strengthening exercises regularly to help strengthen and support the muscles in your back and abdomen.

For most sport-related injuries, rest, ice, heat, compression, and elevation are all tried-and-true remedies that will help get you back on the court. As we mention earlier, it's important to assess the severity of any injury and seek medical attention when necessary.

THE CURSE OF TENNIS (PICKLEBALL) ELBOW

By far, one of the most common injuries plaguing pickleball players is lateral epicondylitis, more commonly known as tennis elbow, or in this case pickleball elbow. You will be hard-pressed to visit pickleball courts without seeing multiple players wearing braces on their forearms.

Lateral epicondylitis is an inflammation of the tendons that connect the muscles of the forearm to the bones in the elbow. It results in an aching or stabbing pain originating from the outside of the elbow that can travel down the forearm and wrist. In more severe cases, you might also notice loss of grip strength or numbness in your hand or fingers. The typical causes of pickleball elbow are overuse, lack of strength, or improper form.

The good news is that you can find a ton of information about how to prevent and treat pickleball elbow. The bad news is that there doesn't seem to be a one-size-fits-all approach. If you ask ten former sufferers how they finally overcame their elbow pain, you will likely get ten different answers. You'll have to find the protocol that works for you.

Here are some of the more popular treatments for pickleball elbow:

- **Rest:** Perhaps the most obvious but least attractive option to many pickleballers is to simply take time off from playing and rest the injured arm. In most cases, rest will be your greatest tool and should be used in conjunction with any of the other treatments in this list.

- **Ice and heat:** Icing the area can help reduce acute pain and swelling. Don't ice right before playing or stretching; save it for after. For long-term care, heat is typically preferred because it brings blood to the area to promote healing and helps the muscles to relax.

- **Stretching:** Doing gentle stretching throughout the day can help improve mobility of the affected muscles and tendons. Stretch both your wrist flexors and extensors by extending the affected arm and then using your other arm to pull your hand toward your body, palm facing in, and then again with palm facing out. Hold for about 15–30 seconds, but not to the point of extreme pain.

- **Strengthening exercises:** After the acute injury phase of your pickleball elbow is over, it's important to begin to build strength in your wrist, hand, and elbow to avoid re-injury. You can work out with small dumbbells or resistance bands. Evidence shows that a particular series of exercises using a resistance twist bar (such as the THERABAND FlexBar) is particularly helpful. You can find videos of how to do these exercises online.

- **Anti-inflammatories:** These can include over-the-counter and prescription medication (such as NSAIDs), topical creams, herbal and nutraceutical supplements, and foods. Consult with your doctor before starting any of these protocols.

- **Massage:** Gentle self-massage of the area feels therapeutic and helps to increase blood flow. Transverse friction massage (TFM) is a more intense type of therapy that applies firm pressure in strokes perpendicular to the tendon. It should be done only by a licensed massage therapist and after consulting with your physician.

- **Acupuncture:** Acupuncture has shown to improve blood flow to injured areas by reducing vascular resistance. It also elicits a localized immune response that can help reduce inflammation. Acupuncture is unlikely to solve the issue in a single session, so be ready to commit to several weeks of treatments if you choose this path.

- **Steroid injections:** Although some sufferers find relief from corticosteroid injections, this remedy is somewhat controversial and is becoming less commonly prescribed. The concern is that repeated injections over time can lead to localized tissue damage.

- **Physiotherapy:** The physical therapist will focus first on pain relief and then on stretching and strengthening exercises to help restore full mobility to the arm.

- **Braces:** When you're ready to return to play, wearing a brace, strap, or athletic tape just below the elbow can help limit the amount your tendon is allowed to flex so that it doesn't continue to tear. Be careful not to wear the brace too tightly or for too long because it can limit blood flow to the area and delay healing. Many people find immediate pain relief from using a brace with a built-in compression pad.

- **Lessons:** It's never a bad idea to take a lesson from a qualified pickleball instructor who can identify any issues with your strokes that could be causing, or aggravating, the injury.

- **Change in paddle:** Some players with pickleball elbow swear by a lighter paddle, finding that heavier paddles cause more arm strain. Conversely, others claim that a heavy paddle is better because light paddles require you to generate more of your own force. Difference in core materials can also affect how much vibration is being transferred from your paddle to your tendon. If you can, try hitting with a variety of paddles and see what feels better.

- **Change in grip size and shape:** Playing with a paddle that has the wrong-sized grip for your hand can lead to improper grip, which puts extra stress on your arm. Many players have benefitted from switching to a contour grip, which is a special type of wrap that has ridges for your fingers to fit into, minimizing slippage. Less slipping means you don't have to squeeze the handle as hard, so your forearm muscles can relax a bit.

WARNING

As we may have mentioned, pickleball is very addictive. Many players simply cannot fathom going a week or more without playing. We totally get it. Pickleball may be your main social outlet in addition to your primary form of exercise. Despite this, it's important to know when to say "when." If you are dealing with a persistent or worsening injury, it's time to prioritize self-care and healing. Take the time off. If you're missing your pickleball pals, meet them for lunch or visit the courts one day just to cheer (heckle) them on. You'll be back to playing — hopefully pain-free — before you know it.

Navigating Physical Limitations

Often you will see players with knee or elbow braces because they have physical limitations or because they are healing from an injury. Many players find that they keep getting older every year (surprise!) and don't run as fast as they used to. Pickleball is a game played on a small court that relies more heavily on strategy and finesse than strength and speed. You can succeed at this sport no matter your physical differences. After all, it was originally designed as a game for grandparents and grandchildren to play together.

Making the best of mobility issues

One of the biggest mistakes we see is that when players have mobility issues, they tend to hang around midcourt and play from there. If you have mobility issues, the sooner you get yourself to the kitchen line, the better. This forward position limits your opponents' opportunities to return the ball where you can't reach it. The farther back you stand, the more court your opponents have available to hit into and the more court you have to cover.

When you're properly positioned at the kitchen line, the only movement required is pretty much just lateral — a few steps to the right or a few steps to the left. Hone your drop shot and dinking skills and force your opponents to play with you at the net. That's fair game for all.

TIP

If you're not the swiftest runner, you can buy yourself more time to join your partner at the line after receiving serve by hitting a deep, lofty return. The extra "hang time" in the air gives you a few added seconds before the other team can hit the ball after the bounce.

Regardless of your mobility, try not to stand flat-footed or with your weight in your heels. Standing in a track stance when you're in midcourt or near the baseline, with your strongest leg slightly back, gives you something to push off of when you need to move quickly. At the kitchen line, transferring your weight just slightly between one foot or the other as you track the ball around the court helps you stay aware of what your feet are doing during the rally. It also makes you more able to accelerate when necessary.

Readiness and paddle preparation are also key for anyone dealing with mobility issues. When you're mentally focused and in the proper ready position (see Chapter 6 for an explanation of ready position), you can anticipate the ball better and save time by eliminating unnecessary movements. If someone hits a short ball to you and you need to move your feet to it quickly, put your paddle out like you're reaching out to catch it, and then move. Figure 10-1 shows what this looks like. You may be surprised how many balls you can actually get when you believe you can.

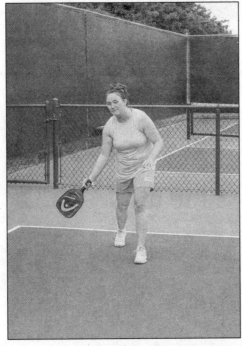

© John Wiley & Sons, Inc./Photo Credit: Aniko Kiezel

FIGURE 10-1: When moving to a short ball, act like you're about to catch it on your paddle.

Equally important when playing with partners or opposing teams is to be respectful of their limitations. Deliberately returning a ball short, for example, when the other player has no way of advancing forward that fast is just poor sporting conduct and not the way to win a point.

Dealing with vision issues

Even if you have issues with vision, you can most likely still play pickleball. Refer to the sections in Chapter 6 about body mechanics and review our advice on playing in the "V." This concept helps you focus on, and deal with, the ball out in front of you, where it's easiest to see. We always recommend keeping your chin up rather than just watching the ball hit your paddle. This way, you can see the ball hit your paddle while simultaneously tracking what your opponents are up to on the other side of the net.

You can team up with a partner who has good vision and use a few small adjustments. For example, as you and your partner move toward the net after your partner serves, you can strategize to hang back a bit to have a wider field of vision so that you can track where the ball is heading. Don't hang back there forever; when you have the opportunity to get all the way to the line, do so. As with many physical limitations, playing strongly right at the kitchen line and focusing on a solid dinking strategy go a long way toward equalizing the playing field for you. Communicate with your partner so that you both play to your best strengths.

Seeing the ball at night is a common issue for many players. Outdoor court lighting is expensive to set up properly, so you will likely find the lighting at your public courts to be lacking. If you find playing at night to be a challenge, you're not alone. Almost everyone over the age of 65 has some amount of cataract in one or both eyes, which impairs night vision. Get your eyes checked regularly and ask your doctor whether you would benefit from having any cataracts removed.

TIP

Wearing bifocal glasses or monovision contact lenses while playing pickleball can often cause problems. Players find they "lose" the ball for a moment as it transitions between their far and near vision fields. Consider purchasing a pair of distance-only, single-vision eyeglasses or contacts to wear when you play. You can even buy glasses specifically made for playing sports that offer fantastic eye protection and a wider lens.

Playing wheelchair pickleball

Wheelchair pickleball, also called para pickleball, is an increasingly growing sport. Players in wheelchairs can play doubles and singles or play a hybrid version with a standing partner. Many wheelchair players are swift, accurate, and competitive.

Here are some ways to get started:

>> **Get the official USA Pickleball Rules.** The latest USA Pickleball/IFP rule book includes Wheelchair Rules.

- » **Connect online and in your community with other para pickleballers.** Networking is the best way to find out who is playing and where.

- » **Reach out to USAPA Ambassadors.** There are USAPA Ambassadors who specialize in wheelchair pickleball.

- » **Consider an adaptive wheelchair.** Adaptive wheelchairs have an extra-wide base for stability while you're going for those winning shots.

- » **Look for ADA-compliant sports facilities.** They should include a ramp, sink, and bathroom. If your community doesn't have an ADA-compliant facility, advocate for getting one built.

Understanding the rules for players with disabilities

There aren't that many exceptions or special rules for those who play with disabilities. That makes it easier for wheelchair users to mix in during recreational play.

Here's what you need to know to abide by the rules of pickleball if you or one of your competitors is using a wheelchair:

- » **The wheelchair user is allowed two bounces.** The second bounce can be anywhere on the playing surface of the court (in or out of bounds).

- » **The server shall be in a stationary position and is allowed one push before striking the ball.**

- » **The moment the ball is served, both rear wheels must be behind the baseline.** They also must be inside the imaginary extensions of the sideline and centerline.

- » **The smaller front wheels may touch the kitchen during a volley.** If the rear wheels of a wheelchair have touched the kitchen for any reason, the player may not volley a ball until both rear wheels make contact with the playing surface outside the kitchen. The playing surface includes the area out of bounds.

- » **Players using wheelchairs may play with either "standup" partners (a.k.a. hybrid doubles) or another wheelchair user.** When a player using a wheelchair is playing with or against a standing person in singles or doubles, the rules of pickleball for standing players apply to the standing players and the wheelchair rules apply to all players using wheelchairs.

>> **Singles play with one or both players using a wheelchair are played on a half court.** The server and the receiver serve, receive, and play the entire point from their respective service and receiving court.

In recent years, competitive wheelchair pickleball has been gaining momentum. Regional and national tournaments that include wheelchair divisions can be found all over the U.S. as well as other countries. (See Figure 10-2.)

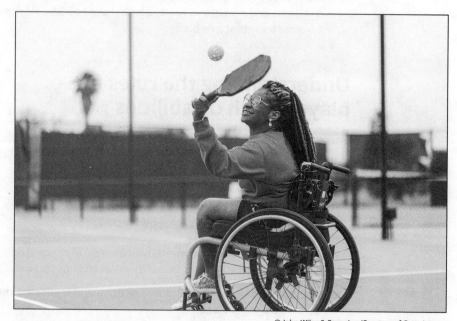

FIGURE 10-2: A pickleball player in action.

© John Wiley & Sons, Inc./Courtesy of Getty Images

3

Mastering Pickleball Strategy

Chapter **11**

Playing Smarter: Basic Doubles Strategies

When players first take up the game of pickleball, they usually focus on just getting the ball over the net and inside the court. As they advance, they begin to strategize more and more. Strategizing is hard to do without having some intellectual understanding of the game. Where you should stand at any given moment, the shots you choose to hit, and how to work well with a partner may feel like huge mysteries at first. No worries; you've come to the right place!

At the beginning of every rally, it's important to have a plan and a vision of how you see that point going. Although many split-second decisions are required in pickleball, you can also make some decisions in advance. The more you can plan in advance, the less you'll have to figure out mid-rally. Even if things don't end up going exactly according to script, at least your goals were clear from the outset. The plan will bring you confidence, and the vision will bring you the motivation to get it done.

This chapter arms you with all the basic doubles strategies you need to start creating and executing those winning plans. If talking strategy sounds serious and intense, we can assure you that building a winning doubles team and learning how to work together is incredibly fun and satisfying. Playing doubles together is a great way to create or enhance a friendship (or marriage!) to last a lifetime.

Recognizing the Four Phases of a Doubles Point

To grasp basic doubles strategy, you need to first understand the phases involved in a point. The rules of pickleball — particularly the serving, Two-Bounce, and kitchen rules — mean that these four phases occur in almost every point. As you progress through a typical rally, it helps to understand what phase you're in, what the goals of that phase are, and which shots you need to succeed there.

If someone were to ask you your goal at the beginning of a point, you might be tempted to say, "To win the rally." Asked to be a bit more specific, you might answer, "Be the last team to hit the ball over the net and inside the lines." (You're a bit cheeky, aren't you?) Although these are certainly sensible goals, this line of thinking doesn't provide much of a road map on how to achieve them. Here's where knowing the phases of the point comes in. By breaking the overall goal down into manageable sections, you'll have a much clearer picture of what's required to navigate your way to victory.

Serving and returning (Phase 1)

Not surprisingly, the first phase of a pickleball point involves the serve and return. Because the pickleball serve is underhand and the Two-Bounce Rule forces a slower, measured rhythm at the beginning of each rally, many players treat the serve and return as perfunctory. They don't put much thought or effort into them, other than getting them in so that everyone can move on to the fun stuff. In fact, this phase of the point is just as important as any other.

Beyond just starting the rally, the goal of your serve should be to force a weak return from your opponent — a return that makes your third-shot drop or drive easier to execute. (Chapter 7 explains third-shot drops and drives.) These shots are difficult enough without attempting to hit them off your opponent's wicked backspin slice or blazing forehand drive. Don't just mindlessly serve up a proverbial "soft ball" that allows the receiver to tee off with whatever speed, direction, or spin they choose. Instead, figure out what your opponents hate the most, and serve that to them. Think of it as being the world's worst dinner party host. ("You simply *must* try my raisin tuna salad gelatin mold! *Bon appetit!*")

For the receiver, the primary goal is similar in that your return should force a weak third shot from the serving team. Your secondary goal is to try to keep the serving team back in the court so that you and your partner can dominate from the line. You want to hit a deep return rather than a short one — the deeper, the better! A short return invites your opponents to immediately come up to the net. An especially tasty treat for the serving team would be a short, high-bouncing return. If you hit one of these, expect it to be driven back extremely hard!

After you've hit your nice deep return, hustle up and join your partner at the line. Go as fast as you safely can and still be able to make a gentle stop at the line. Try to get there before the ball comes back to your side of the court so that you and your partner both have a chance at volleying the next shot. By getting all the way to the line, you shrink the amount of court your opponents have to land their third-shot drop. Should your opponent hit a drive, you're far better off dealing with it above your waist than down at your feet. Get to the line and let the net do some of the job of protecting your feet.

If you are the receiver's partner, you also have a few important jobs to do:

>> **Look big and scary.** Consider the visual you're presenting to your opponents. Are you standing way off the court, paddle down, hand on your hip, like you're waiting in line at the post office? Or are you in ready position with your paddle up, taking up space on the court and staring down the server like a pro wrestler ready to rumble? Visuals matter.

>> **Call the lines.** Watch the serve carefully and call it out or short if necessary. Your partner is busy trying to hit and can't call the lines as well as you can.

>> **Evaluate the return.** You want to actually turn your head and watch your partner hit their return so that you can anticipate what comes next. Did your partner just get pulled off the court, trip over their shoelaces, and shank the ball high in the air? You need to know! Don't stare straight ahead when all the action is happening behind you.

>> **Cover the middle.** As your partner is scurrying up to join you at the line, be extra ready for the ball to come back to the middle. If the next ball comes anywhere within reach, pounce on it! That's your ball.

REMEMBER

The server's partner certainly has the least to do during this first phase, but don't mentally check out. Remember to stay back behind the baseline and avoid creeping into the court after the serve — you might just get a deep return and end up backpedaling to let it bounce. Be actively planning your third shot based on what your opponents are doing. That's happening in Phase 2, and it's coming up next!

Transitioning to the line (Phase 2)

In most cases, after the serve and return have occurred, you'll see the receiving team up at the kitchen line and the serving team back at the baseline. Because of the Two-Bounce Rule, the serving team is not allowed to "serve and volley," meaning that they can't serve the ball and immediately rush the net. They must hang back and wait for the ball to come back and bounce on their side of the court.

Meanwhile, the receiving team has already let the serve bounce, so they are allowed to come to the kitchen and volley their next shot. Just two shots in, and the serving team is stuck with a major positioning disadvantage. No fair! The second phase of the point is all about overcoming this disadvantage. The serving team must find a way to safely move through the middle of the court (known as *the transition zone*) and meet their opponents at the line.

The best way to accomplish this transition is through drop shots. (Chapter 7 goes into more detail on how to hit them.) An effective drop shot is a ball that is unattackable, meaning that it forces your opponent to swing up on the ball and hit back another drop or dink. When you see your opponent having to get low and lift the ball, you know it's safe to come a few steps forward. If you see your opponent with their paddle held high, ready to slam, don't come forward. (Figure 11-1 shows you what each of these poses looks like.) If you're ever wondering, "Was that drop shot any good?" just watch what your opponent is doing for the answer.

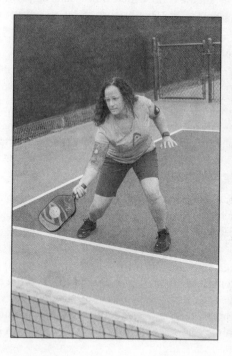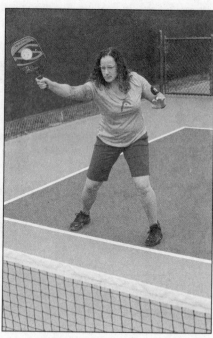

FIGURE 11-1:
A player swinging up at an unattackable ball (left) and down on an attackable one (right).

© John Wiley & Sons, Inc./Photo Credit: Aniko Kiezel

TIP

Don't expect to get to the line with just one drop. It may take two, three, or even more drops to work your way up. Be patient and stay confident that you can keep hitting as many drops as necessary. If you hit a poor drop, don't panic and give up! Stay where you are and be ready to field an attack. Block or reset the ball as best you can and then go back to dropping. See the section "Staggering," later in this chapter, for more advice on how to move through the transition zone with your partner.

Drop shots are the tried-and-true method of transitioning to the line, but they're not your only option. As pickleball evolves, we're seeing the third-shot drive utilized with increased frequency, especially by younger and more aggressive teams. Driving the ball is fun and may feel easier than attempting to finesse the perfect drop, but it doesn't always help you achieve your goal of getting to the line. When you drive the ball right at your opponent, you're essentially giving them an opportunity to volley. They might block it back hard at your feet, or angle it off the court for a winner. Test your opponents early in the match to see how well they handle your drives. Continue driving the ball only if the drive has been successful. It's never smart to hit all your third shots as drives just because you don't have faith in your drop. If you do decide to drive the ball, you may still have only enough time to advance a few steps, so be ready to keep fighting your way to the kitchen.

Now, how about when you're on the receiving team? Your goal during this phase is to keep the serving team from accomplishing their mission of getting to the line. Punish any high balls by smashing or blocking them back deep in the court, ideally at or behind your opponents' feet — or better yet, off the court for a clean winner. If you're comfortable hitting a *roll shot* (described in Chapter 14), that's another great offensive option for balls that are about waist high. Keep pushing the other team back as long as possible, and perhaps they won't even make it to the next phase.

Dinking (Phase 3)

If you've made it this far in the point, congratulations! You've successfully navigated Phases 1 and 2 without a fault, and now you get to enjoy one of the very best things about pickleball: dinking!

In this phase, all four players are standing at the line. They take turns trading unattackable balls called *dinks*, which are soft, low-bouncing shots that bounce in or near the kitchen. A successful dink is one that your opponents can only dink back, which is done by swinging low to high and gently lifting the ball back over the net. A poor dink is one that your opponents can speed up and convert into an attack, either off a high bounce or by volleying from above the waist.

To an outside observer who knows nothing about pickleball, dinking looks like a very strange ritual. It almost appears as if players are just standing there politely tapping the ball back and forth instead of trying to win the point. If you've read Chapter 8, you know that this is far from the truth. Dinking is actually a complex battle of skill and wits, requiring tremendous precision, patience, and strategy.

The goal in this phase is to force an error from your opponent before they do the same to you. To borrow from a famous television show, your personal motto while dinking could easily be "Outwit. Outplay. Outlast." To force your opponents to make an error, we recommend dinking toward players' feet or making them reach or move. Use varied dinking patterns so as not to let your opponents get into a rhythm. Try to slowly back them off the line so that you have more access to their feet. Try dinking several times in a row to the same person, and watch their partner out of the corner of your eye to see whether they lose focus; then surprise them with an offensive dink or a speedup.

During this phase, you'll be totally absorbed in carefully placing your dinks and plotting out your next few moves. However, somewhere deep inside your calm, patient, calculating self, a tiger sits perched and ready to pounce. All that dinking strategy ultimately leads to one goal: forcing an error from your opponent so that you can move to the next phase of the point — the attack! *Grrrrrr!*

Attacking, counterattacking, and resetting (Phase 4)

You're approaching the thrilling conclusion of your well-planned battle strategy. You've set your team up well with an effective serve or return, moved yourself to the kitchen line, and traded dinks with your opponents until one of them finds themselves off-balance, reaching, or pulled out of position. They accidentally send the ball up a little too high, and *whammo!* You attack the ball by smashing it down toward the ground.

WARNING

The scenario just described is classic pickleball, and, in many cases, the end of the point. In others, depending on the defensive skills of your opponents, you might be surprised to find the ball coming back over the net! Your smug satisfaction is quickly replaced with panic as you realize that the ball is still in play. You should be aware that rather than end with a single attack shot, this phase of the point can go on for many shots and contain many exciting twists and turns. Be ready to hang in there!

Knowing exactly when in a rally to move to Phase 4 takes experience and practice, and not knowing the right time still trips up many advanced players. Impatience with dinking and a desire to be offensive often cause players to prematurely attack the wrong ball. The result is usually a ball hit very hard into the net, out of bounds, or straight up to their opponent's waiting paddle. Regrets are had and inner curse words are muttered. (But it's all part of the game we love.) Do your best to wait for the right ball — the "sure thing" ball, or at least a high-percentage ball — before initiating an attack. See the section "Selecting the Right Shot," later in this chapter, for some advice on how to wait for the right time to attack.

TIP

Not all attacks are slams. One of our favorite attacks is something we call "medium speed up the middle." Through your careful, strategic dinking, you've parted your opponents by drawing one or both of them out wide, and a large hole has opened up between them. All you need to do to finish the point is to hit a low, moderately-paced shot down the middle of the court. Although not flashy, this attack can be as demoralizing as it is effective. See the section in Chapter 14 about relishing the attack for a few more ideas. If something's not working, really, really resist the urge to think, "Maybe if I just hit it a little harder . . . ." Try a different tactic instead.

You may find that after attacking, your opponent is able to return it with a counterattack, suddenly putting you on defense. Be wary of trying to "body shot" players above the waist who have quick reaction times. Unless you can pinpoint weak spots — such as their dominant-side armpit or hip — you are essentially giving them an easy block volley that they can choose to angle downward, or away from you, for a winner. This type of shot is often referred to as a Big Bummer. (It's important to know the right terminology.)

If your first attack is unsuccessful, your odds of winning the point actually decrease if you commit to attacking every ball that follows in the same way. Don't throw good after bad; you always have the option to *reset the point*, which means to revert back to Phase 3 and start dinking again. Slow down the pace by hitting a dink or drop shot that your opponents can't possibly attack (see the section in Chapter 14 about controlling the pace to find out how). Start working your dinking strategy again, and wait until you get another "sure thing" ball before you attack again.

Just remember that it's okay. You're just going through a phase (or four).

Getting into Position

In pickleball, getting (and staying) in good court position is probably the most important thing you can do aside from striking the ball with your paddle. Your opponents are constantly looking for open court, so leaving too much open real estate will quickly spell disaster.

At any given moment during the rally, if you aren't hitting the ball, you should be getting yourself into better position. You should always be busy doing something that helps your team. We like to say, "Never be doing nothing," or just to make our English teachers crazy, "Don't you never not be doing nothing." Observe what your partner and opponents are doing, anticipate what comes next, and close off any available angles or open court by occupying space and squaring to the ball. Save the spectating for when you're off the court!

In this section, we detail some of the best court positioning techniques in doubles pickleball. You need to be sure you're working in tandem with your partner, so give them a copy of this book so that you're both literally "on the same page." Nothing in pickleball is written in stone, so feel free to adapt these plays based on your team's strengths and abilities, as well as your opponents'.

Staggering

This section isn't about having one too many at the bar; it's about how a doubles team should move forward in the court. For many years, pickleball coaches taught that the two partners on a team should move in parallel, as though they're tethered together on the same foosball stick. Eventually, the great minds of pickleball figured out a better way — a slight staggering of the players. This means that as a team begins to move forward through the transition zone, one partner advances slightly ahead of the other. Figure 11-2 shows you exactly what this looks like. This way, if the ball comes to the middle, the player in front has room to slide over for a very cool-looking poach shot. (We're all about looking cool!)

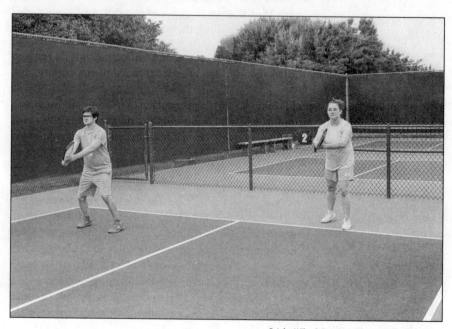

FIGURE 11-2: A team in the staggered position.

This technique frees up the middle so that the players have room to work (and by "work" we really mean "play!"). If both players are right next to each other, confusion can ensue over who will take the middle, or even result in a clashing of paddles (and knuckles). Be sure to check out the Drop and Hunt play described in Chapter 12. It's fun and effective, but it works only if the partners are slightly staggered.

To implement the staggering technique, the player on the serving team who is not making the third shot should take a few steps forward as their partner is hitting. Turn and observe what your partner is doing. If it looks like they are hitting a good shot that is unattackable, you're safe to keep striding forward. If not, definitely don't move forward. That's called "chasing garbage." Do not chase garbage! (This is also great dating advice.)

After your partner finishes their third shot, they should begin walking forward as well. Often, the player hitting the third shot immediately knows that their shot isn't good. If that's the case, they might say something like "stay back!" in order to keep you from moving toward the inevitable attack. (In truth, your partner may say something a bit more colorful than that.) No matter how many shots it takes for your team to get to the kitchen line, try to maintain that slight stagger. Stagger gives you swagger!

Funneling

In Chapter 6, we talk about squaring your body to the ball whenever it's on your opponent's side of the court. Squaring to the ball is critical when using the funneling technique. *Funneling* is essentially imagining that you have a giant funnel out in front of you. (In case it's not obvious, the funnel's purpose is to collect pickleballs!) If you square your body to the ball and open your arms in a "V" shape, that's your funnel.

If the ball is traveling toward your funnel, you take it. If the ball is traveling toward your partner's funnel, they should take it. This technique ensures that the player who is most squared to the trajectory of the ball is the one hitting it.

You and your partner both need to position yourself so that your funnels can collect almost any ball that comes your way. If a breakdown occurs in the funnel system, you need to adjust accordingly. For example, if your partner has been pulled out wide and left the court, your funnel needs to get *really* large! Back up a few feet, move to the middle, and direct your funnel toward the opponent hitting the ball.

The funneling technique really helps your team cover the middle. You may hear this same concept described as the "X" strategy. The diagrams in Figure 11-3 show that if the ball were to come back diagonally through the middle, it would be headed toward the crosscourt player's funnel. The other player should be funneling straight ahead in case the ball comes down the line. Note that this technique applies only if both partners are relatively even with each other in the court. See "Figuring out who's got the middle," later in this chapter, for more on covering the middle. (Figure 11-3 shows how players' funnels change based on the ball's location.)

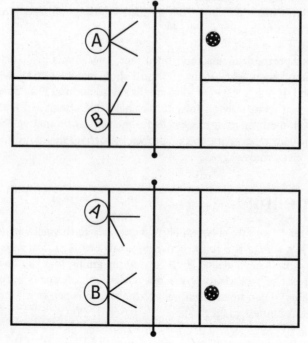

FIGURE 11-3: How players' funnels change depending on where the ball is coming from.

Paddle tracking

When considering court positioning, you need to think about more than just where to stand. Simply taking up space on the court doesn't guarantee that you'll be able to successfully return the ball. Your upper body and paddle need to be in optimal position as well. If you're standing in the right spot but facing the wrong direction, the right spot isn't going to do you much good!

Paddle tracking is a technique that the amazing pro player and coach Sarah Ansboury taught us early on. It has made all the difference in our games. Paddle tracking means constantly keeping your paddle up and pointed at the ball. Keep your paddle out in front of you, preferably holding it with both hands, and stalk the ball as it moves around the other side of the court. When you're first learning this technique, it can be helpful to use the index finger on your nondominant hand to actually point at the ball (see Figure 11-4). However, it's fine to place your nondominant hand anywhere on the paddle that feels comfortable.

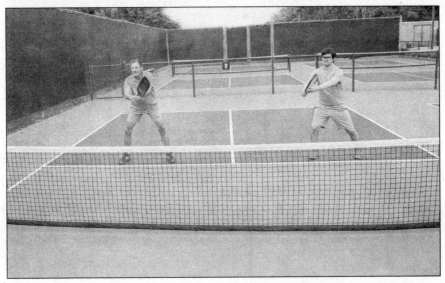

FIGURE 11-4:
The game-changing paddle tracking technique.

© John Wiley & Sons, Inc./Photo Credit: Aniko Kiezel

This technique works beautifully in combination with funneling. It prevents your paddle from dropping down by your side and makes you more ready. If you're paddle tracking, you're keeping your major joints square to the ball, and you're playing with a heightened degree of attention. You simply cannot lose focus while paddle tracking. When the authors are at the end of a long tournament day and all we can think about is tacos, we shift our attention back to our paddle tracking. Even when mentally exhausted, you can use this technique to keep focus and power through to the medal stand. With luck, the taco truck hasn't already left by then!

Staying in your lane

When we talk about staying in your lane, we're giving some fantastic driving advice as well as solid pickleball instruction. Combined with our attempt at dating advice earlier in this chapter, we'd say this book provides great value!

If, at the end of a rally, you find that you and your partner are standing right next to each other in the middle of the court, this should tell you something. You're not really covering the middle if you're both standing in it, because neither of you has any room to hit. (You're more likely to hit each other than the ball.) You're also leaving the sidelines wide open for your opponents to easily hit a passing shot or angle.

REMEMBER

Basic pickleball strategy is "make a hole and hit through it." Effective court positioning means minimizing any holes and maximizing your total court coverage. Only two of you are responsible for the entire court, so if you're standing too close to your partner, you are not making the best use of your bodies and paddles.

Figure 11-5 is a road map showing where each of your lanes are on the court. There is no carpool lane, so you and your partner should never be sharing! For beginner or intermediate players, we recommend that your lanes run directly through the middle of each service box. For more advanced players, try shifting your lane slightly more to the outside of the court. This leaves the middle looking a bit open, which will tempt your opponents to try to attack there. Knowing this, you'll be ready to jump in with a counterattack and punish them for taking the bait!

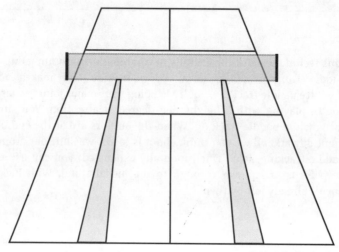

FIGURE 11-5: The lanes you should travel through up the court.

As you move forward in the court, be mindful of your lane. Carefully walking with big dynamic steps will help you shift directions faster (and more safely) if you suddenly need to leave your lane. Many players are in the habit of making a bee-line for the center of the court and then parking it there. Often, this habit comes from following your shot (running in the same direction in which you just sent the ball), a habit you may have developed playing tennis. In pickleball, the court is much smaller, so following your shot is not necessary. Instead, maximize your court coverage by staying in your lane.

Of course, sometimes you need to leave your lane in order to hit the ball. That's fine — just move to the ball and then return to your lane. Think of your shot as being incomplete until you've repositioned yourself well for the next one.

Keeping forward pressure

If you have ever faced a team that just seems to mercilessly march forward toward the net in a constant state of readiness, you know very well what *forward pressure* looks like. You might feel as though a tsunami wave, or maybe that giant boulder that chased after Indiana Jones, is coming toward you — it's absolutely terrifying! (We would never resort to hyperbole in this book.)

As we describe earlier in this chapter, Phase 3 of a pickleball point involves transitioning to the line. You can't dink until you are there, and your attacks will be less effective from deeper in the court. As best you can, try to keep your team moving forward at all times using your great drop shots, drives, and smart court positioning. Whenever you are back in the court, *forward* is your goal.

If you're midcourt and have the option to step backward or forward into a ball, always step forward. Stepping back to let it bounce may give you more time, but it gives your opponents more time, too. It also increases the likelihood that you'll have to awkwardly deal with a ball bouncing at your feet, inside your hoop (see Chapter 8 if that term doesn't ring a bell). Constantly applying forward pressure will make you hit more balls out of the air as volleys, which is much more offensive. It also guarantees that you're putting a forward weight shift into your shots instead of leaning backward (which is a good recipe for a pop-up).

A team applying forward pressure limits their opponents' options. If you're hanging back in the court, you're leaving way too much open court for your opponents. You might as well be saying, "Have at it; the court is your oyster!" Shrink the amount of court in front of you, as well as the available angles, by getting all the way to the kitchen line.

Be the team that is moving forward, steadily and in balance. It will strike fear in your opponents. More important, it will make you and your partner look calm, cool, and collected.

Figuring out who's got the middle

You commonly hear players reminding each other before the game even starts that "forehand has middle." This statement makes pickleball coaches cringe a little. Perhaps, with all other things being equal, you should defer to having the forehand take the middle. However, there is much more to sorting this situation out.

We recommend using the following order of priority to determine who should take middle:

1. **The player in front.** If you are the player closest to the net, you're in the more offensive position because you have a greater chance of volleying the ball. Whether you're using forehand or backhand, taking time away from your opponent and hitting down on the ball is always the better choice. Go ahead and leave your lane if you see a high, middle ball you think you can reach! Don't politely let an attackable ball float by just because it wasn't on "your half" of the court.

2. **The player who is more ready.** The player who just hit the last ball is often the least ready for the next ball. Be constantly aware of what your partner is currently doing and whether they are in a state of readiness. If they are still finishing their follow-through, or recovering position after their last shot, you need to be extra ready to take the next ball. If they have fallen flat on their face and their last word before they pass out is "You!" then by all means, take the next ball.

3. **The player whose funnel the ball is coming toward.** As described earlier in this chapter, if the ball is heading toward your funnel, you are the player most squared to that ball. If both players are positioned evenly in the court and are equally ready, let this player take a middle ball that is coming crosscourt.

4. **The player with the stronger stroke in the middle.** If both players are even with each other and the ball is coming straight down the middle of the court, the player who can make the stronger stroke (typically forehand) should take the ball.

Communicating with Your Partner: Great Minds Dink Alike!

Who doesn't love a good mystery? People love the suspense, the speculating on what comes next, and the final surprise twist at the end. All those facets are great when they're part of the novel you're reading, but not during a pickleball rally.

Communicating effectively with your partner can help eliminate some of the guesswork and surprises for your team. Clear, consistent communication helps you and your partner play the same game rather than two separate games on one side of the net. Solid communication builds trust between partners and helps you find your rhythm as a team.

Few things are more disheartening on the court than when you and your partner just look at each other as a ball is hit right down the middle, without any movement from either of you. Then you get the dreaded, "Was that mine? I thought you were going to get it" and then the reply of, "I thought *you* were going to get it." Ugh! Imagine if you had a way to tell each other your intentions. Oh, wait — you do! Talk to each other. Mystery solved.

Calling the ball: "Me! You!"

So you've decided to use your language skills to improve your team's performance. Great choice! Partner communication will make your life much easier after you get used to it.

The moment you see a ball that you feel you should be taking, call out loudly and proudly, "Me!" If you feel that a ball should be taken by your partner, let them know with a shout of "You!" Communication should be loud, clear, and prompt. Use single-syllable words whenever possible. "Mine" and "yours" are just as acceptable. It's not helpful to hear your partner say things like, "I'm pretty much almost certain that I should be the one to retrieve this particular ball" as it sails past you both. Nor is it helpful to yell "You, me, you, YOU, ME!" Keep it short and decisive.

We hope that you and your partner are both familiar with the general strategies for who takes middle balls (see the "Figuring out who's got the middle" section, earlier in this chapter). Those strategies will help you both avoid shouting "Mine!" at the same time. It will still happen sometimes, but as you improve your pickleball knowledge and instincts, the sense of who should be taking which ball will become much clearer.

TIP

Whoever is the first to yell "You!" is off the hook. We recommend selecting a partner who is at least ten years younger than you. We also recommend invoking this unofficial rule whenever your opponent sends a lob up over your head.

It's important to call the ball throughout the rally, not just at the baseline. We often see dinking rallies fall apart because of poor or nonexistent communication. The communication not only tells the team who intends to hit the ball, but also releases the nonhitting partner so that they can use that time to get themselves in a better position. Remember, if you're not busy hitting, you should be doing something else to help your team, such as paddle tracking, repositioning, or looking for openings on the other side of the court.

"Let it go!"/"Bounce it!"

When playing doubles, you should take advantage of the fact that there are two players on your side of the net. Both players are watching the flight of the ball and will have slightly different perspectives on it from where they stand. Use that fact to your advantage by guiding each other on when to let a ball go out, or at least to let the ball bounce because it *might* be going out.

REMEMBER

The easiest way to win a point in pickleball is to let the ball go out! Don't miss opportunities to win points by failing to help your partner identify "out" balls. One of coauthor Reine's favorite qualities in a doubles partner is someone who tells her when to let the ball go.

If you see your partner starting to go for a ball that is clearly going out, cram all three syllables of the phrase "Let it go" into one syllable and yell out, "Letitgo!" You can also just yell, "No!" (Unless your partner's name is "Mo.") Yell whatever it takes to stop your partner in their tracks. Some players prefer to just yell, "Out!" You should know that it's legal to say "out" for the purpose of partner communication as long as the ball has not bounced. If the ball has already bounced and you say "out," it's considered a line call and the ball is dead. For this reason, we recommend choosing a different word when communicating with your partner versus making a line call, so as not to cause confusion.

TIP

If a lofty shot looks like it's about to land near the sideline or baseline, often the nonhitting partner has a better view of it than the player who is busy chasing it down. In this case, it's a good idea to yell, "Bounce it!" This tells the hitting player to wait and hit it *after* the bounce, just in case it lands out.

"Switch!"/"Stay!"

Things can get a little wild and wacky in pickleball rallies. Anything can happen, and the partners of a good team will guide each other to avoid leaving the court wide open. When chaos or scrambling occurs, you want a way to tell your partner whether they should switch places with you or stay put.

For instance, if one player runs back to retrieve a lob, the nonhitting player might tell them "Switch!" because they can see that the hitting player will wind up on the opposite side of the court from where they started. That way, as soon as the hitting player finishes their shot, they don't have to try to scramble back over to their original position. The nonhitting player has already moved over to that side and the hitting player can stay where they are.

On the other hand, if the lob lands in the middle of the backcourt or on the same side as the lob retriever, the nonhitting partner might yell "Stay!" This tells the hitting player to stay on the same side of the court where they were originally playing.

If you're stacking or using hand signals (see Chapter 12 for details on those strategies), it means that you've planned in advance whether you and your partner will be switching sides at the beginning of the rally. Sometimes things don't go according to plan, and you need to let your partner know that it's time to terminate. For example, if you're stacking on a receive of serve and your partner gets pulled out wide by the serve, they might yell "Stay!" to let you know not to slide over as originally planned. Otherwise, this rally would be a total disaster for your team.

Strategizing and connecting between points

Coauthor Reine was in a tournament several years ago when she and her partner, Laurie, lost their first match. Reine's sister, who had watched them play, pointed out that as soon as they lost the first few points, they had stopped interacting with each other. They had let their discouragement break down their usual teamwork. For the rest of the tournament, Reine and Laurie made a conscious effort to connect between every point with eye contact, paddle tapping, and words of encouragement. They went on not only to beat the team they had lost to in the first round but to eventually take gold. It was an important lesson in partner communication.

Good doubles teams develop their strategy and chemistry by communicating between every point. Communication can be both verbal and nonverbal. Partners commonly stay connected with each other through just a simple paddle tap. In pickleball, we don't shake hands or high five; we paddle tap. A paddle tap can mean "Hey, we got this!" or "Nice job!" or "Don't sweat it." Most of all, it means "We're connected." Connection is paramount to playing good doubles. Otherwise, you just have two individuals doing their own thing, not a team working synergistically.

If you or your partner notice weaknesses, strengths, or patterns in your opponents, take a few seconds between points to talk about them. One of the quickest ways to lose a pickleball match is to enter with one single strategy and never deviate from it, even when it's not working! (This mindset doesn't work well for life, either.) Most people dislike being bossed around, so get to know your partner's personality and be mindful of your tone. Try phrasing your suggestions as observations, such as, "Pssst . . . the guy in the unicorn t-shirt keeps leaving the sideline open." (Classic unicorn behavior.) You might also present them as ideas to experiment with: "Let's try a third-shot drive to the gal who keeps dropping her paddle." If you've established yourself as team captain and your partner is cool with it, that's fine; otherwise, make it a collaborative effort.

It is extremely critical to not be critical! Both partners need to feel supported by each other. Do not coach your partner in the middle of a game. Coaching is for lessons and clinics, not game time. Mid-match coaching between partners usually does much more harm than good. Your partner most likely already knows what they've done wrong, and the last thing they need is to hear it from you. That will dig them into a mental hole that is very hard to climb out of.

REMEMBER

Your number one job as a doubles partner is to lift up your partner. If they make a mistake, tell them "No worries! We got this!" Share a laugh or a smile between rallies. It's just pickleball, not life or death. People are more important than points.

Calling time-out

In competitive pickleball, you are allowed to take *time-outs* in order to pause the game. You can and should use all your available time-outs for a variety of reasons. In most games, each team is allowed two time-outs that can last for up to one minute.

Use your time-outs wisely. If your opponents are running away with the game and have all the momentum, call a time-out. A time-out is a great way to change the vibe of the game and give your team the mental reset you need. Sometimes just breaking a server's rhythm will cause them to make an unforced error rather than continue to run up points.

You may also want to use a time-out to discuss strategy with your partner whenever you need more than those few seconds between points. Outside coaching from spectators is not allowed during game play but is allowed on time-outs. A trusted coach or friend nearby may have some outside perspective on what's happening.

Are you absolutely exhausted and can't catch your breath? Call a time-out. Are you or your partner emotionally imploding? Call a time-out. Are you bleeding from any body part? That's an automatic medical time-out! Whatever the reason, don't forget that time-outs are yet another useful tool in your toolbox.

TIP

Sometimes you might be at a loss as to what to do to turn a match around. Even if you don't have any brilliant strategic ideas, call a time-out and then try changing one thing. Start (or stop) stacking. Toss up some lobs. Hit third-shot drives instead of drops. Force more dinking rallies. Give your opponents something new to deal with, and it might just throw them off long enough to get your team, and your groove, back in the game.

Selecting the Right Shot

When you play pickleball, you must make hundreds of small decisions. At first, you may feel that you have no time for decisions. You're simply reacting to a ball flying your way and hoping you can get it back over the net. As you gain more skill and experience, you can begin to be more proactive than reactive. A big part of being proactive is learning good shot selection; that is, deciding on the best shot to hit given the current circumstances in the rally, game, or match.

Context matters. If you have just won the first game of the match 11–0 and you're now up 10–0 at match point, you can probably get away with taking bigger risks than you should if it's 19–18 in the third game of the match. Sure, it's still match point, but you have some room for error. We're certainly not telling you to be a bad sport by doing foolish things or grandstanding when you're way ahead; that would be insulting to your opponent. What we *are* saying is that there are better times than others to take risks. Practicing smart shot selection will really boost your game by leaps and bounds. (Just make sure your shots are carefully thought-out, practical, and well-timed leaps and bounds.)

Visualizing the upside-down traffic signal

A popular visualization technique with many players and coaches is that of an upside-down traffic signal superimposed on your own body. The purpose is to help you decide whether to attack a ball that you receive when standing near the kitchen, and it can really help by evoking smart choices during rallies. Here's how it works: Because it's an upside-down traffic signal, red is on the bottom, yellow is in the middle, and green is on top. Figure 11-6 shows you how to visualize this in relation to your body:

>> **Red light: Feet to knees.** Red light means *Stop* — don't attack. You are contacting this ball very low, which means you have to swing upward and lift the ball in order to clear the net. Because of that upward trajectory, you must swing very slowly and be careful not to add too much energy behind the ball. If you swing too fast and try to speed it up, the ball will pop up or go into the net. "Red light" balls require you to stop attacking and wait for a higher ball that you can do more with. It is definitely dangerous to speed through a red light!

>> **Yellow light: Knees to ribcage.** A yellow light signals *Caution* and should cause you to evaluate your options. Are your opponents in perfect position, looking super ready to pounce on whatever shot you might send their way? If so, consider yielding and hitting a soft, unattackable ball. Wait for a better ball to come later. However, if your opponents have left a swath of court wide open, go ahead and hit through it. Don't pass up this chance. It might also be a great time to flick a ball at an opponent who has let their paddle drop down by their knees, lost their balance, or looks unready in any way. The idea here is that your shot will depend on what's going on in front of you, so keep your chin up. You shouldn't be whipping through a yellow light while checking your cellphone, so don't drop your chin down when you get a "yellow light" ball, either. You need to see what's in front of you!

>> **Green light: Chest and above.** Green means *Go!* Finally, you have the ball you've been building the point toward and hoping to receive — the beloved "green light" ball! This ball arrives at chest height or above, which means you can swing from high to low, sending the ball on a downward trajectory. This ball deserves to be punished — as long as you're in balance (nose over toes) and ready. You have earned this ball, so take it. Don't take a giant swing and overhit it, but be assertive and accurate, and have fun with it.

REMEMBER

If the ball is coming at you high in your green zone, it might actually be traveling out of bounds. Pay attention to the speed, trajectory, and spin of the ball. It takes some court time to develop your skill in accurately identifying "out" balls. If you never let any balls go past you, you'll never learn which ones were about to land out.

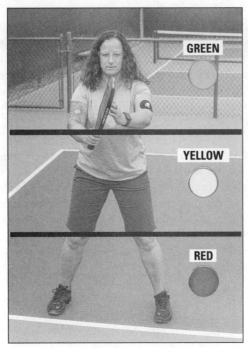

You might discover some similarities between your driving habits and your pickleball play. Yellow-light balls in particular can function as a bit of a personality test: Are you more apt to "punch it" through every yellow light, or do you play it safe and slow down every time? Feel free to be your unique self (we wouldn't love you any other way), but if you want to win more, try not to get tempted into overly risky choices. Dealing with red- and yellow-light balls with calm and patience will earn you plenty of green-light balls while also minimizing errors. Self-discipline is the most important skill when it comes to good shot selection.

Understanding time and space: Depth, angles, and moments of opportunity

A pickleball court is relatively small, but you still have a lot of choices of where to hit the ball. A lot of players focus too much on trying to blast the ball through their opponents and ignore the fact they are all standing in a rectangle with many other places to aim. If you aren't constantly looking for open court and angle opportunities, you're missing out on tons of points. Understanding time and space on a pickleball court is critical to good shot selection.

In many ways, pickleball is a game about depths. As we mention earlier in this chapter, there are times to hit deep shots (such as on serve and return), and times to hit shallow shots (third-shot drops and dinks). Where you want to hit next depends entirely on where your opponents are standing. If your opponent is deep in the court, you don't want to hit a midcourt ball that they can easily drive. On the other hand, if your opponents are both at the kitchen line, you want to hit a shallow, unattackable ball.

To hit angles, you need enough open court in front of your opponents. As best you can, keep them deep in the court for as long as possible by using deep serves, deep returns, and punch volleys that pin players back near the baseline. Keeping your opponents deep in the court opens up angles and gives you many more options. Meanwhile, your goal is to get your team to the line and shrink the amount of available court in front of you. The more acute you make the angles available for your opponent, the more difficult it is for them to hit them accurately. Make the needle harder to thread!

Another key tenet of good shot selection is to take time away from your opponent and buy yourself more time when needed. Ideally, you always want to hit the ball as early as possible so that your opponents will be less ready to deal with it. If you're in trouble, you might want to slow things down so that you have more time to recover. (Just know that whenever you give yourself more time, your opponents get to take advantage of those extra moments, too.)

Here are some ways to use timing to your advantage:

>> **Volley whenever possible.** Try to take balls out of the air as volleys rather than let them bounce. As you're waiting for the bounce, your opponents are busy recovering and getting in perfect court position.

>> **Use forward pressure.** While transitioning to the kitchen line, if you have to decide between stepping forward or stepping back, always choose forward. Not only will you be hitting the ball earlier on its flight path, you can also usually take it at a higher contact point.

>> **Attack the nearest opponent, resetting to the farthest.** When on offense, your goal is to overcome your opponent with surprise and speed, so hit the ball to the opponent closest to you. On defense, your goal is to buy yourself more time, so hit the ball to the opponent who is the farthest away.

>> **Take advantage of the Two-Bounce Rule.** Your serve return must bounce before your opponents are allowed to touch it. Knowing they can't volley it, you can hit a return that gives you plenty of time to arrive at the line in good balance. Sometimes you may not want to take time away from yourself by hitting a fast, low return that will come back before you're ready. If you struggle to get to the line quickly, hit a lofty, deep return to give you more time to get there safely.

TIP

Altering your frame of mind from the goal of "beating my opponents" to "placing the ball wherever I want" can help tremendously. No matter how good your opponents are, you'll always have open spots, angles, and moments of opportunity. Prevent your opponents from playing their best by consistently placing the ball in undesirable locations. (See more tips in this vein in Chapter 12.) Instead of making it about you versus them, make it about you versus the ball. Can you be the boss of the ball and consistently make it go where you want? Yes, you can!

Playing the odds: High-percentage pickleball

We all do it. We see a ball that we might be able to do something really dazzling with, and a titillating idea comes to mind. "I hit that sweet backhand drive down the sideline last week at 100 MPH, and it was glorious! I'll keep doing that as often as possible from now on!" Or maybe you've missed every single lob you've hit today, but you think that surely the odds have to tilt in your favor at some point. "I watched a pro player hit a tweener lob to the back corner in that video the other day; how hard could it be?"

This all sounds like a recipe for disaster. Was that the first time you've ever made that backhand drive go in? Have you ever successfully hit a tweener, let alone a tweener lob? Playing high-percentage pickleball means selecting shots that are more likely to be successful and less likely to result in an error: low risk, high reward. It doesn't mean your play has to be boring, scripted, or passive. You can still play around with many different shots and mix them up. Just be sure to pay attention to which ones are actually winning you points. (If you find these pointers a bit too much to process while playing, ask a friend to video or chart some of your matches; see the section in Chapter 16 about self-assessment tools.)

At beginner and intermediate levels, the majority of points are lost through unforced errors. You can quickly advance your overall skill level by learning how to avoid being the first person to make an error.

A number of shots are generally regarded as having a lower percentage of success for most players:

>> **Lobs from the baseline:** These must be struck almost perfectly so that they are higher than the players' reach but short enough to land in bounds. Lobbing from deep in the court means that your opponents have plenty of time to see the lob coming and get into position to smash it. We do not recommend this type of shot. Your partner probably doesn't, either.

» **Drives down the sideline:** Successfully hitting a ball very hard down a narrow lane is tough to do, even for advanced players.

» **Serving or returning to the actual baseline:** Although you definitely want to serve and return deep, don't attempt to aim precisely for the back line. You will likely miss as many as you make.

» **Attacking while off-balance:** You might be tempted to punish a green-light ball whenever you see one, but attacks struck while off-balance frequently go awry. You will also be even less ready if the shot gets counterattacked right back to you.

» **Overswinging on an overhead or volley:** Sure, it feels great to crush the ball with all your might, but too often these go straight into the net (or into the back fence).

» **"Dribbling" back over a dribbler:** You dove into the kitchen and managed to get a ball that barely dribbled over the net. It would seem natural to barely lift it straight back over the net, forcing your opponent to perform the same daring feat. However, this is an extremely difficult shot to pull off, and you're better off dinking it a bit harder crosscourt, over the lowest part of the net.

» **Fighting spin with spin.** When you see a player adding a lot of "junk" to the ball, you might attempt to either add to, or counter, this spin with your own. Doing so requires a high degree of precision and often results in a mis-hit. Instead, use a flat stroke with a tiny bit more lift than usual. Really hit *through* a heavily spun ball.

Of course, you have a lot of room for individuality in your choice of shots. The shots that you're comfortable with and know you can rely on are *your* high-percentage shots. With practice and determination, you can develop your lower-percentage shots into higher ones.

In general, some recommendations for high-percentage play include:

» **Aiming about a foot or two inside the lines:** This target gives you a nice margin of error while still utilizing most of the court.

» **Hitting over the lowest part of the net:** A pickleball net is 2 inches lower in the center than on the sides. If you're in a sticky situation, it can often be easier to hit over the middle of the net.

» **Resetting the point when you're stressed:** If you are out of position, off-balance, or not ready, hit an unattackable ball to your opponent and then use that time to recover. Try to stay in the point rather than finish it.

>> **Resisting the urge to attack from midcourt:** Unless the ball is a clear pop-up or high floater, focus on getting yourself to the line before trying to end the point. Most balls you encounter in the transition zone are too low to effectively attack, and you are too far away from your opponents to overcome them with speed.

>> **Hitting with only 60–70 percent of your full power:** There is really no reason to ever hit a pickleball with 100 percent of your might. "Precision over power" is the name of the game. For most players, the higher the miles per hour, the lower the chance of success.

Sometimes the percentages change based on your opponents. It's important to know their strengths and weaknesses as well. If I have crazy fast hands at the kitchen line, it won't be a very high-percentage behavior for you to try to flick a ball at my chest. If I flinch and squeal when someone flicks a ball at my chest, the percentages go way up for you. Look for your opponents' weaknesses and try to exploit them with your strengths.

TIP

A great tip for practicing good shot selection is to play at least one game per session with this thought in mind: "I am going to do only what is necessary to win the point. No more, no less." You'll probably start eliminating those big windups and flashy finishes. Play smart, high-percentage shots only. You'll eventually want to play this way more and more, because winning turns out to be very fun! Medals are heavy but they're good exercise for your neck.

When you feel ready to challenge yourself beyond this chapter's techniques and strategies, go to Chapter 12 for a deep dive on intermediate and advanced doubles play. Our recommendations aren't about achieving pickleball perfection, but rather learning new skills to improve your game. Always!

Chapter **12**

Diving Deeper: Intermediate to Advanced Doubles Strategies

After you have played pickleball for a while, you might notice that some opponents find ways to win points against you even though they aren't any more skilled at hitting the ball than you are. Is it because they have a more expensive paddle, or nicer shoes? Is your partner worse than you thought? Are they mind readers? No, they are just using strategies, targets, and plays that you haven't learned yet.

This chapter aims to help you gain the upper hand over your opponents by showing you how to control the action whenever possible. Some of these concepts may seem complex at first, but they are really just different ways of creating a hole to hit through, or forcing a pop-up from your opponent. These are just a few tried-and-true techniques that you can adapt to your own game. As you feel more confident, feel free to get creative and design your own! You might write the next great pickleball book.

Using Dinking Patterns

Using intentional patterns in dinking rallies is critical to your success as an intermediate or advanced pickleball player. A series of well-struck targets can create space for you to attack, or make your opponents hit off-balance, giving your team a nice pop-up to put away. If you're just dinking aimlessly, you aren't being offensive. Most likely, your opponents are busy executing their plan, and you've fallen right into their trap.

We hope that you've devoured Chapter 8, "Dinking: The Game within a Game," and committed it to memory. You have practiced and honed your dinks into beautiful works of art, hitting your targets precisely every time. No? That's okay; our dinks aren't always perfect either! This section can still help you.

Dinking patterns are specific combinations of dinking targets that can help force an error from your opponent. They aren't necessarily 20-shot patterns that need to be memorized like football plays. Rarely do our opponents stick to *our* plan long enough to finish executing a series that long. Rather, you're looking for opportunities that allow you to insert a specific combination of dinks, usually three to six shots at a time, into a rally (and repeat them as necessary).

Here are a few examples of smart dinking patterns created by fellow Evil Dinking Geniuses:

>> **Outside-Inside Isolation** (*Courtesy of Evil Dinking Genius Sarah Ansboury*): Hit two dinks deep (near the kitchen line) to the outside edge of the court, and then dink once to that same player's inside foot (the foot closest to the centerline). Next, dink a shorter ball to the outside edge of the court with backspin, and then dink deep to the middle again, followed by a topspin dink to the outside edge of the court. If your opponent is teetering off-balance, gradually moving out of position, or appearing stressed, you know it's working. (See Figure 12-1 for the Outside-Inside Isolation pattern.) Keep repeating the pattern until your opponent does something desperate and makes an error, such as attempting to attack a low inside ball simply because it's a forehand and they're tired of moving back and forth. You'll be waiting there in the middle to pounce on it!

>> **Pop-up Generator** (*Courtesy of Evil Dinking Genius Robyn Penwell*): When dinking to a right-handed player who is in the odd court, hit your first shot shallow and close to your opponent's inside foot. The next dink will be slightly deeper, between their feet. The third dink should be slightly deeper again but to their outside foot. (Figure 12-2 shows this pattern.) Try to make these changes subtle enough that your opponent stays rooted in place, allowing themselves to become flat-footed by the second or third dink. Finally, hit a

fourth dink that is behind their left foot. As they reach for the backhand, their weight will go back into their heels and their back will be pointed toward the court. The path of least resistance for them will be to dink straight up the line, but because their weight is falling backward, they will unintentionally lift the ball — right up to your partner, for an easy put-away!

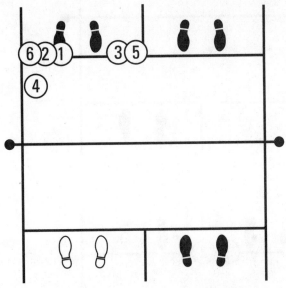

FIGURE 12-1:
The Outside-Inside Isolation pattern causes stress for your opponent.

>> **The Erne Setup** (*Courtesy of Evil Dinking Genius Morgan Evans*)**:** To set up a fun Erne opportunity for yourself (see Chapter 14 if you don't know what an Erne is), start by dinking one or more balls toward the middle of the court. Wait for the opponent straight across from you to leave their home position or shift their weight too far in toward the middle. Steal time away from them by taking the next ball out of the air and dinking it out wide, toward that same player's sideline. Immediately move over to get in position for the Erne. More than likely, they won't be able to cut the ball at a steep enough angle to avoid your waiting paddle. Figure 12-3 shows the Erne Setup.

WARNING

Be careful not to overcommit to any pattern you had in mind. Remember, the three other people on the court may not be cooperating with your genius plan. If you find yourself off–balance or out of position, stop the pattern and get back to a neutral state before attempting to become offensive again. You'll need to pivot to a new plan or manipulate the situation so that you can return to the original pattern.

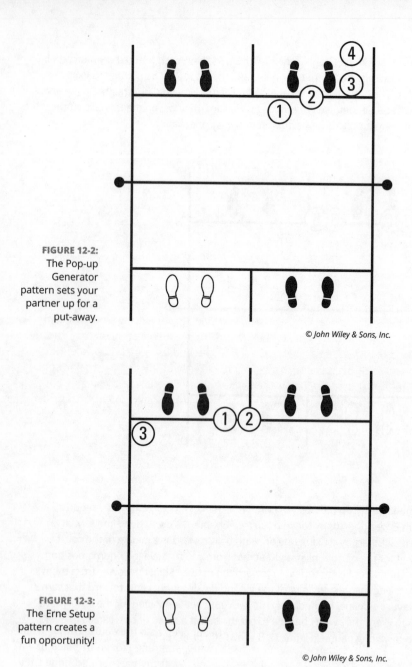

FIGURE 12-2:
The Pop-up Generator pattern sets your partner up for a put-away.

© John Wiley & Sons, Inc.

FIGURE 12-3:
The Erne Setup pattern creates a fun opportunity!

© John Wiley & Sons, Inc.

Sometimes a dinking pattern is completely spontaneous: You make it up as you go along. The main goal is to never let your opponent get into a dinking rhythm. Keep your opponent moving as much as possible. Move them left, right, forward, and back. Dinking is hard enough standing still, so forcing your opponent to dink while on the move makes it even more difficult for them. Adding different spins to the ball forces them to deal with a ball that is accelerating (topspin), decelerating (backspin), or jumping to the right or left (sidespin) after it bounces. That is a lot for an opponent to cope with. Remember, they might have a dinking pattern in mind, too, so do whatever you can to disrupt it.

Keep track of what types of dinks your opponents struggle with the most and include those shots frequently in your patterns.

If you're able to keep the ball low, be sure to put plenty of extra pressure on your opponents by dinking deep, toward the kitchen line. It has to be low because you don't want your opponent to be able to easily reach forward and attack the ball. Aiming low is especially important when playing against tall players with albatross-like wingspans.

A lot of dinking rallies end up with two players dinking to each other crosscourt. If you're one of these players and want your partner to get more involved in the rally, try changing it up by hitting to the middle or straight across the net. A middle ball is most likely to come back to the middle, which allows either you or your partner to hit next. Hitting straight across will likely inspire your opponent to hit crosscourt to your partner; just be very careful not to hit this ball too close to the sideline, or too high. Either of these shots often results in your team's being on the losing side of a forehand attack or an Erne.

Try to be the calm, patient dinker with a plan. Be ready to hit 30 or more dinks in an advanced-level pickleball rally. Be the one who can last all day and waits for their moment to speed up the ball. Patience really does win points in pickleball. Build the point. Watch for your moment. When it arrives, take it. Don't speed up the ball just because you're bored with dinking. Keep dinking and allow the pressure in the point to build. This is exciting! Never boring.

Retrieving Lobs Successfully

Drat! My opponent just sent a lob over my head, deep into the court. Hmm, what to do? I know . . . I'll panic and yell "YOU!" while standing frozen in place like a statue. After we lose the point, I'll shrug sheepishly at my partner and hope they find it endearing.

If this scenario is hitting a little too close to home, you should probably consider finding out a bit more about dealing with lobs. You have a couple of different ways to do it. You and your partner need to consider your strengths and weaknesses and agree on what will work best for your team. This is best done *before* the first lob comes your way!

Safety is the top priority. No ball is worth getting injured over. If you can't retrieve a lob safely, just say "nice shot" and move on.

If only one player in your partnership has good mobility, you may choose to assign all lob retrieval to that one person. That person may wind up using both of the methods (straight-on and diagonal lob retrieval, described in the upcoming sections) in order to cover their own side of the court as well as their partner's side. That's a totally valid option. Just be sure to sort that out before the game starts.

No matter how your team decides to handle lob retrieval, the first order of business is to call the ball, loudly and clearly: "Mine!" or "Yours!" Calling the ball minimizes the confusion and chaos that is often created by a lob. Next, you need to quickly assess whether to take this ball as an overhead smash rather than let it bounce. If you think you can reach the ball in the air by drop-stepping and shuffling back one or two steps, an overhead is the much better play. If attempting to smash requires any amount of hasty backpedaling, don't do it!

As mentioned previously, the two main approaches to lob retrieval are the straight-on and the diagonal retrievals. We take a look at these two methods next.

Straight-on lob retrieval

In the straight-on lob retrieval, the player closest to the ball will be the one to retrieve it. As you see the ball going over your head, immediately open the front of your body toward it, like a door opening on a hinge. So, if the ball is going up over your right shoulder, quickly turn on your left foot (the hinge) and step back with your right foot. You should now be sideways to the net with your right toes pointing in the direction of the ball. The next step is a pivot step: Your left leg crosses over your right and your left toes also point toward the ball. Now you can take off running!

If the ball goes over your left shoulder, do the opposite: Hinge on the right foot, step back with the left, and cross over with the right. If the ball is going directly over your head, you need to make a choice. It's easiest if you opt to turn toward your paddle side, which sets you up to hit with your forehand (assuming that's your preferred shot).

That initial step and pivot are very important. If your first step is aggressive and quick, and you point your toes in the correct direction, you'll have more time to get to the ball. If you stumble around, taking extra steps before you even get out of the blocks, you'll have to really hustle.

WARNING

Please do not rock back on your heels as the ball goes over your head. If you do, definitely yell "You!" and have your partner run back for it. If you're on your heels, there's no way you're getting that ball in time. Please, don't ever backpedal to get the ball. Running backward leads to hard landings and bruising your butt, your noggin, and certainly your pride. Coauthor Carl ripped his favorite pair of bell bottoms as a result of backpedaling.

As you're running back for the ball, your partner should be retreating a few steps back in the court as well. You don't want to end up with too much space between you. Your partner should adopt a more defensive stance (getting a bit low, with paddle out in front) in case your shot ends up being attacked.

Diagonal lob retrieval

The diagonal lob-retrieval method sends the player who is on the opposite side of the court to get the lob. If the ball is going straight over your partner's head, you should run diagonally behind them to get it. If it's straight over your head, your partner should get it. The same aggressive footwork you use in the straight-on method described in the preceding section still applies here. Open your hips toward the ball and point your toes in the direction you want to run. You have to turn and push off quickly to get there. There is no time for hesitation. Call it ("Mine!") and go!

The diagonal lob-retrieval method has some pros and cons. It's easier for you to track a ball that's going over your partner's head than it is for them. You can quickly assess where the ball is going to bounce and position yourself correctly to hit it. This method's main disadvantage is that the retrieving player has to take more steps to get to the ball because they have a longer distance to travel.

TIP

Don't run directly at (or under) the ball when retrieving a lob. You need to get behind it so that you have space to hit through the ball, with a forward weight shift. Your path will look a bit like a question mark or an upside-down J. If you run in a straight line, your back will still be to the court when you arrive at the ball. The only shots you can possibly hit are a between-the-legs "tweener" or an over-the-shoulder "shovel" shot.

As you're running back for the lob, your partner should keep an eye on the situation and call "switch" if you've completely crossed over to your partner's side of the court. If the ball is more toward the middle, your partner might tell you to stay, indicating that you should return to cover your original side of the court. It's a good idea for your partner to move back deeper in the court so that you don't have a giant gap between you. Your partner should get their paddle up and be extra ready in case the next ball comes back hard.

Hitting a lob recovery shot

Now that you've successfully arrived behind the ball, what shot should you hit? If you're off-balance, late, or otherwise in a bad way, just keep the ball in play any way that you can. Ideally, though, what you want to hit is a quality drop shot. That way, your opponents cannot attack the ball, and you and your partner can work your way back up to the line again. Hitting a good drop shot off a lob isn't easy and will take plenty of practice. Even if you don't end up eventually winning the rally, if you manage to hit a good drop off a lob, you should feel proud of yourself!

Don't go too big on your shot and try to drive the ball hard, or hit an angled winner. You're under duress, so just aim for an unattackable ball toward the middle of the court, reducing your chance of hitting it wide. Recognize that your team is now on defense because you're deep in the court and your opponents are (presumably) still up at the kitchen line. The most important goal is to buy yourself time to recover from the chaotic situation you and your partner just dealt with. You can buy time by making sure your next shot is unattackable.

Some players choose to respond to an offensive lob with a defensive lob. In some situations, this can seem helpful because it buys your team a lot of extra time. However, this is statistically a very low-percentage shot. More often than not, the return lob is poorly executed and ends up getting smashed back. Return a lob with a lob only if you are especially good at them (and if perhaps your opponents are both under five feet tall) — or if it truly is your only "Hail Mary" option.

Practicing an ounce of prevention

If the methods described in the previous sections for dealing with lobs just seems like way too much work (we're exhausted just writing about it), why not try preventing players from lobbing you in the first place? Nobody enjoys being lobbed, not to mention it sends your team back to the baseline when you'd rather be up at the kitchen line. You might be in the middle of working one of the awesome dinking patterns from earlier in this chapter when suddenly your opponent decides to ruin the whole thing by sending up a lob. No fun!

Fortunately, you have a few ways to try to reduce the number of lobs you're forced to deal with. As the old saying goes, an ounce of prevention is worth a pound of cure.

Try the following tips to prevent your opponents from sending lobs:

>> **Dink deep.** Avoid shallow dinks that are easy to get under and lob from. It's very difficult for your opponent to hit a lob off a dink that is bouncing at their

feet. The easiest balls to lob are the ones that land mid-kitchen, where you can step in with one foot and use your knees to lift the ball into the air.

>> **Stay on the balls of your feet.** Letting your weight rest back and into your heels will cause you to be very slow. You're signaling to more observant players that you're not ready to turn and run after a lob. Bending over at the waist or adopting too wide of a stance are common causes of improper weight distribution.

>> **Stand tall.** No matter what your actual height is, try to look as tall as you possibly can. Smart opponents know that lobbing over a tall player is a risky move. By bending over or crouching down, you're clearing tons of air space for your opponent's lob to travel through.

>> **Keep your paddle up.** Don't let your paddle drop between shots. A dropped paddle makes punishing a weak lob with an overhead smash nearly impossible. If your paddle is hanging down by your knees, by the time you raise it up over your head, you'll be too late. The more lobs you punish with overheads, the fewer your opponents will keep hitting.

Going Hunting: Drop and Hunt

There are many great plays to set up in a pickleball point. Drop and Hunt is one of our favorites, and we hope you have fun with it, too. This play outlines a specific method for the serving team to transition to the kitchen line that's a little more offensive than the traditional method (which we describe in Chapter 11).

As you may have guessed, this play begins with a third-shot drop. (See Chapter 7 for our tips on how to execute a great drop shot.) For the Drop and Hunt play, you hit your drops crosscourt. Doing so puts the ball in front of your partner and increases the likelihood that it will come back crosscourt, through the middle.

REMEMBER

It's always easier for players to send the ball back from whence it came, rather than change the direction of the ball. Use this knowledge to help predict where your opponents will hit next.

The partner not hitting the drop shot needs to get into the mindset of a hunter. Picture Elmer Fudd carefully stalking his prey: "It's wabbit season!" Okay, maybe that's not the best visual for pickleball. How about something slightly cooler: Jennifer Lawrence in *Hunger Games*, armed with her bow and arrow. No? Okay, fine, just picture *yourself*, armed with your paddle and nondominant hand out in front of you, stalking *your* prey, which in this case is an attackable pickleball.

Every good hunting team needs a plan. Follow these steps to put the Drop and Hunt play into action:

1. **Serve the ball to your opponents.**

2. **Watch where the return goes and prepare for the next shot:**

    a. **The partner who is in the best position to hit the next shot will prepare to be the "dropper."**

    b. **The other partner (the "hunter") takes a few steps forward into the court.**

    This positioning creates a slight stagger, with one player standing a little bit forward of the other. (See Chapter 11 for more on staggering.)

3. **The dropper hits a beautiful crosscourt drop (see Figure 12-4, top).**

4. **As the dropper swings, the hunter watches carefully in order to determine as quickly as possible whether the drop is a good one.**

    If the drop isn't quite as stunning as your team had hoped (say, it popped up too high and will probably come back hard), the hunter retreats back near the baseline. If the drop looks good, the hunter continues striding forward with slow, measured, steps.

    The hunter is now poised to pounce on any middle ball that comes back too high.

5. **POW! The hunter pounces with a poach volley (see Figure 12-4, bottom).**

    If your team doesn't get an attackable ball, no worries. The dropper should be joining the hunter at the kitchen and continuing with the rally. Even if your team doesn't get the reward you were hoping for, you've still applied plenty of forward pressure on your opponents. Just the visual of your team walking into the line with your paddles up, super focused, may intimidate your opponents enough to throw off their next shot.

This play works only if the player who didn't hit the drop shot starts slowly moving forward first. This player positioning creates the space needed to poach across the middle, if necessary. It also clears up any confusion about who is taking the middle. You can't poach if you're both exactly even with each other. That results in awkward collisions and certainly won't win you any rallies.

The traditional way of transitioning to the line can feel a little defensive. You are carefully hitting drops, inching together toward the kitchen, praying that you don't make a mistake. The receiving team knows they have the upper hand based on their starting positions (one up and one back). This confidence can sometimes lead to a lazy fourth shot that they hit without much thought. These are the shots you're hunting for, and you can catch many opponents off guard because they aren't used to worrying about two opponents who aren't yet at the line.

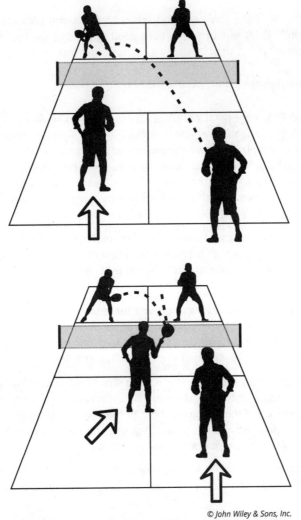

FIGURE 12-4: In the Drop and Hunt play, the dropper sends a drop shot (top) and then the hunter finishes off the opponent's fourth shot (bottom).

Go out and try this play and have some fun with it. Explain it to your partner and ask them to hit crosscourt drops if the serve return goes to them. Then, go hunting!

Shaking It Up with Shake 'N' Bake

Another very fun play you can try is called the Shake 'N' Bake. (Is anyone else suddenly craving 1960s chicken?) This play begins when one partner hits a hard drive (often as a third shot) with the goal of eliciting a pop-up. Meanwhile, their partner hurries in toward the kitchen line in the hope of putting the pop-up away.

The Shake 'N' Bake can be a high-risk, high-reward play, depending on your team's skill set. If one of you is very good at driving the ball and one of you is quick-footed with a strong put-away, this recipe was made for you!

Here's how to set up and execute the Shake 'N' Bake:

- » Either before the game or before your team serves, make a plan with your partner. Decide whether one or both of you has a strong enough drive to attempt the play. You can also pick out which opponent you think the drive should be directed to. This might be a receiver who is slow to come in to join their partner at the kitchen line. It's especially difficult for a player who is still moving forward to deal with a drive coming at them. Or, it might be to the player already at the net, if you feel that the player's blocking abilities are weak.

- » When the return comes back, assess whether this is a good ball to drive. If the return is very deep, it's probably best to just hit a drop shot instead. If the return is short, go ahead and "shake" things up by driving it hard and low at your chosen target.

- » Your partner should be watching where the return lands and reading your body language to see whether you're about to drive it. You can also verbally communicate your intentions by saying something like "Go!" if you're about to drive. This tells your partner to go ahead and charge the net.

- » As you're hitting the drive, your partner should rush in and take position at the kitchen line, slightly toward the middle of the court. Your partner should be ready to "bake" the ball by watching for the pop-up and putting it away. Doing so often involves a poach, so watch closely and switch sides behind them if necessary. (Be sure to call out "Switch!" if you do change sides.)

- » Both players should finish the Shake 'N' Bake by getting into good position, ready for the next shot, just in case the "baked" ball comes back.

TIP

"Shake 'N' Bake" is slang for anytime one partner hits a hard drive that is popped up and then put away. You can even hit both the "shake" and the "bake" yourself if the pop-up happens to come back your way. After driving the ball, be ready to pounce on a pop-up that your partner can't reach.

If you're playing against a team who likes to Shake 'N' Bake, here are a few ways to defend against it:

- » **Hit deep returns.** The easiest ball to drive is a short, high-bouncing return. Pay extra attention to the depth of your returns if you find yourself on the receiving end of a lot of hard drives.

» **Direct your returns to the opponent with the weaker drive.** It usually doesn't take long in a match to figure out which opponent favors their third-shot drives over their drops. If one of your opponents has an amazing forehand drive, keep the return away from their forehand!

» **Get all the way to the line.** You may need to hustle just a bit more, or hit a loftier deep return, to ensure that you get all the way to the line before the ball comes back to your side of the court. You are much less likely to pop up the ball on your fourth shot if your feet are set and you're in a balanced ready position.

» **Stop stacking.** If your team has been stacking on the receiving side and getting repeatedly burned by your opponent's third-shot drives, you might need to consider stacking only on serve. When in a full stack, the service receiver must run very fast diagonally to get to their position at the line. Also, while crossing behind your partner, you can visually lose track of the ball for a moment, which makes you very vulnerable to a hard drive. See the next section for more on stacking.

» **Plan your fourth shot.** If you know that the third shot is probably going to come at you hard, have a plan already in mind for your fourth shot. The best shot would be a soft drop volley into the kitchen, which prevents the "baker" from having anything to attack. Obviously, this type of shot is easier said than done. You may not be able to successfully reset the ball, but you can at least try to angle your block far away from the player who is charging toward you.

Stacking and Switching

Chapter 2 tells you the rules of serving and receiving, as well as the typical player starting positions. Based on the current score, there is always one correct server and one correct receiver. The serve must also be struck from the correct side of the court (right or left) and land in the diagonal service box. If you just served the ball and your team wins the point, you switch places with your partner and serve from the other side.

If you've ever observed pro matches or other advanced play, you might have witnessed something strange. Rather than lining up in the traditional starting positions (one partner standing on each half of the court), some teams line up with both players on the same side. Or they line up in a seemingly normal way, only to suddenly rearrange themselves into a new configuration after the serve. It's quite mesmerizing to watch them crisscross and dart about, like a halftime show featuring a four-person marching band. What is going on here? Is this tomfoolery even legal?

When two players line up on the same side of the court rather than in the traditional starting positions, it's known as *stacking,* in which both players are "stacked" up next to each other. The designated server and receiver line up in their usual positions. The server's partner stands right next to the server, but on the opposite side of where that partner would normally stand. After the ball is served, the server shifts over to the other side of the court and the partner slides into the spot just vacated. For the receiving team, the partner who is up at the line stands outside the court on the same side as the receiver. After hitting the return of serve, the receiver runs diagonally up to the kitchen line on the opposite side of the court. Figure 12-5 illustrates what these positions look like.

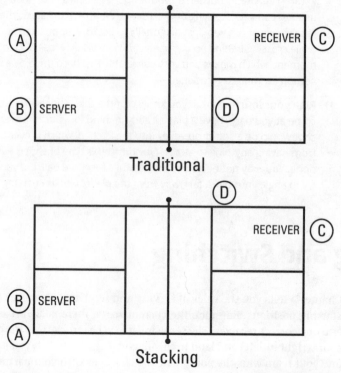

Traditional

Stacking

© John Wiley & Sons, Inc.

FIGURE 12-5: Traditional starting positions versus two teams that are stacking.

So what's the point of all this crazy choreography? Stacking helps teams "stack the deck" in their favor by allowing each partner to spend more time on their preferred side of the court. You might find that you can win more points when you're on the right and your partner is on the left. You can start the game this way, but as soon as you win a point, you are forced to switch places. Boo! After you win a second point, you're back where you want to be — yay! Until you win another point . . . drat! And so on. With traditional court positioning, if you haven't won a point in a while, you can get stuck playing most of the game on your "bad" side. Stacking lets you play in the same position every rally, no matter the current score.

In case you're still wondering, yes — it's all perfectly legal. No rule says that players must stay on any particular side of the court during a rally. They just have to make sure that when the next point starts, the correct players are serving and receiving from the correct sides.

REMEMBER

Only the server's starting position is restricted by the rules. The server must be standing behind the baseline, on the correct side, and between the imaginary extensions of the sideline and centerline. The other three players on the court may legally stand anywhere they want on their team's side of the net.

Stacking has many benefits as well as some disadvantages. You can choose to stack only in certain situations, and in a few different ways, depending on your team's strengths and weaknesses. We cover all these points in the upcoming sections.

Choosing your types of stacking

Stacking doesn't have to be an all-or-nothing deal. You can start and stop stacking as often as you like throughout a match. You can choose to stack only when your team is serving, or only when receiving. Here are some of the different methods you can try:

>> **Full stack:** In a full stack, your team is stacking on both serve and return — 100 percent of the time. Ideally, you'll have two mobile players and at least one partner who is good at keeping track of the score to pull off this method.

>> **Half stack:** A half stack means your team is stacking only on serve. Stacking on serve requires a lot less running (and, most people would agree, less thinking) than stacking on both serve and receive. So if you're just getting the hang of stacking, you might want to start out with a half stack. Pro tip: The "half stack" is also a more sensible choice when ordering pancakes. Let's face it: Pancakes are carb heavy and often followed by regrets.

>> **Three-quarters stack:** This style is less common but is a great option if one player has mobility issues. With a three-quarters stack, you always stack on serve but only half the time on return, depending on who is receiving serve. The player receiving serve needs to really hustle to get up to the line. If one of you is struggling to make it quickly enough, don't worry about stacking or switching when that person is returning serve. Just play the point the "normal" way.

You might also try a few fun variations on traditional stacking:

>> **Shadow Shift on Serve:** This is a fun, deceptive strategy created by Tony Roig from the In2Pickle YouTube Channel. When your team is stacking on serve, have the nonserving partner stand directly behind the server (as if that partner were the server's shadow). Be sure to allow enough room for the server to hit so no one takes a paddle to the face. After the ball is served, as your opponent sets up to hit the return, the shadow player quietly tells their partner whether to go right or left. Your opponents will have no idea which player is going where. If one player has been repeatedly isolated because of a weak third shot, this strategy prevents the opponents from targeting that player with all their returns. Sneaky!

>> **Switch on Receive:** This method is an alternative way for the receiving team to line up before swapping places as they would in a regular stack. Rather than standing outside the court on the same side as the receiver, the kitchen-line player stands in their normal position but quickly slides over after the return is hit. This version of stacking is becoming increasingly favored over the traditional "off the court" starting position because it allows the forward player to cover the middle of the court while the receiver is on their way up to the line. Visually, the court looks much less open than if the kitchen-line player is standing out of bounds. This method also opens up the possibility of concealing from your opponents whether you plan to switch; you achieve this concealment through the use of hand signals. (We explain more about these signals in the later section "Using hand signals.")

Knowing the pros and cons of stacking

Many people think of the stacking-and-switching technique as being strictly for advanced players to use. However, after you get the hang of it, it's really no more complicated than using the traditional positioning. Stacking can benefit many teams in a variety of situations. Here are the most common reasons players choose to stack:

>> **Opposite-handed players:** The most common reason for stacking is when a right-handed player teams up with a left-handed player. By stacking so that the left-handed player is always on the right and the right-handed player on the left, you've now positioned both forehands up the middle. This makes the middle a very dangerous place for your opponents to hit to!

>> **Highlighting strengths:** If one of you has a particularly great forehand or backhand, you can stack to always feature that shot in the middle court. Or, if one of you is an amazing backhand crosscourt dinker, you might want to position that player so that their backhand is toward the sideline.

>> **Difference in skill level:** If one partner is playing at a significantly higher skill level than the other, you might want to position the stronger player so that their forehand is always in the middle, allowing them to cover more court and a higher percentage of balls. If your opponents have clued into your skill gap and are attempting to isolate the weaker player, this strategy can help the stronger player get more involved.

>> **Poaching abilities:** If you are better at recognizing and seizing poaching opportunities than your partner, you might want to position your preferred attack shot (forehand or backhand) up the middle so that you can take advantage of high middle balls.

>> **Mastery of one position:** Like baseball players who spend their career perfecting their chosen positions, you and your long-term partner might opt to each choose a side and become expert at it. You would then have to deal with only 50 percent of the possible situations your team might encounter. This approach can really help your team develop your "pickleball telepathy" — the ability to predict exactly what your partner is going to do without verbal communication. Silent, but deadly!

Stacking has some potential pitfalls, so it's not necessarily the best choice for every team; otherwise, the traditional starting positions would not be what they are. It's important to evaluate both the pros and cons as you decide whether these strategies are right for you.

Consider the following drawbacks when deciding to stack:

>> **More mental stress:** Stacking requires additional brainpower to remember where you're supposed to be at all times. You can easily get confused as to who is supposed to be serving or receiving, and from what side. Even the pros get mixed up and frequently ask the referee, "Am I the correct server on the correct side?" Having the wrong player serve or receive causes an automatic fault, and your team loses the rally. That is definitely not the way you want to give up points. If you're feeling mentally tired or struggling to keep track of things, you might want to limit your stacking or save it for another day. Your primary focus should always be on playing well and winning points, not trying to keep track of the score and your stack.

>> **More physical stress:** When stacking on the receiving side, the player who hits the return will need to run diagonally up to the kitchen line rather than walk in straight ahead. It's a longer distance to travel, so you need to really hustle to get there before the ball comes back. This can become very tiring over the course of many matches. If you have mobility issues or are running out of energy, stacking on your return may not be for you. You can still use the half or three-quarters stack, though.

>> **Higher-stakes returns:** During those moments after you hit your return and are running diagonally to the kitchen line, you'll leave a giant hole on one side of the court with nobody covering it. Given the opportunity, your opponents can easily drive their third shot down the line for a winner. You'll need to put some careful thought into your return and make sure it's a great one. The safest return to hit while stacking is either straight ahead (putting the ball in front of your partner) or to the middle of the court (reducing the number of available angles). It's imperative to hit your returns deep, not only to make the drive less tempting but also to give yourself more precious time to get to the line.

>> **Getting served out wide:** If you're receiving a serve and get pulled out wide, you have a very tough time getting all the way over to the other side of the court after you hit your return. When you're the player in front and you see this happening to your partner, yell "Stay!" and quickly move over to the other half of the court. Doing so lets your partner know they're off the hook for running diagonally into position. (Be sure to keep this in mind when you are playing against a team that is stacking. Being able to target your serves in ways that cause stress to the stacking team is very helpful.)

>> **Blind spots:** Any time you are crisscrossing behind your partner, you create the potential for momentary blind spots that cause you to visually lose track of the ball. Smart opponents will know how to exploit this. Pay attention to whether this is negatively affecting your game, and change your method of stacking if necessary.

>> **Middle confusion:** If a righty and lefty are stacking so that both of their strong forehands are in the middle, you become less clear on who should take the middle balls. Be sure to call the ball — "Me!" or "You!" — to avoid a collision. Before you play together, review Chapter 11 and discuss middle coverage strategies with your partner to make sure you're on the same page.

The best way to know whether stacking will benefit your team is to try it! Experiment with a few different methods of stacking, trying both sides of the court, and see how it goes. Don't try it for the first time on tournament day. Stacking needs to be practiced many times before you can rely on it, especially in a high-nerves situation. Keep in mind that your success depends a lot on your opponents. What works during one match may not work in another. Be ready to adjust your stacking plan, and don't get too stuck in your ways, especially if it's not helping you win games.

Using hand signals

When it comes to stacking or switching, you'll often find it smart to reassess your strategy before every point. Depending on the situation, staying on your assigned side may be better than switching. For example, you might want to choose your position based on the current positions of your opponents. Say you've noticed that every time you engage in a crosscourt dink battle with a certain player, you win the rally. You might choose to either switch or not switch with your partner so that you will always end up diagonally from that opponent. Or perhaps you've been stacking the entire game and the score is currently 0–9. Yikes! Time to try something else. Sometimes just giving your opponents something different to deal with for a few points will disrupt their rhythm and force them to come up with new strategies.

When using the "Switch on Receive" stacking method described in the "Choosing your types of stacking" section, earlier in this chapter, you have the option of deciding whether to switch or stay on each point. Pickleballers use hand signals to communicate the plan to their partner while hiding it from their opponents. Who doesn't love a secret plan? The receiver's partner, who is standing in their normal position at the kitchen line, will display one of the following signals behind their back (see Figure 12-6), making sure that only their partner can see it:

>> **Closed fist:** "Stay on your side."

>> **Open palm:** "Switch sides with me."

>> **Flashing between open and closed:** "I'm going to fake." This signal means that the front player intends to take a step or two over, as if they were switching, but then quickly return to their side. This fake-out is meant to trick the opponent into hitting the ball right to them, thinking that the space was going to be left vacant while the switch was occurring. Time to break out your devilish grin!

After one partner displays the hand signal, the partner in back must verbally acknowledge that they have seen, and accept, the signal. That partner can say something like "got it," "yep," or "yessiree Bob" to affirm. If they don't like the play that was called for some reason, they can say "no," and both partners should plan on doing the opposite of what that signal conveyed. If your partner doesn't say anything, you have to assume they didn't see your signal. At that point, it's probably best to call out "switch!" or "stay!" after the rally starts, to avoid confusion.

TIP

If you're using hand signals, make sure you continue to use them on every play, not just when you want to switch. Your opponents are smart enough to catch on if they see you put your hand behind your back only when you are planning to switch.

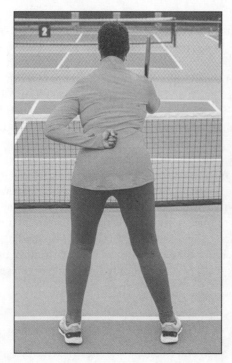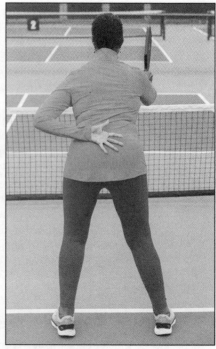

FIGURE 12-6:
The hand signals for stay (left) and switch (right).

KEEPING TRACK OF YOUR STACK

When you first learn to play pickleball, it takes some mental effort to figure out where you and your partner are supposed to be standing at the start of each point. After a couple of play sessions, you notice it becoming easier. Soon enough, you find yourself automatically standing in the right place. It isn't something you have to think about; your body just does it! Remember this feeling when you're learning stacking. It might seem confusing at first, but it will eventually become just as natural.

As you're practicing this new skill, here are a few tricks to help you keep track of your stack:

- **Position yourself in relation to your partner.** Rather than trying to memorize different configurations, just look for your partner. If you're stacking on the left side, you should always be on the left side of your partner. You should only ever see the left side of their face. Just for fun, pretend they have an embarrassing tattoo on the right side of their face that they don't want you to see ("No Regerts!"). If you ever find yourself lining up on the right side of your partner, you'll instantly know you are in the wrong place.

- **When your score is even, things are normal.** When the game started, the score was zero (an even number) and you were (presumably) standing on your preferred side. You switched places after you won a point, and then switched back when you won a second point (an even number again). Whenever your team's score is even, you should be back on the "good" side. You don't need to stack whenever your score is even. You just play it like a regular point.

- **When your score is odd, things get odd.** Whenever your team's score is an odd number, that's when things get weird — meaning that it's time to stack. Normally, after scoring one point (an odd number), you'd be standing on the opposite side from which you started the game: your "bad" side. Instead of playing out the point from there, you're going to stack and slide back over to your "good" side. Whenever your team's score is odd, that's when you have to remember to put your stacking into action.

Stacking is not as hard as it may seem. You've got this! Just don't overthink it. Practice stacking the way you would any other pickleball skill and you'll pick it up in no time.

Beating Those Bangers

The term *banger* refers to a player who hits everything hard. Nothing is wrong with hitting the ball hard; in fact, it's an important part of the game. But every rally includes times you should hit softly and times you should hit hard. A banger either doesn't know or doesn't care about using good strategy, relying instead on brute force. This brutal tactic often works up to a point, but they will never get past the intermediate level using this approach.

So how do you deal with bangers? This is one of the most common topics on pickleball social media and is often asked about in pickleball lessons. It's a huge source of frustration among intermediate players. They say, "We never get to dink because the ball is always zinging around the court at 100 miles per hour." It's always fun to watch the light bulbs go on over our students' heads when we make a few suggestions about how to turn things around in their favor.

Here are some tips for defeating bangers:

>> **Keep it low and slow.** The best way to beat a banger is by not being one. Bangers want a high ball that they can hit down on — so don't give them any! A slow ball that is dropping at their feet doesn't give them the opportunity to smack it back down your throat. If all you hit to them are drops and dinks, their attempts to attack will result in the ball going into the net or sailing way out of bounds.

» **Keep it out of the middle.** Bangers live in the middle. They want high-floating middle balls right in their strike zone that they can drive into oblivion. Aim your shots more to the outside of the court, using plenty of angles. It will be more difficult for bangers to drive a ball while they are on the move, as opposed to just planting themselves right in the middle of the court and teeing off on it.

» **Hit lofty, deep returns of serve.** Bangers want a shorter ball that they can drive and then move in behind. Hit them a return that keeps them deep in the court, hitting off their back foot, using mostly their shoulder. This type of return also gives you plenty of time to get up to the kitchen line. You'll have a much easier time blocking a ball above your waist while standing at the line, as opposed to digging one at your feet in the transition zone. If you're at the line and they're still back in the court, you have many more options than they do for the next shot.

» **Don't get hypnotized into playing their game.** Banging begets more banging. It's their game, not yours, so they're much better at it than you. Don't get sucked into their game! Hit unattackable balls and reset the pace of the rally. Turn it into your game. Play the soft game and invite them to try it. You'll surely come out on top.

» **Be ready to let their shots go out.** Lots of bangers hit balls that would go out if you didn't intercept them. So practice letting "out balls" go out. Never hit "out balls" in warm-up or drill sessions. You're inadvertently practicing losing points. Drill with a friend by having one of you hit very hard while the other tries to call the ball in or out as early as possible. Watch for the tells — subtle clues of what's to come. If the player is outstretched, on the run, or taking a huge windup, those may be indicators that their shot is likely to go out. It is fine to let a ball go and be wrong once in a while. Test your opponent's shots early in the match. Do they hit hard, but with enough topspin so that the ball lands in? Or are most of their hard shots heading for the gas station across the street? This early test will help you to intelligently play the odds for the rest of the match.

» **Take responsibility.** Don't just blame bangers for doing what they enjoy most. If it's working, why would they stop? If you are dishing up their favorite balls to bang, you are essentially feeding the beast. Instead, hit shots that take them out of their comfort zone (such as angles, lobs, drop shots, dinks, and so on). Put the beast on a restricted diet! See "Making Things Awkward," later in this chapter, for more ideas on how to take players out of their comfort zone.

These tips sound easy enough, right? It won't feel easy until you learn good paddle control. You have to be able to take pace off the ball and hit reset shots that change the rhythm of the rally. Gaining these skills takes a lot of practice! When fielding hard shots, relax your body as best you can. Grip your paddle lightly and try to absorb power off of an incoming ball, as if you were about to catch a water balloon. Hit a soft drop volley near the kitchen that will be impossible for the banger to attack. (See Chapter 9 for tips on executing this important shot.) Changing up the pace and beating bangers is very satisfying. You will look calm, cool, and collected, while they'll look sweaty and frustrated.

TIP

Find someone who is a good player but doesn't like you very much. Don your eye protection and ask them to hit really hard shots right at you while you're standing at the kitchen line. They'll be delighted at this request! Meanwhile, you'll get in some great practice on absorbing power and resetting the ball.

Making Things Awkward

Most of us understand what it's like to feel awkward at a stuffy dinner party or business function where you don't know anyone. Some of us have even embraced the fact we feel socially awkward every time we leave the house —and there are more of us than you might think! If you can relate, that's okay, because now is your chance to turn the tables. It's a strategy we like to call Make It Awkward, and it can apply to every aspect of your pickleball game.

Earlier in this chapter, in the section "Beating Those Bangers," we talk about taking bangers out of their comfort zone. Everyone has certain shots they love to hit, or a style of play that allows them to dominate. No matter how skilled or intimidating your opponents may seem, remember that they don't get to play alone in a vacuum. You and your partner are on the court, too. Your opponents can hit the shots they love only if you feed them the right balls. Should you helpfully give them everything they want and allow them to shine? No, you're here to stifle their talents and dreams by denying them the chance! (Gee, that sounds a little harsh . . . but hey, this is a competitive sport.)

Your goal is to make things awkward for your opponents by sending balls that make it difficult for them to execute clean shots. Basically, this means keeping the ball out of their strike zone, which is out in front of their body, about knee height (see Chapter 6 for more about the strike zone). Instead, force them to dig balls out from their feet, contort for balls that land behind them, reach, lunge, or perform other awkward movements — a far cry from the graceful, athletic shots they would prefer to be hitting. Graceful athleticism is *your* thing!

Although the concept behind Make It Awkward is simple, this strategy requires precise targeting and placement. You also need the ability to track where your opponents are standing, and which direction they are currently moving or shifting their weight toward. When you first start playing pickleball, you focus primarily on what you're doing on your side of the net. Being able to also see what your opponents are doing takes court time as well as confidence in your own shot-making abilities. For these reasons, Make It Awkward is considered a more advanced strategy. However, it's never too early to start encouraging more awkward moments in your opponents' games by using the skills you currently have.

Here are several different ideas you can try to make things awkward:

>> **Change the pace.** If you're facing an expert dinker, try surprising them with a speedup — even if it's a "red light" ball (explained in Chapter 11), which we don't normally advise attacking. In this case, the element of surprise can work in your favor. If your opponents like to hit hard, turn every rally into a soft game. Drop shots, dinks, and maybe a lob or two might be in order. If you find that your team tends to lose every volley battle at the line, don't get sucked into those battles. After one or two volleys, reset the ball softly into the kitchen, or at least hit an off-speed volley that's a little slower than expected. You will throw off your opponent's timing just enough to cause an error.

>> **Hit to their feet.** Very few players can do anything offensive with balls hit right to their feet. Even better is to hit slightly behind the foot on their nondominant side. These shots don't have to be particularly hard. A series of medium-speed balls "dumped" to your opponent's feet almost always results in an eventual error. Be persistent and let your opponent become frustrated. When players are frustrated, they often beat themselves through poor decisions.

>> **Hit in the opposite direction of their momentum.** If you see a player moving to one side, perhaps to poach, hit the ball to the opposite side. Changing direction quickly is very awkward for a player, even when making smaller movements, such as when dinking. If you see a player taking a step in one direction, or shifting their weight toward one foot, dink to the opposite foot.

>> **Keep them in motion at the kitchen line.** Use the dinking patterns you learned earlier in this chapter to keep your opponent dancing from side to side and backward and forward while at the line. The more awkward the choreography, the better for you!

>> **Watch for poor paddle position.** If your opponent drops their paddle, hit them a higher ball that forces them to quickly jerk the paddle upward. This awkward motion will almost always get you a juicy pop-up.

>> **Aim for the dominant shoulder and hip.** If you're in a volley battle at the kitchen line, an excellent target is the opponent's dominant shoulder or hip. This can cause your opponent to do the dreaded "chicken wing" motion that typically results in a mis-hit. Sexy!

>> **Hit a lofty serve or return.** A lofty serve or return results in a high-bouncing ball — way out of most people's strike zones, forcing them to hit with a pitiful-looking "T-Rex arm." High-bouncing balls can also really mess up a player's timing. Many players lack the patience or experience to wait an extra beat and allow the ball to drop lower before swinging.

>> **Hit to the Awkward Spot.** Figure 12-7 shows a specific spot on the court that tends to win a lot of points. It's right between and slightly behind two players, leading to momentary confusion over which partner should go for the ball and causing the hitting player to react late. That player can't achieve a forward weight shift and has to swing using mostly their arm and wrist, resulting in a weak shot. If the two players are currently moving forward together (especially if they're running at full speed), even better! Bounce it between them for an easy winner.

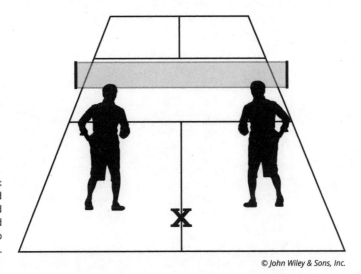

FIGURE 12-7: The Awkward Spot is located behind and between the two players.

© *John Wiley & Sons, Inc.*

Chapter **13**

Going Solo: Singles Strategy

You may have noticed that most of the information you find about pickleball, including in this book, focuses mainly on doubles. The vast majority of pickleball players play only doubles. Why is that? Well, if you try playing singles, you'll quickly realize that it feels like a very different game.

A pickleball court is quite short at only 44 feet from baseline to baseline, so you don't have much time to react to a ball that is flying your way. In contrast to tennis, the width of a pickleball singles court is exactly the same as a doubles court, and now you're responsible for all of it. The stopping, starting, changing direction, and lunging are particularly tough on the knees and back, so if you're "joint-compromised," you may want to proceed with caution.

Singles rallies tend to be shorter and more aggressive. You have to gain the advantage early and keep your opponent moving. Playing singles requires great stamina, footwork, anticipation, precision, and power. Did we mention stamina? If you want to get in shape quickly but hate treadmills as much as we do, singles pickleball might just be the ticket.

The one thing that is easier in singles than in doubles is scoring. It involves only two numbers! If the server has a score with an even number, they serve from the right (even) side. If the server's score is odd, they serve from the left (odd) side.

The receiver always lines up diagonally from the server. Easy breezy, right? Everything else about singles may not be so easy, but it can be a lot of fun and can definitely improve your doubles game as well (more on that later).

In this chapter, we break down the four phases of a singles point and compare them to the four phases of a doubles point described in Chapter 11. We also discuss some basic strategies you can start using right away to launch your new singles career. This chapter can't make you faster or more fit, but when you see how to play smartly and place the ball well, you'll find playing the solo game much easier.

Understanding the Phases of a Singles Point

Just as in doubles, a singles point has distinct phases. Assessing your opponent and creating a good plan for every phase helps to slow the game down. You need to have clear goals for navigating your way through each point, game, and match — taking you all the way to the medal stand, to the first rung on your club's ladder, or to being the top dog at your local park.

Serving and returning (Phase 1)

In singles, play tends to be more aggressive. It's all about making your opponent run. You need to get the ball past your opponent before they get the ball past you. With no partner to back you up, you're responsible for covering the entire court, and after the ball is past you — it's over! The first two shots are critical to putting yourself in a dominant position early and for the rest of the point. Both players will be trying to get an advantage right out of the gate with a fantastic serve or return.

You're playing a game over a net, which means you want to keep your opponent back and away from the net for as long as possible. You want to make both the serve and return hard and deep. Short serves invite your opponent to the net and make it easy for them to drive their return. Short returns set your opponent up to easily pass you with a third-shot drive. Strive to send the ball deep into the court, even if it means occasionally making an error and hitting the ball too long.

Compared to doubles, you'll see serves in singles that are much more weaponized. Your goal is to force a weak return from your opponent, and a conservative serve won't achieve that. Make the receiver struggle to hit the return they had planned to hit. (Later in this chapter, in "Go big on your serve," we suggest some serving strategies and targets to help you do that.) Another difference from doubles when serving in singles is that you want to stand close to the centerline. Standing close to the centerline puts you in the best position to cover the entire court for your next shot because you don't know where the return will end up going.

Hitting a hard, deep return is equally important. As the receiver, your number one priority is to force a weak third shot from your opponent, which usually means hitting a crisp drive deep to the corner on their weaker side (usually their backhand). Make sure to put enough *pace* (meaning plenty of speed behind it) on the ball so that your opponent doesn't have time to run around their backhand and hit a forehand.

Take some risks when hitting the return in order to set the point up well. Playing it safe is really not very safe at all, because you put yourself on defense for the remainder of the point. A good return allows you to safely move up to the kitchen line, where you can intercept the ball sooner and hit more offensive angles. Keep in mind that you're also vulnerable up there without a partner to help you cover the entire width of the kitchen. That's why the return of serve is so important! A strong return makes it much more likely that the next ball you intercept at the kitchen line is one you can not only reach, but put away.

Transitioning to the kitchen line (Phase 2)

Just as in doubles, being first to the kitchen line in singles will allow you to dominate the point. What's the best way of getting yourself there — a drop shot, a drive, or a lob — and when should you make your move? As with almost everything in pickleball (and life), it depends.

You have many factors to consider when attempting to transition to the line:

>> Whether you are in good court position and in good balance

>> Where your opponent is standing

>> Which direction your opponent is moving

>> How your dinking skills compare to your opponent's dinking

>> How tired you are, and how tired your opponent is

You have a lot to think about! Transitioning to the line is a little more complicated in singles. When you have twice the court to cover, you can get passed much more easily if you blindly run in after a weak return or third shot. Taller players can often move in behind weaker shots, but players who don't have as much reach should quickly assess the situation before they move in.

You can't guarantee that you'll be able to transition immediately after your return or third shot. You might find yourself stuck at the baseline for longer than you'd like, waiting for a good opportunity to move forward. To be a great singles player, you need to develop accurate, powerful groundstrokes that will keep your opponent deep in the court and moving from side to side.

If your opponent has beaten you to the line, hit your transition shot with pace only if you can direct it away from them. Otherwise, you are setting them up for an easy put-away volley. As you move in, follow the flight path of your shot rather than running straight toward the middle of the court. Doing so keeps the ball directly between you and your opponent and puts you in position to cover the side of the court nearest to them. To get the next ball past you, they will need to hit cross-court, which gives you more time to react because the ball has to travel a longer distance.

If you aren't set up well to hit your transition shot as a drive but need to get to the line because your opponent is already dominating at the kitchen, consider hitting a drop shot. Don't hit a drop shot to an opponent who is still deep; you're just inviting them up to the line.

WARNING

Beware that drop shots tend to lead to dinking rallies. Dinking rallies in singles are exhausting! If you are incredibly fit and fast, and great at hitting sharp-angled dinks, this is a good option. If you're gasping for air and your legs feel like jelly, try to end the rally quickly instead with a passing shot or well-placed topspin drive.

The lob is also an option for your transition shot, but it had better be a great one! Lobbing from deep in the court is generally considered a low-percentage shot. If you're the rare individual who has honed your lob into a masterpiece, it can be a way to send a forward opponent back to the baseline, resetting the rally.

Dinking (Phase 3)

Not every pickleball point involves dinking, and this is even more true in singles than doubles. However, it helps to know what to do if you find yourself in a one-on-one dinking situation. You have a 20-foot-wide area of court to cover all by your lonesome, and only 14 feet between you and your opponent. Gulp! It's time to make some smart choices.

Say you've made it to the kitchen line, but so has your opponent. You need to keep the ball soft and low to avoid being attacked. Your opponent knows this, too, so the two of you start battling it out with dinks. Why does it suddenly feel like you're running a marathon at high altitude? It's because you have to field dinks that are intended to make you move as much as possible. Even when you're not busy hitting, you must keep the ball in front of you and anticipate where you should be standing next. Otherwise, your opponent can easily hit a ball right past you. You have to stay in constant motion while trying to hit accurate dinks. That's tough stuff.

You need to dink with the goal of moving your opponent around and making sure they get worn out before you do. A tired, lunging dinker is more likely to make an error. Dinking is where stamina really comes into play. Did we mention that you need to make your opponent move? This is what singles is all about!

You can put additional pressure on your opponent by dinking to uncomfortable locations, such as behind their nondominant foot. Dink out wide to open up more court, but beware of dinking *too* wide and inviting an Around the Post (ATP) shot (explained in Chapter 14). You should always be dinking in the opposite direction of your opponent's momentum. If they are moving or shifting their weight to their right, hit to their left. Then hit the next dink to their right. Keep repeating this obnoxious pattern until they throw up their paddle in disgust (or more likely, throw up a pop-up by mistake).

TIP

Be sure to use every type of dink in your toolbox to prevent your opponent from getting into a rhythm or being able to anticipate your next move. Add some deception to your dinks by using an inside-out stroke, or by looking in the opposite direction of where you intend to hit. Dinking in singles requires great anticipation skills and a certain amount of guesswork, like a soccer goalie deciding which way to jump in order to block a penalty kick. The more you can hide your true intentions, the more often your opponent will guess wrong.

Attacking (Phase 4)

You've put in a lot of hard work so far. When the moment is right, be sure to attack! We don't mean hitting a ball faster than the speed of light, right on the back line. We mean hitting the ball into the open court, or in the opposite direction of your opponent's momentum. Often, this shot involves more of a medium-speed ball, as long as it's one your opponent can't reach. It might even be a slow dink! Just the two of you are on the court, which means that you can *always* find some open court or angle that your opponent cannot possibly cover.

If you get an attackable ball and are in position to hit a winner, that's great! You'll want to aim toward the corners or sidelines, but no less than a foot inside the line. Do only what is necessary to win the point. Now is not the time to impress your buddies with overly fancy or powerful shots. Save the flexing for your next body-building competition. (Nobody likes puddles of baby oil all over the court, anyway.)

If your opponent is a baseline player who likes to hang back and drive the ball at you, you can try absorbing their power and hitting a devilish drop volley into the kitchen. This shot works best when they are *back-footed* (on their heels) or pulled out wide in the opposite corner of where you plan to drop it. Even if they manage to scramble and get to the ball in time, there's a good chance they'll pop it up. Now you have an easy put-away shot against an opponent who is already off-balance. This strategy may not work against opponents who are particularly swift-footed. You will learn early in a match whether this type of attack can be effective.

WARNING

Whatever you do, don't get sucked into hitting the ball back and forth mindlessly to your opponent. You're not playing catch; you're playing singles pickleball! Adopt an aggressive mindset in which you move in toward the kitchen, close in on your opponent, and stay there until you finish them off. Look for every opportunity to hit where your opponent is not.

Winning Singles Strategies

This section delves into the nitty and the gritty of singles strategy. First, do some assessment in order to come up with a solid plan. What are your strengths? For singles play, it helps if your strengths include fitness, the ability to anticipate, a solid drive off the forehand and backhand sides, great footwork, a variety of serves, and deep, aggressive returns. If you don't have all these skills, don't despair; you can develop all of them with training and practice, and in the meantime, you can use smart strategy to help compensate for some of your weaknesses.

In addition to your self-assessment, you need to assess your opponent. Often players assess each other quickly, during warm-up. When you warm up opposite your opponent, you can watch for how well they hit their backhand. Do they try to run around it to their forehand? Also assess other traits: Can they move well to a short ball? Do they favor certain shots over others? Are they left-handed? What types of serves can you expect? You're essentially scouting while also warming up your own game. Remember that they're scouting you, too, so don't give too much away.

After you size up your opponent, you can put some strategy into play. In this section, we outline some basic singles strategies that work for the majority of players. Have fun experimenting with all of them to see what works best for you.

Go big on your serve

For many years, traditional pickleball-serving wisdom decreed, "Just get it in." (As you already know, we think you're better than that.) Many people feel that missing their serve is the greatest pickleball *faux pas* imaginable. For playing singles, you need to let this notion go because just getting your serve in won't help you win the game. Expect to make some service errors as you take bigger risks and get a bit more aggressive. Your serve is your opportunity to take charge and dictate the point from the very beginning.

Here are some suggestions on how to make the most of your serve in singles:

>> **Serve deep:** A back-footed opponent is less likely to get to the net before you do. Hit deep serves that are difficult for your opponent to time correctly. Pushing them back also forces them to run a longer distance to get to the kitchen line.

>> **Serve to their weaker side:** Typically, the weaker side is their backhand, but it depends on the opponent. Try to assess early in the match whether they prefer their forehand or backhand for returns, and then avoid serving to that side.

>> **Serve toward the centerline:** This target cuts off the sharp angles your opponent can hit with their return, meaning that you won't be sent scrambling off the court and way out of position for your next shot.

>> **Vary your serves:** Don't become too predictable with your serves. Make your opponent stay hyperfocused and unable to guess what you'll serve next. Maintaining this level of focus is mentally taxing and will tire them out over the course of the match.

Beat your opponent to the net

In singles, just as in doubles, the player who gets to the net first has a distinct advantage. The net position is where players can hit down on the ball and access more angles. A player standing at the line can close off a lot of court with their body and reach, limiting their opponent's shot options. Generally, if you're first to the kitchen line and your opponent can't get the ball past you with their next shot, you have a very high likelihood of winning that rally.

After your beautiful deep return that you hit with a solid forward weight shift and a fabulous, photogenic follow-through, hustle up to the kitchen line and try to intercept your opponent's third shot.

If you're the server, hit your sweet third-shot drive (or drop) and try to get in at least a few good-sized steps to shrink the amount of court available to your opponent. Then, at your earliest opportunity, finish coming to the line. Most likely the receiver has beaten you there. If not, you should be able to make them pay for their hesitation.

TIP

Immediately after you get to the kitchen line, expect a passing shot and try your best to intercept it. Get your paddle up and square yourself to the ball. If possible, volley it to the open court, or behind the player if they're on the move. If the ball is too low to attack, dink it to a spot as far away from your opponent as possible.

Hit to your opponent's weaker side

An opponent's weaker side is usually, but not always, their backhand side. In fact, many players these days have an amazing two-handed backhand drive that might even be stronger and more dependable than their forehand drive. Whatever their weaker side turns out to be, figuring it out gives you solid-gold intel!

If you can't hit your targets, however, picking on your opponent's weaknesses will be tough. You can improve your aim and really improve your game by using targets in practice. We've used some pretty unusual objects as targets. Everything from yoga mats and pool noodles, to old towels and shopping bags all work perfectly fine. Also, it's a great idea to practice hitting serves and returns in a fan pattern. Hit one serve to the sideline, one to the middle of the service box, and one near the centerline. Be sure to practice serving to these targets from both the right and left sides of the court. Do the same with returns, fanning them throughout the court.

Of course, your opponent may use the same strategy of hitting to your weaker side. To neutralize this strategy when used against you, work on developing strong forehands and backhands. Singles is a great equalizer. With no partner by your side to compensate for your weaknesses, you have to become a strong all-around player. If you try to run around your weak side to avoid having to hit those shots, you wind up leaving a great deal of open court for your opponent. Build your shot catalog and your confidence at the same time.

TIP

Along with identifying an opponent's weaker side, pay attention to how well they handle low-bouncing versus high-bouncing balls. Their skill in this regard will depend on the quality of their footwork. Some players have a tendency to reach and "scoop" under low balls, resulting in more pop-ups. Others have difficulty with high-bouncing balls because they allow the ball to get in too close to their body, jamming them up. Practice a variety of serves and groundstrokes so that you can exploit any weaknesses you find — high or low, right or left, topspin or backspin.

Make them move

Singles pickleball is all about movement. Winning points comes down to who can move better, and who can make the other move just a bit beyond their ability to hit a good shot. When trying to make your opponent move, think about open space and angles.

Hitting where your opponent isn't standing seems obvious, but it's natural to want to hit the ball back to the person opposite you, as you did if you played catch in the backyard. Or maybe your mind is still stuck on warm-up, where you courteously traded shots back and forth with your new pickleball friend — before you two officially became arch nemeses during the match. To force your opponent to move, you'll need to resist the temptation to keep the rally going and instead hit the ball as far away from your opponent as possible. Yearn for those wide-open spaces where the buffalo roam.

Even if your opponent happens to be your pickleball best forever friend (PBFF), it's time to turn up your Rude Dial and make it your mission to get rid of them. You'd like for them to leave the court (and venue) if possible (I said, "Good day, Sir!") When they have exited the boundaries of the court, they've left lots of open space behind them, giving you a lot of time to select the perfect (rude) shot before they can get back to cover things. It seems mean, but you can always treat them to fro-yo after the match to make up for it.

To open up the court in this way, you need to use angles. Ideally, setting up for angles begins with the serve and return. As the server, you have two options. You can serve at a wide angle, immediately opening up a lot of court. However, know that the most likely shot to come back is an equal and opposite angle. If your opponent has a wicked crosscourt return, this strategy could backfire on you. Your second option is to serve closer to the centerline. This target will make it more difficult for your opponent to hit a wide-angled return, especially if it's on their weaker side. You may have to wait until you get the right ball to start hitting your big angles.

TIP

To keep your opponent on the move, just think "corner to corner." Sending your shots from one corner to the other keeps your opponent back and constantly on the move while also creating opportunities for your eventual passing shot or angled put-away.

Recover quickly

Logically, both singles players attempt to stay toward the center of the court so that they can cover more court. Also, if you're running up the side of the court, you can't transition to the line without getting passed by the ball. Be sure to return to the centerline quickly after each shot. Proximity to the centerline puts you in the best position to deal with the next ball, plus it forces your opponent to hit more accurate shots. This strategy puts more pressure on your opponent and can sometimes be enough to force them to take bigger risks, therefore forcing more errors.

In addition to recovering your court position, you want to recover to good ready position after every shot. Keep your paddle up and out in front of your body. Square your major joints to the current location of the ball. Keep your chin up and watch your opponent's body language and paddle movement carefully. This is where fitness and mental stamina really come into play. If you drop your paddle or drop your guard, you will certainly anticipate the next ball late.

Improving Your Doubles Play through Singles

Singles pickleball is an extremely exciting game that demands athleticism, precision, and speed. If you haven't tried it, consider it. You never know . . . it might be your thing!

Playing singles can also benefit your doubles game. It forces you to hone shots you might not otherwise spend much time developing. The baseline game, consisting of serves, returns, and groundstrokes, is the most obvious example of how singles improves your doubles play. Singles players typically become masters of the topspin drive and can place the ball deep into either back corner. Singles will also improve your fitness, endurance, and footwork. You have no time to kick back and daydream in the middle of a singles point! You have to move constantly, and every step counts. Talk about a great workout!

Passing shots, though hugely important in singles, are often forgotten about in doubles. In doubles, players commonly focus too much on the middle of the court. You have two opponents to track who happen to be very interesting to look at — perhaps more interesting than the open court on either side of them. (Mismatched argyle socks are hard to stop staring at!) When you're this focused on your opponents and all the action happening in the middle, you may not notice when one or both sidelines suddenly open up. The more you play singles, the more you will start to recognize when your opponents are pinching the middle, leaving the sidelines wide open.

Many doubles players also lack confidence in their down-the-line shots. Hitting there can feel too risky because you might miss wide. Players often direct all their shots to the middle to play it safe. By playing singles, you build confidence in your down-the-line shots because you must quickly learn to rely on them. You can't pass an opponent who's constantly recovering to the centerline of the court if you only ever hit to the middle.

Singles is also incredibly helpful for building mental toughness. You alone are responsible for everything that happens on your side of the net. If you yell "You!" no one is coming to help you. If you lose a rally, you have no one to blame but yourself. It's up to you to quickly analyze what's going wrong and come up with a new strategy. Toughest of all, you have nobody to lift you up with a paddle tap or encouraging words. This means you must become the world's greatest pickleball partner — to yourself! Negativity only makes things worse, so stay positive and speak to yourself only in the way you'd speak to your favorite doubles partner. See Chapter 15 for more on the mental side of pickleball.

TIP

Even if you have no desire to ever play singles, we recommend watching it. It offers a lot of thrills for the competitors and spectators alike. Check out some major pro tournaments (most are streamed online), or cheer on your local singles players next time you see them battling on the court. They'll appreciate it!

SKINNY SINGLES

Skinny singles is a game for very thin people. Okay, maybe not. Skinny singles is actually another term for half-court singles. It offers a fun way to practice when you don't have enough people to play doubles but don't feel like covering the entire court yourself. In skinny singles, you play on only one side of the court (right or left).

You have a few variations of skinny singles to choose from (see the figure in this sidebar for a diagram of each type):

- **Straight-ahead skinny singles:** In this version, you and your opponent will always line up on one side of the court across from each other and hit only to that side of the court. You have to serve straight ahead rather than crosscourt, which might feel a little strange!

- **Diagonal skinny singles:** You serve crosscourt as usual, and the receiver must likewise return the ball crosscourt. You can serve from the same side the whole game or alternate serving from the right or left based on your score (as you would in regular singles). The receiver always lines up diagonally to the server.

- **Score-based skinny singles:** This version is really the best of both straight-ahead and diagonal singles because you'll be playing both straight-ahead and crosscourt throughout the game. When the server's score is even, the server stands on the even (right) side of the court. The receiver also stands on the side that matches their score (even or odd). So, depending on the two players' scores, some points are played straight ahead and some diagonally.

(continued)

(continued)

- **Three-Person "Cutthroat":** This game is a hybrid of singles and doubles that you can play when you have three people. In this scenario, you play two against one. To make it fair, the single player can hit anywhere on the court, but the doubles players can hit only to one half of the court. Typically, the single player is the server and is the only one with the opportunity to win a point. When the server wins a point, they switch sides and continue serving from the other side. After the single player loses the rally, everyone rotates one position and a new player serves. Keep track of your own points and announce your score before you serve. (Don't worry about keeping track of all three players' scores!)

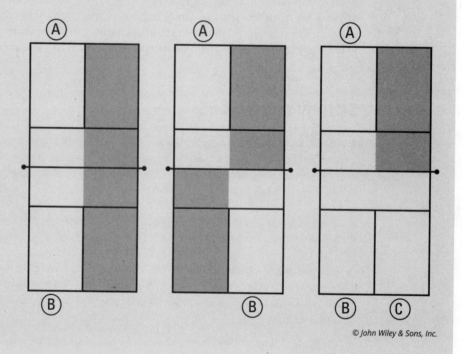

© John Wiley & Sons, Inc.

In each of these variations, you need to mentally draw an imaginary line down the middle of the kitchen. A single player isn't expected to cover the entire kitchen unless they're playing regular singles. Because none of these formats is an "official" style of pickleball, you get to make up your own rules. You're on a pickleball court, playing with your friends, so relax and enjoy. Be creative and have fun with it!

Skinny singles can be great for improving your accuracy because you have only half the court to land the ball. Your opponent takes up most of that available space, so you need to really thread the needle to get the ball past them. With so little open space on either side, controlling the ball's depth becomes even more crucial if you want to avoid being attacked. It's a fun way to improve your doubles game, or ease into the idea of playing full-court singles.

4

Improving and Competing: Living with Obsessive Pickleball Disorder (OPD)

Chapter **14**

Leveling Up: Advanced Skills You'll Need

M any intermediate-level players find that they reach a plateau in their game at some point. Even if they play several times a week, they don't see the same rapid improvement they experienced as a beginner.

Court time and repetition will certainly improve your muscle memory and anticipation skills. If you were mostly sedentary before taking up pickleball, you'll see your fitness level continuing to increase as well. Not to mention, you're meeting people and having tons of fun! However, if your goal is to advance past the intermediate level, you need to cultivate some additional skills and knowledge. Otherwise, you may keep practicing bad habits without realizing it. Fortunately, you've come to the right place. This chapter is all about "leveling up!"

Even if you haven't passed the beginner stage, you may be well "served" (pun definitely intended) to read about some of these more advanced skills and tactics. Knowing what's to come can help you to begin to build toward it. Be careful, though. Just because you read about a subject — such as the various spins that you can apply to the ball — doesn't mean you should start trying to spin every shot. Start working on more advanced skills only after you've built a good, solid foundation to your game.

Don't rush through any of it. Learn it. Practice it. Try it out a few times per game whenever you play recreationally. Then, see what you need to do to improve upon it. Pickleball can take a lifetime to master, and there's no pressure to go pro next week. It takes patience. If you've been reading this book up to this point, you already know all about patience in pickleball!

Preventing Pop-Ups: Six "Scientifically" Proven Causes

A *pop-up* happens when a player accidentally lifts the ball too high in the air, allowing their opponent to smack it down hard. Although your opponents may enjoy receiving pop-ups (and even write you a nice thank-you note), we assume you would prefer not to hit them. Our students are always asking us how to deal with being attacked after hitting a pop-up. Like many unfortunate situations in life, the key is prevention!

To reduce your number of pop-ups, you first need to understand what causes them. There are currently six major "scientifically" proven reasons that players pop up the ball. (Confession: Our "scientific" method results from years of teaching and observing students. Hey, that doesn't mean the six reasons aren't true.) Read on to find out what causes pop-ups.

>> **Standing in an improper ready position:** Figure 14-1 shows a player who is definitely not ready, and possibly not even awake. If an opponent hits a ball toward her chest, she'll have to quickly raise her paddle up to intercept it. This rapid raising of the paddle means the ball can go in only one direction: up! If you ever see a player standing like this, hit the ball right to them. Meanwhile, keep your own paddle up and stay in the good ready position described in Chapter 6.

>> **Dropping your paddle head:** Dropping the tip of your paddle down toward the ground so that your paddle is mostly vertical, as shown in Figure 14-2, is another major cause of pop-ups. First, it encourages "wristiness." You won't find that word in a dictionary, but in pickleball talk, it means you're using your wrist too much. When you flick at the ball with your wrist rather than use your larger joints, you struggle with accuracy. Dropping the paddle head also encourages you to swing upward in a "scooping" motion instead of pushing forward through the ball. This scooping motion makes it difficult to get any topspin on the ball. Instead of a nice, low shot that arcs over the net, you get a shot that flies straight up into the air — a tasty treat for your drooling opponents looking to slam. See the section in Chapter 6 about upper body mechanics for more tips on how to add topspin to your shots.

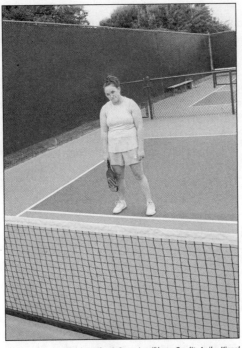

FIGURE 14-1:
A player who is definitely not in a good ready position.

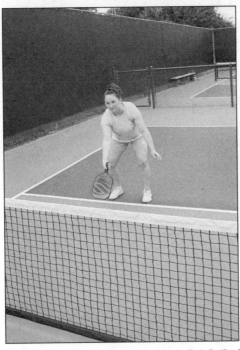

FIGURE 14-2:
A player who has dropped the paddle head vertically.

» **Hitting behind you:** The only time you should be hitting the ball behind your body is when you're dazzling the crowd with a trick shot. Otherwise, you want to hit every ball out in front of you. (Go to Chapter 6 to find out about your strike zone and playing in the "V.") After the ball gets past your "V," you're already late and will have to use your wrist to make up for it. At that point, your odds of hitting an accurate shot are very slim. Starting from a good ready position, with both hands out in front of you, makes intercepting the ball earlier and out in front much easier. Figure 14-3 shows a player trying to deal with a ball that has gone past her strike zone. Her wrist will have to do some real heroics here to make this shot!

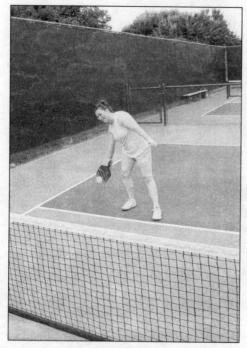

FIGURE 14-3:
A player attempting to hit a ball from behind her.

© John Wiley & Sons, Inc./Photo Credit: Aniko Kiezel

» **Swinging too fast:** When you swing too fast, especially at a low "red light" ball (see Chapter 11 if you haven't yet read about the upside-down traffic light), you add too much energy to the ball. The ball continues to rise as it crosses over the net rather than dying (running out of energy) and dropping low.

A ball on the rise looks a lot like a pop-up — because it is one! Remember this phrase: "When it's low, go slow." Most players don't need nearly the amount of power they bring to each shot. Swinging too fast (depicted in Figure 14-4) is the most common cause of pop-ups at intermediate and advanced levels. Slow down and hit carefully, guiding the ball to your intended target.

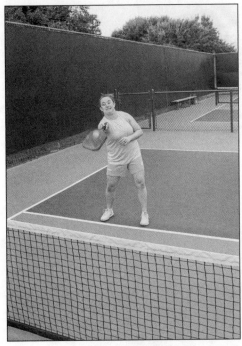

FIGURE 14-4: A player swinging too fast.

>> **Incorrect paddle face:** Using too "open" of a paddle face (see Figure 14-5) on volleys and groundstrokes can cause the ball to rebound off your paddle with too much loft. As you can see in the photo, an open paddle face points up in the air, so that's exactly where the ball is going to go. Try to keep the paddle face mostly flat at the point of impact so that the ball travels forward instead of upward.

>> **Running through your shot:** If you were trying to catch an egg thrown at you, would you sprint toward it as fast as you can? We hope your answer is "no." (We also hope nobody in your life has a habit of tossing eggs at you.)

If you want to stay in control of your shots, you need a pause in momentum. Hit your shot with a forward weight shift and *then* move in behind your shot. If you combine running forward with trying to hit your shot at the same time, you'll probably deliver an out-of-control pop-up. A ball that you've hit with your entire body mass traveling at high velocity simply has too much momentum behind it. (Oops, we promised earlier there would be no more physics talk.)

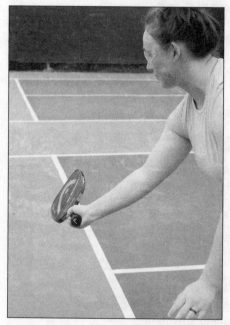

FIGURE 14-5:
An "open" paddle face.

Often, players run through their shots because they're already thinking about getting in position for their next shot. Remember, there's no shot like the present! If you hit a pop-up, or dump the ball into the net, there won't *be* a next shot. So set up properly in relation to the ball, pause, execute your beautiful shot, and *then* move forward. Figure 14-6 shows a player who is running through her shot. If she took the time to focus on her current shot, she'd be a pretty darn happy player. We want you to be happy with all your shots, so stay present in the moment before worrying about the future.

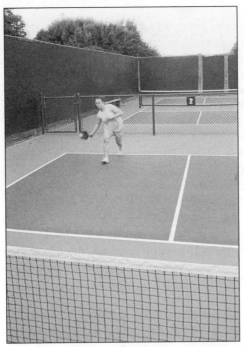

Controlling the Pace

As you advance in pickleball, your success is directly proportional to your ability to control the pace of the ball. When you can control the speed of the ball, you get to dictate the tempo and rhythm of the rally. Your opponents will be forced to play the game *you* want to play, rather than your having to constantly react to *their* game. Adding, absorbing, and changing speed are all important skills for you to master as you begin to play better opponents.

Sending unattackable balls

If your opponent isn't attacking you, that means you have the time and opportunity to move forward in the court. You want to be the player at the kitchen line, hitting down on the ball. You *do not* want your opponents doing that! If you keep finding yourself stuck deep in the court, unable to move through the transition zone, or constantly feeling like you're on defense, you're probably hitting too many attackable balls.

You can keep balls from being attacked by hitting *low* and *slow*. That should be easy to remember, because "low and slow" is also the key to great barbecue. (Is anybody else hungry all of a sudden?) Hit low-energy balls that your opponent has to reach down for and lift over the net. Make the ball land at their feet, or better yet, completely out of their reach in an open area of the court. An opponent who is off-balance, crouching down low, or swinging from low to high is not in good position to attack.

Drop shots are a perfect example of the "low and slow" concept. A good drop shot has to be lifted up by your opponent. Refer to Figure 11-1 in Chapter 11 to see what this looks like from across the net. When you see your opponents swinging from low to high, move forward a few steps. Stay calm and balanced, and don't rush. If your opponent sees you wildly running in, they may try to attack the low ball anyway because you're clearly not in a state of readiness to deal with even a poorly executed attack. Instead, confidently approach the line in measured steps, with your paddle up and a menacing look on your face. Attacking will be the last thing on your opponent's mind!

We realize it's easy for us to say "just keep the ball slow and low." In practice, every pickleball player knows it's much harder than it sounds. Here are some tips on how to bring your shots closer to earth to prevent them from being attacked:

>> **Swing through the ball:** Your hitting sensation should be one of pushing forward toward your target. If you jab or scoop at the ball, it will travel more upward than forward — a nice high pop-up for your opponent to slam!

>> **Hit through a window:** It can help to imagine that you're hitting the ball through a window or picture frame floating 6–18 inches above the net. This target feels more attainable than one that's several feet past the net, on the other side of the court. Focus on guiding the ball through the window rather than up and over the window.

>> **Use a long follow-through:** The follow-through is critical to keeping the ball low because it provides all the topspin, as well as all the information about where it should go. If you just poke or jab at the ball, it won't have enough information. It needs more time on your paddle to be influenced by the directional forces you are applying.

>> **Swing slowly:** To hit the ball slowly, swing slowly. It's not rocket science! (Thank goodness.) Take a compact backswing, contact the ball out in front of you, and swing slowly through the ball. If your shots are going too high or too far, swing slower. If they're not going far enough, swing faster. We don't want you to have to learn 50 different swings for 50 different shots. Learn one swing and execute it at different speeds depending on how deep or hard you want to hit the ball.

We often see players who, upon finding that their shots are traveling too high or too far, eliminate part of their swing and start jabbing at the ball, decelerating at impact. Sadly, the part of the swing they take off is typically our beloved follow-through. Such players are then dismayed to find that they've made the problem worse! The correct adjustment is to keep the follow-through and just swing a little slower. The less energy you add behind the ball, the more it will drop low instead of zinging up into the air.

TIP

During your warm-up, be sure to calibrate height and distance by trying to land some balls near the baseline and some near the kitchen. Adjust your swing speed or the size of your "window" if needed. On any given day, your shots can be thrown off by a variety of conditions such as wind, altitude, fatigue, or ball composition and condition. Be sure to get this information dialed in before you start your match.

Resetting the rally

When a rally starts getting frantic and out of control, or isn't trending in your favor, your best option is to *reset* the rally by hitting an unattackable ball. When you reset a rally, you momentarily neutralize your opponents' ability to be offensive. A reset puts both teams back on more equal footing and buys you and your partner time to get into a better position.

Resetting can involve a few different actions, but typically it entails slowing down the pace. It may also involve changing the depth or direction of the ball. Resetting is one of the more difficult skills to master in pickleball, but with time and practice, you can do it. No worries; you've got this!

In fact, having no worries is the key. We want you to relax and do almost nothing. Huh? That's right, when things are not working in your favor, it's time to relax your body, including your grip, and absorb power off the ball by using a very minimal swing. Try to hit it softly into the kitchen as a low, slow, unattackable ball. Your goal is to force your opponent to have to lift the next ball. Don't panic, tense up, or get jumpy. Be calm, steady, and stable. Don't try for a crazy-hard, low-percentage shot as a means of bailing out of the situation. Just because your opponents are attacking you doesn't mean you need to freak out and give up on your smart strategy! It just means you need to take control of the pace again.

Depending on where you and your opponents are positioned in the court, you have a few different options for your reset shot:

>> **Drop volley:** When a volley battle starts while all four players are up at the line, this shot is your best bet for a successful reset. Start by holding your

paddle in a relaxed continental grip. (See Chapter 6 for details on this grip.) On a scale of one to ten, your grip pressure should be about a four. Hold your paddle out in front of your chest, your arms slightly bent and your elbows at about a 45-degree angle from your body (not sticking straight out). Most block volleys are backhands, unless the ball is well over on your dominant side. With a slightly open (tilted upward) paddle face, push forward a few inches, with a downward "feathering" motion, as if brushing along the back of the ball. This motion gives the ball a little backspin, which causes it to decelerate even more when it bounces. See Chapter 9 for more on how to execute this incredibly useful shot.

>> **Lob:** If necessary, you can use a lob to reset the point as well. If you find that things are getting a little crazy and your opponents are having too much fun dominating at the kitchen, kick them out of there by making them run back for your sweet lob. This shot is especially effective on a sunny day. Making your opponents look into the sun can definitely reset the rally in your favor. We'll leave the ethical judgments to you and your conscience. (We sleep fine at night, thank you.) Lobs can be pretty low-percentage shots, though, so be sure you've read Chapter 9 and practiced a ton before you rely on them.

>> **Drop shot:** If you've retreated to deep in the court (or perhaps never made it forward to begin with) and your opponent is attacking with balls toward your feet, you need to reset by hitting a groundstroke or half-volley (short hop) drop shot. Although you may feel like you're in a hopeless situation, remember that a drop shot isn't that different from hitting a third-shot drop. If you're the serving team, you have to begin every point from this same undesirable position; that is, your opponents are up at the line while your team is back. Don't make being deep in the court any bigger in your head just because you're in the middle of the point and things haven't gone your way so far. See Chapter 7 to review our tips on hitting great drop shots.

REMEMBER

Just because a rally speeds up doesn't mean it has to stay that way. Some of pickleball's most exciting points involve long rallies that include multiple speedups followed by multiple resets. As fun and tempting as the fast game is, after two or three hits, nobody is really in control anymore. After things get totally out of control, your odds of winning the point are basically 50/50. Be the hero for your team by stopping the madness and taking charge again with a well-timed reset.

Defending against attacks

"I feel personally attacked!" It's pickleball, so you're probably not wrong. Like a good therapist, we're here to validate your feelings. Getting attacked is not much fun (unless you're into that sort of thing, which is a subject for a different book). So, how do you deal with it? First, try to prevent it by not popping the ball up. Be sure to read and memorize the "Preventing Pop-Ups: Six "Scientifically" Proven Causes" from earlier in this chapter; write them on the back of your hand or the inside of your eyelids if necessary. When you play, try to pay attention to which of the six may be causing most of your problems. If you still aren't clear why you're popping the ball up, enlist a coach or friend to observe you playing, or record a video. (See Chapter 16 to read more about self-assessment tools.)

Although preventing an attack is always the best option, this is real life, and none of us is perfect. (This goes for your partner, too.) You can, and will, get attacked throughout a match. You should probably know what to do besides panicking!

Here are our tips for improving your defense when under attack:

>> **Square yourself to the ball:** If you're always squared to the net, you will struggle to cope with attacks coming at you from awkward angles. The attack should always seem as though it's coming right at you. Imagine you're a baseball catcher ready for a fastball pitch. Square yourself confidently toward the opponent hitting the ball and think, "Bring it!" When your eyes, paddle, and torso are facing the ball, an attack is much easier to deal with. (See Chapter 11 for more information on this technique, called paddle tracking).

>> **Do not squeal and turn away:** As long as you are wearing your trusty eye protection, your opponent can't do much to you other than possibly leave a small bruise. That's fine. You will live through it, and pickleball bruises are cute because they have little polka dots in them. Fun!

>> **Get low:** If your team has popped the ball up high and the attack looks like it's coming down hard, it's time to get low. Attacks are most often hit toward your feet. Get ready to protect your feet as well as your entire "hoop" (explained Chapter 8). Lean forward, crouch down slightly, and lower your paddle. Figure 14-7 shows a player in good position to defend against an oncoming attack.

>> **Consider a counterattack:** If the attack is just a speedup during a dinking rally, you may be able to counterattack it. Try to be offensive whenever possible. Being offensive doesn't necessarily mean fighting fire with fire by adding more speed to the ball. An offensive counterattack may simply mean redirecting a volley down toward your opponent's feet, or angling it away from them to where they didn't expect it.

>> **Get your paddle out in front of you:** If you keep your paddle well out in front of you, as if your elbows are resting on a bar, you will have more time to take an offensive shot with the ball rather than just defensively react. However, if your ready position is collapsed with your elbows touching your ribs, you will be late and probably mis-hit the ball because you're jammed up.

» **Stay ready:** If your paddle is out of position, you'll really struggle to deal with a high-speed attack. You simply don't have enough time to move your paddle up from lazily dangling by your side, swinging in the breeze, to meet a ball hurtling toward your chest at 50 MPH. When your paddle is up, you can use it as either a sword or a shield. By sword, we mean hitting an offensive counterattack (usually a forehand volley). As a shield, your nice flat paddle face will be executing solid, defensive block volleys. Either of these options certainly beats taking a ball to the belly button!

» **Relax:** Whether you're on offense or defense, try to relax your body. Being relaxed helps you to absorb some of the power from the ball, allowing you to reset the rally. Counterintuitively, it also makes it easier to hit the ball hard. Tense people don't tend to use their full range of motion, which means they generate less power.

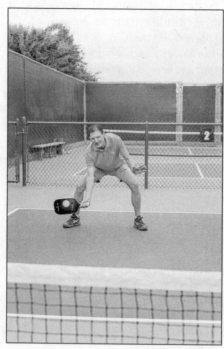

FIGURE 14-7:
A player in good defensive position to field an attack.

© John Wiley & Sons, Inc./Photo Credit: Aniko Kiezel

» **Retreat a few steps:** We talk a lot in this book about the importance of forward pressure and holding the kitchen line. If you have amazing reaction time, try not to retreat because you'll be giving up your hard-fought forward position. Stay in there and show everyone your amazing hand speed.

However, if you don't have the fastest hands in the West, you may find retreating a step or two beneficial. A retreat gives you a little more time to react to the incoming attack. Please do this safely; absolutely no backpedaling allowed. Bend your knees, put your weight forward, and shuffle back. If your weight is forward, you can't fall backward. After your fabulous reset shot, don't forget to move back up to the line.

TIP

One of the best ways to improve your ability to handle attacks is to practice hitting block volleys. This practice will pay significant dividends because the block volley shot is a great way to reset the point back to neutral after an attack. The block volley is a pretty fun shot to drill. You stand at the kitchen line and have someone hit hard shots at you, which you block softly into the kitchen on the other side of the net. Next, do the same thing from the middle of the transition zone. Have a player hit balls toward your knees and feet. Practice getting low while holding your paddle face slightly open, and then block the ball with a slow push on your follow-through. If you can't take this ball out of the air, don't worry. Just get your paddle right behind where you expect the ball to bounce; now your block volley has magically become a half-volley. It's really the same shot, so don't overthink it. See Chapter 9 for more tips on how to execute these shots.

Another good way to practice dealing with attacks is create a gameplay scenario, with you and your drill partner dinking across the net from each other. Follow this pattern: dink, dink, dink, pop-up, attack, reset. Take turns being the attacker and resetter. You can also try this pattern without including an obvious pop-up so that the attack comes as more of a surprise. Try experimenting with counterattacking rather than always resetting. These more realistic gameplay drills are great for improving your real-life game reactions. You're much less apt to panic if you've seen and practiced the scenario a hundred times before.

REMEMBER

Many players tend to over-hit their attacks, so be ready to let them go out. Attacks are especially prone to go out if the player attacks while on the move, off-balance, or hitting too low of a ball. Attacks generated from less-than-ideal conditions often land beyond the boundaries of the court.

Using Spin Effectively: Spin It to Win It!

Putting a nice spin on things isn't just for politicians and record players. (We're showing our age now, aren't we?) Spin is for pickleball players, too! Using spin in your pickleball game is a fantastic idea, but reading your opponent's spin is equally important. The more you understand various spins and the swing paths that generate them, the easier it is to predict the bounce of a ball coming toward you. Anticipation is key in the fast-moving game of pickleball, so understanding spin can be very helpful. If you can watch your opponent's backswing and follow-through to predict how the ball will bounce, you're ahead of the game. Figure 14-8 illustrates some different kinds of spin and the resulting bounce of the ball.

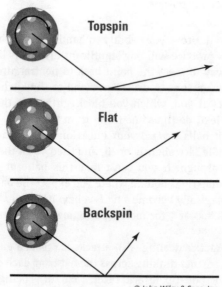

FIGURE 14-8:
Different spins to apply to a pickleball.

© John Wiley & Sons, Inc.

Students often ask us to help them add more spin to their game. We approach this request with caution. For the most part, the main spin you need to worry about is topspin. Chapter 6 tells you a bit about topspin and possibly dazzles you with our knowledge of physics. When you're playing a game like pickleball or tennis, in which you must send a ball over a net and then get it to drop into the court, you need topspin. It makes the ball rotate forward over itself so that even a hard-hit ball will arc over the net and then fall within bounds. Other spins are useful, but be sure to master topspin before venturing into the world of other spins. Don't get too fancy before you master the basics!

Serving with spin

As you may recall from previous chapters, we encourage you to have a variety of serves in your arsenal. One way to add variety is through various spins. The serve is a great place to start playing around with spin because it's hit under the most controlled conditions. You don't have to worry about counterspinning a ball that's already spinning thanks to your opponent. You can "tee up" the ball exactly as you like, either with or without applying spin using your nondominant hand. The receiver is required to let your serve bounce, which allows you to observe the results of your various spin attempts.

Generating topspin

The first spin serve to master is the basic forehand topspin serve. To hit this serve, you need to avoid dropping the paddle head completely (pointing the tip of the paddle at the ground). This is known as the *bowling serve*, and the biggest problem with this serve is that you can hit the ball only upward toward the sky, with almost zero spin. It also uses just one side of the body, with mostly just the arm doing the work. If you hit more out to your side, as you would a regular forehand, you can get your wrist to lead your paddle until just before it contacts the ball. Leading with your wrist creates some tension and allows you to hit through the ball and follow through upward. Your body can now rotate and open up your hips toward your target. This motion creates generous amounts of topspin and pace.

Whether you're using the traditional out-of-the-air serve or the drop serve, as long as you contact the ball out in front of you (near or even with your forward-most leg) and follow through upward, you will generate topspin. You can strike the ball quite hard if you so choose; it will start to drop after it reaches its apex. When it bounces, it will accelerate, making it even more challenging for your opponent. You'll have to play around with it until you figure out how hard you can hit it and still keep it in the court.

TIP

After you've figured out your service motion and can get your topspin serve in 85 percent of the time, practice aiming for specific targets. One particularly great weapon is a topspin serve that hits the closest part of the service box, near the sideline, and pulls the opponent out wide. You have just forced your opponent to leave the court, which means they have left plenty of open court behind them and will be scrambling to get back into the rally. Nice work!

Creating sidespin

Now you're ready to move on and challenge yourself to hit other types of spin serves. Coauthor Mo has a favorite evil serve that she hits from the odd side of the court. She hits it softly, with tons of sidespin, and lands it just past the kitchen, near the sideline. Because it is hit softly and with sidespin, it barely bounces as it lands. The trickiest part about this serve is that it is disguised to look like any other serve that normally has pace on it. This disguise is very helpful when hitting serves. You don't always want your opponent to know what you've got up your sleeve. Is it a rabbit? No, but it may be an ace!

You create sidespin when you strike the ball on its side as opposed to its backside. When hitting the sidespin or "cut" serve, you brush the side of the ball with your paddle, making the ball spin around itself, like a top. You adjust your paddle face with your wrist and follow through forward, but somewhat off to one side, instead of upward like the topspin serve. When a ball with sidespin lands, it bounces either to the left or the right, depending on which direction the paddle struck the ball.

To make the ball bounce to your left when it lands, hit a counterclockwise sidespin. Your backswing looks almost like you're brushing something off your thigh with your paddle, and then your follow-through wraps around toward your left side a bit. Your paddle face brushes the right side of the ball, causing it to spin counterclockwise.

To spin the ball clockwise, start by taking your backswing with your paddle face slightly open. At contact, brush your paddle face against the left side of the ball. The follow-through will cross in front of your body and extend forward.

Adding backspin

Hitting a backspin serve is very difficult to do. When hitting a traditional serve, out of the air, you're required by the rules to swing in a low-to-high motion. This motion can't create backspin. When hitting a drop serve, this rule doesn't apply, but you have to squat down extremely low to be able to hit from high to low (the swing path required to create backspin). The ball just won't bounce high enough to make it work well. If you're the player who likes to experiment with different serves, go ahead and try it, but backspin just isn't a very practical goal when serving. You have plenty of other options, so don't worry.

Returning with spin

Just as in serving, spins can help you add more variety to your serve returns. You never want your opponent to get into a rhythm, always knowing what to expect from you. Being predictable will make their third shot start to feel very easy! Instead, make their third shot feel like a new challenge every time. With this in mind, it's good to hone a few different types of returns. As with serves, returns are a great way to start experimenting with spin because your opponent is required to let it bounce. You'll get feedback every time on how well you applied your desired spin.

Make sure you have developed a good topspin return before trying other spins. Hit the ball out in front, about even with your front leg, following through forward and upward to give it that sweet topspin we all love. You can also try some sidespin if you find yourself playing against someone who struggles when dealing with spin shots. See the previous section to get a feel for hitting sidespin.

Many players like to return serves with backspin because it makes their opponent's third shot much trickier. You achieve backspin by hitting the ball with a high-to-low swing motion. You take the paddle up to about the height of your ear and then extend it downward, striking the ball on its backside with a slightly open paddle face, and follow through forward. It involves a bit of a chopping motion, but be sure to also swing through the ball, finishing forward, so that the ball goes over the net. For many players, backspin comes more naturally on their backhand.

When you apply backspin correctly, the ball travels through the air fairly straight and then decelerates after it bounces, skidding a bit on the court. It's this funky bounce, or lack thereof, that makes backspin tough for your opponent to deal with. If you're struggling against a team who hits killer drives on their third shots, try a backspin return. The lower bounce of the ball makes it more difficult for anyone to drive the ball from high to low. A low-bouncing ball can also make a third-shot drop tricky because the player has to add extra lift to get the ball over the net. You may get your opponent to hit a number of third-shot drops into the net before they figure out how to deal with your backspin return.

Watch for these pitfalls when hitting spin returns:

>> **Lack of forward momentum:** If your swing path is too vertical (straight down), the ball won't have enough forward momentum. Ideally, you still want your return to land deep in the court, so you will need to use enough forward motion.

>> **Jabbing at the ball:** Whenever you jab or poke at the ball, you make controlling the depth and direction of your shot difficult. The ball needs more information on where you want it to go and which direction to spin. Keep the ball on your paddle as long as possible by using a full follow-through.

>> **Overdoing it:** Spin shots can cause strain on your arm, especially your elbow, so don't try to get the most spin that has ever been imparted onto a pickleball in the history of the sport. Your goal is to keep your opponents guessing and having to make last-second adjustments, not to spin the ball so much that it causes them to "whiff" every shot. Hone some nice consistent spin shots and use them intermittently. They are important tools in your pickleball toolbox, but not your only tools.

Dropping with topspin or backspin

After you gain a pretty good command of spin shots, especially topspin and backspin, you can start integrating spin into your drop shots. Putting spin on a drop shot is a great way to really "level up" your game because you're turning a fairly defensive or neutral shot — the drop — into an offensive weapon, a.k.a. the Drop of Doom! Few things are sweeter in pickleball than winning a point off your drop shot. Many players hit all their drops either with topspin or backspin and argue about which technique is better. We encourage you to learn and use both.

Topspin on drop shots allows you to add more pace. Topspin enables you to hit a harder ball, but one that still drops low after the apex. Whenever you can add pace to the ball, you take time away from your opponents. With a faster-traveling drop shot, you may be able to catch your opponents out of position. They will also have less time to analyze the situation and select their next shot. When you hit a good drop, your opponent has to bend low and get under the ball. If they have to do this with a faster ball, they will definitely have more difficulty controlling it and may accidentally pop the ball up.

Backspin drop shots are one of our favorite shots, especially when hit crosscourt with a backhand slice. This is a fantastic shot because after it clears the net and drops on the other side, it bounces low and usually skids a little. Backspin is typically easier to do with your backhand, but you can experiment with forehands, too. Take that paddle back, up by your ear, lay your paddle face open a little, and swing through the ball. The paddle face must be slightly open at contact. Don't forget your forward follow-through and weight shift, and don't try to hit backspin if your weight is on your back foot. Hitting off your back foot with an open paddle face usually results in a pop-up!

Spinning your dinks

We talk a lot in this book about dinking offensively, which primarily involves using targets and preventing your opponents from getting into a rhythm. You can't hit dinks with much pace, so there's only so much variety you can add there, but you *can* spin them. Mixing up your dinks with different spins and targets will keep your opponents guessing and show them that you simply cannot be trusted! You force your opponents to think on the fly rather than several moves ahead. You also demand better footwork from them as they adjust to each unique bounce.

When dinking against players who tend to let the ball bounce too close to themselves, add some topspin to really jam them up. The ball will bounce and then accelerate into their body. This technique is great for encouraging your opponent to back away from the kitchen line. To dink with topspin, hit over the top of the ball with a flat or very slightly closed paddle face. Think of it as a slight brushing motion. Be sure to finish with a long, pretty follow-through that guides the ball toward your target. Keep applying pressure to the player who is backing up until they make a mistake.

If you want your dink to die a little when it bounces, hit it with backspin. Hit under the ball, swinging slightly high to low with an open paddle face. This shot is particularly useful if you're playing against someone who is proficient at the

Around the Post (ATP) shots (explained later in this chapter). Put backspin on any dinks that you're hitting toward the sideline to help prevent the ball from traveling so wide that they can slide over and hit an ATP. Backspin dinks are also a great tool for resets. If a dinking rally isn't going your way, hit a shallow, backspin dink toward the center of the kitchen. Your opponents can do very little with this ball besides hit a neutral dink back. This strategy can buy your team some much needed time to recover and get back into ready position.

Adding some sidespin to your dinks also helps keep them unattackable. Neutral, flat dinks are like blank canvases that invite your opponents to take control by placing their next dink exactly where they want (and with any type of spin). A spinning dink, on the other hand, limits your opponent's options. They will have to concentrate a little harder on analyzing the ball and not allowing your spin to mess up their next shot. Sidespin also pairs well with inside-out forehand dinks, which involve adding some deception to your shot by facing one direction and then hitting in the opposite direction. If you see your opponent pinching the middle of the court, hit a sidespin dink toward the sideline behind them and watch them scramble!

REMEMBER

Again, it's important not to overdo your use of spin. Don't attempt to add a ton of "junk" to every ball before you've become proficient at basic dinking. Whenever you strike the ball with an open or closed, rather than flat, paddle face, you are effectively shrinking the sweet spot found in the middle of the paddle. This means you need to be incredibly accurate with your contact point. If you're off-balance, out of position, or otherwise in a defensive position, that's not the time to get fancy!

Handling your opponent's spin

To deal effectively with spin coming your way, you first have to learn to anticipate it. Carefully watch what it looks like when players hit with different spins. Is their swing going from high to low? That's backspin, so the ball's not going to bounce much. Are they swinging from low to high? That's topspin, and the ball will bounce high and then accelerate. Is it a sidespin? It's going to bounce left or right, depending on how it was struck. If you find a player who hits these spins, ask them to drill with you. Spinners love to play around with spin, so they will probably really enjoy it!

TIP

You can also practice dealing with the actual bounces of various spins by using a ball machine that can produce spin. The disadvantage of a ball machine is that you're not practicing anticipation skills because you're not seeing the player generate the spin with their stroke.

Here are some tips on how to handle balls hit to you with spin:

>> **Lift the ball a little more.** You'll typically have to open your paddle face slightly to absorb the spin and give the ball some added lift. This lift will help you to stop hitting those pesky spin shots into the net.

>> **Take the ball out in front of you.** If you let the ball get in too close to your body and too far back in your stance, you will find that your paddle gets pushed back by the spin instead of neutralizing the spin by hitting through it.

>> **Keep your chin up.** Dropping your chin often leads to inadvertently closing your paddle face, which causes your shot to go into the net.

>> **Hit the ball sooner, on the rise.** The farther you let the ball travel after the bounce, the more of the spin effect you'll see. It will travel into, or away from, your body more and more the longer you delay.

>> **Bend your knees.** You need to really get under those low-bouncing backspin shots.

>> **Take a short backswing.** Committing to a big backswing makes it difficult to adjust quickly. Spinning balls often require last-millisecond adjustments.

>> **Don't set your feet too early.** You delay setting your feet for the same reason you don't take that big backswing: You need to be able to make adjustments. Dealing with spin on the ball is very much like playing in the wind. Keep those feet light and nimble.

>> **Take a firm approach.** Hit through the ball with a lot of forward momentum, a bit of extra lift, and a long follow-through. Gently tapping at the ball doesn't give it enough guidance or energy to counteract any spin.

>> **Don't let it get in your head.** Spin can make shots more challenging, but not unmanageable. You can do this! Hit confidently *through* the ball with your solid strokes. We believe in you!

WARNING

It can be tempting to try to match or counter the spin of an oncoming ball. If you're a strong spinner yourself, countering the spin may work for you. However, for most players, this tactic doesn't typically end well. A neutral drive with some added lift is the highest-percentage shot to use against heavy spin.

Relishing the Attack

You had to know that there would be the occasional pickle pun in this book. (We feel we've been pretty good at restraining ourselves thus far.) No need to get sour or make a big dill out of it. In this section, we encourage you to "relish" (in case you missed that one) your attack, meaning that as you advance in skill level, we want you to capitalize on attackable balls in as many different situations as possible. Going for attackable balls, however, does not mean letting your eyes get wide as the drool gushes from your gaping mouth, taking a huge windup, and blasting the ball into the fence. That's just giving away points.

We hope you've committed Chapter 11 of this book to memory, or at least skimmed it while learning to speed read. Chapter 11 has a great deal of information about when and when not to attack. As you read this section, assume that it's time to attack — and these are some of your options!

Poaching: Not just for eggs

If you look up "poaching" in a dictionary, you find a couple different definitions. One is a delicious way of preparing eggs. Another, less savory definition involves trespassing on another person's game preserve in order to hunt. In pickleball, *poaching* refers to crossing over to the other side of the court to attack a ball. In that sense, it's about "hunting" in an area that may appear to be your partner's property (meaning, their side of the court). Poaching is neither illegal nor unsavory in pickleball! In fact, it's a great idea.

Here are the main reasons you may want to poach:

>> **Positioning:** You're closer to the net than your partner and therefore in a more offensive position. You can take balls at a higher point than they would be by the time they reach your partner standing behind you.

>> **Reach:** You're taller and have a longer reach than your partner, so you're able to strike balls from a higher point and swing down more.

>> **Skill level:** You're a better player than your partner, or at least have stronger attacks.

>> **Surprise:** Your opponents have fallen into a pattern or are attempting to isolate the weaker player on your team. Start poaching at unexpected times to throw them off their game plan.

>> **Greed:** You're a bit selfish and feel the need to hit every ball. This last one is *not* a good reason to poach!

The centerline exists only to mark the right and left service boxes — not to divide partners. Pickleball is not meant to be played by two people operating independently inside adjacent rectangles. You can, and should, cross the centerline whenever it will benefit your team. If you watch professional or other high-level pickleball, you may be surprised by how often players cross and switch. Free yourself from the confines of your rectangle and watch your game soar! Just be sure to communicate with your partner before, during, and after the rally. The more you can play with a regular partner, the easier crossing and switching becomes. Figure 14-9 shows a player poaching. Notice how happy he looks. Poaching can be really fun!

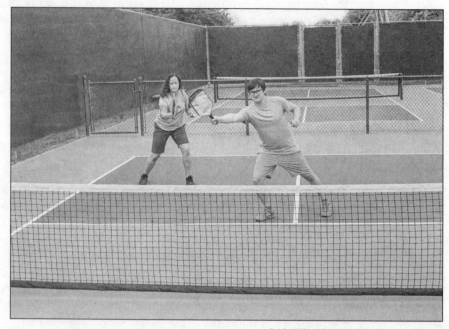

FIGURE 14-9: A player poaching from a good position and in good balance.

For many beginner or intermediate players, poaching doesn't come naturally. As a beginner, you may have felt you had enough on your plate just trying to cover "your" side of the court. With pickleball being such a social sport, you are probably also concerned about how other players view you and don't want to be seen as an inconsiderate ball hog. However, more advanced players know the value of poaching and recognize that you're only doing what's best for the team. A well-executed poach is often celebrated enthusiastically by the poacher's partner. Don't be shy about adding this great strategy to your game!

Here are some tips on how to poach effectively:

>> **Look for the right ball.** You perform a poach using a lateral movement toward a ball that is above the net and heading toward the opposite side of the court from you. It must still be an attackable ball by the time you actually get to it — not a ball that has since dropped below the level of the net.

>> **Be sneaky.** Just as in any other type of hunting, poaching is best done as a sneak attack. If you broadcast your intentions to your opponents, all they have to do is hit the ball in the opposite direction from what you expected, where nobody is home! If you move to poach at the last second, the opponents cannot hit such a great anticipatory shot.

>> **Poach from a strong position.** The ideal area in which to poach is just a bit behind the kitchen line. You need to be forward in the court so that you have enough room to hit down on the ball without sending it straight into the net.

>> **Step off from your outside leg.** If you are poaching from left to right, push off from your left foot and move toward the right. If you are poaching from right to left, take off with a push from your right foot. Try your best not to cross-step. If you're crossing your feet, one in front of the other, you are more likely to commit a kitchen violation or wind up off-balance.

>> **Keep at least one foot on the ground.** Poaching is done with quick, careful, well-balanced footwork. It is *not* a flying leap through the air! A sideways leap will make timing your swing extremely difficult and guarantee the need for a few seconds to regain your balance and position should your shot be well defended and returned to you.

>> **Don't over-hit it.** Use a compact, authoritative volley aimed at an area of open court or the nearest opponent's feet. Your attack shot can also be very effective if hit to the nearest opponent's dominant hip. Don't overdo your attack, especially if you're still in motion at the point of the contact or it's likely to go out or in the net.

>> **Communicate.** If you've committed to going all the way over to the opposite side of the court, it's best to stay there after your shot and let your partner switch to cover the other side of the court. Either you or your partner should yell "switch!" or "stay!" to let the other know what to do.

REMEMBER

Poaching doesn't have to be viewed as a selfish act. In fact, it can be a great way to help your partner. Say you made it to the kitchen line, but your partner is stuck deep in the court. By intercepting a ball coming toward them, you're giving them the opportunity to keep coming forward instead of having to stop and deal with the ball. If you're a sneaky team, your partner may just *act* like they are slowly and lazily moving forward after their serve return. This act pretty much guarantees that the third shot will be hit in their direction. You pounce over for a poach while your partner moves diagonally behind you to occupy the space you've just left. You may even call this fancy play in advance by using hand signals. (See Chapter 12 for more on stacking, switching, and signaling.)

THE ETHICS OF POACHING

We hope we've convinced you that poaching can be a positive addition to any team's playbook. Keep in mind, however, that many recreational players don't care for poaching. They may feel that a shot is being stolen from them, or that you are implying you're a far superior player who needs to "take over" the entire court. People have a right to their feelings, so please respect them. When heading out on the court during a casual drop-in session, you may ask your partner, "How do you feel about poaching?" or "How do you like to handle balls to the middle?" Or any other questions that may help you and your new partner connect as a team and enjoy your time on the court as much as possible.

If your partner indicates that they don't like players coming onto "their" side, adjust your behavior accordingly. If they make broad statements such as "forehand takes middle," be aware that they may not use the same strategies as you. That doesn't mean you should give them a lesson. Just relax and play, making adjustments to your game as needed. If they want your advice after the game, you can tell them about this great book you read (hint, hint).

It's certainly fun when you and your partner are on the same page and can play as a well-oiled team, but even highly skilled players sometimes have different opinions on how the game should be played. Right or wrong, we can all learn from each other — and have a fantastic time doing it!

TIP

If you're just getting used to the idea of poaching, try this fun play whenever your partner is receiving serve and you're up at the kitchen line: After your partner hits their return, and just before the serving team hits their third shot, take a half step (slide) toward the centerline. Look for a ball that comes back to the middle anywhere you can possibly reach, and punish it with an offensive volley. It's important that you don't make the move too soon. If you do, the serving team will just hit their third shot down one of the sidelines. This "light" edition of poaching doesn't require you to fully commit to changing sides and involves very little risk. It will, however, help train you to start looking for those high, floating balls that are within your reach but not necessarily on "your" side of the court.

Surprising your opponents with an Erne (or a Bert)

One of the best strategies you can employ in pickleball is to take time away from your opponents. If they have less time to react, they are less likely to hit a good shot and much more likely to hit a ball that sits up nicely for you to pounce on.

A very popular time-stealing shot is the *Erne* (pronounced like "Ernie"). This shot is named after Erne Perry, one of the early top players who first used it regularly in competition. Although considered an advanced move, it can be done with a little practice. Many players view it as a milestone the first time they successfully execute this shot in a game. ("Dear Diary, today I hit my first Erne, and it was marvelous!")

So what the heck is it? You do the Erne by stepping around, or jumping over, the corner of the kitchen and hitting a volley just after the ball has crossed over the net. This shot is legal because the player is technically not contacting the kitchen. (As we describe in Chapter 2, the out-of-bounds area next to the kitchen is not considered part of it.) Figure 14-10 shows a player who has stepped around the kitchen to hit the Erne. Both of his feet are out of bounds, so this player is not committing a kitchen violation despite standing very close to the net.

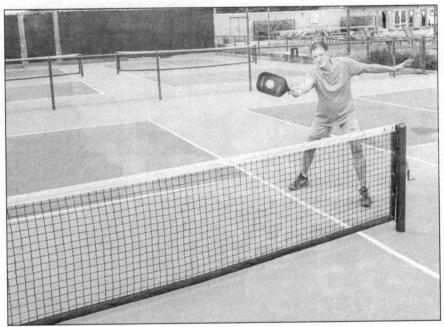

FIGURE 14-10:
A happy player hitting a perfectly legal Erne.

© John Wiley & Sons, Inc./Photo Credit: Aniko Kiezel

The time to hit an Erne is when your opponent has sent the ball down the sideline near you and floated it up a little too high. This scenario most commonly occurs during dinking rallies. You can patiently wait for your opponent to make this mistake on their own, or you can set yourself up for an Erne by using the dinking patterns we cover in Chapter 12. Wait until your opponent contacts the ball before making your move. Step outside the kitchen and then move forward, toward the net post. Strike the ball out in front of you with a crisp volley aimed sharply downward. As you do this, your partner should move over to cover the middle because you've left the court. If all goes well, your shot is a winner and your team doesn't need to worry about recovering back into position after your bold move (but be ready either way)!

Even if you don't get the high ball you hoped for and don't wind up hitting the Erne, you have let your opponents know that you *may* hit one. It is not uncommon to see fake Ernes, when a player steps around and straddles the corner of the kitchen but doesn't actually take the early volley. Players fake an Erne to make the opponents uneasy about hitting any balls down the sideline. You've effectively closed off that part of the court simply by threatening an Erne.

The biggest challenges with this shot are recognizing which balls are "Erne-able" and, of course, avoiding a kitchen fault in the process. You'll want to drill this new skill a few times to get a good feel for the footwork before attempting to use it in a game. Otherwise, you'll probably end up watching your feet instead of the ball. The Erne tends to be a little easier to do on the forehand side. It is certainly doable on the backhand side as well, though. Both sides require practice.

Here are a few things to watch out for when hitting the Erne:

>> **Don't leave the court too early.** If you leave too early, you lose the element of surprise and your opponent has time to react and hit into the space you just left behind. Instead of looking super cool with your sweet Erne put-away, you may end up feeling a bit silly! Failed Ernes usually lead to a lot of giggling. (We promise we're laughing *with* you, not *at* you!)

>> **Don't leave too late.** You may miss the ball entirely and watch it sail right past you! Timing is everything on this shot.

>> **Don't do it too frequently.** This shot should have an element of surprise to it. Also, your partner may not appreciate being pulled over to the middle constantly to cover the entire court every time you "leave the building."

>> **Don't drag your foot through the kitchen.** After either foot contacts the kitchen, you'll need time to reestablish both feet outside the kitchen before you're allowed to volley. If you can avoid touching the kitchen at all (by stepping or jumping over it), you won't have to worry about reestablishing your feet outside the kitchen again before you hit.

>> **Don't step or land in the kitchen after your shot.** You can't touch the kitchen until after you have regained your balance from your volley. Remember that the kitchen rules dictate not touching the kitchen in the act of volleying, but after you've regained your balance, your momentum from that

prior shot ends. This means that after your Erne put-away, you can calmly turn around and walk through the kitchen without fear of being called for a foot fault. If the ball is still in play, we recommend that you come back *around* the kitchen to get in position. Otherwise, your wise opponent will just tag you with the ball as you're strolling back through the kitchen (oops).

To defend against an Erne, you can try to hit the player's body with the ball, or lob it over them. The best way to deal with an Erne-loving player is to avoid dinking near the sidelines in the first place. This is often a good chance to practice your misdirection skills. Try to look like you're going to dink right into their Erne "sweet spot," and wait for them to make their move. Then hit the ball right to the open space they've left behind.

The *Bert* is much less common than the Erne. It's a crazy shot that is basically a combination of a poach and an Erne. Like an Erne, it involves leaping the kitchen, but is done by the partner on the far side of the court leaping in front of their partner and over their half of the kitchen. It's like an Erne on four shots of espresso! Figure 14-11 shows you a diagram of what the Erne and the Bert look like on the court.

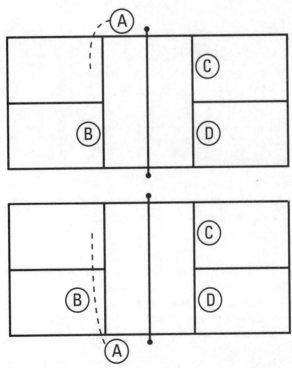

FIGURE 14-11:
A player's path of travel when hitting an Erne (top) versus a Bert (bottom).

Hitting the Around the Post (ATP) shot

The *Around the Post* or *ATP* shot is another fun and interesting attack shot. The name is pretty self-explanatory: You literally hit the ball around the net post instead of over the net. This shot is legal, fun, and exciting! To be clear, we don't just hit this shot because it's fun, but because it's also a very difficult shot to defend against.

A player typically hits the ATP shot during a dinking rally, after an opponent has sent a dink way out wide at a sharp angle. Figure 14-12 shows a player who has moved out wide and is directing the ball around the net post, rather than over the net. She will hit her shot so that it travels very low to the ground, giving her opponent almost no chance of hitting it before it bounces twice.

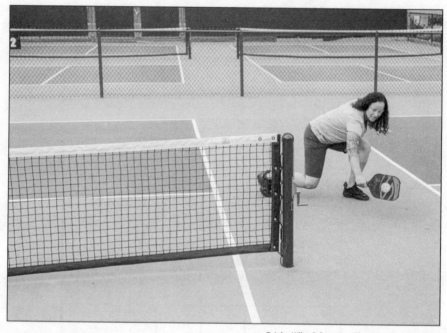

FIGURE 14-12:
Hitting an Around the Post (ATP) shot.

© John Wiley & Sons, Inc./Photo Credit: Aniko Kiezel

Notice that she has waited a beat for the ball to drop down low. You should hit the ATP just before the ball bounces a second time. This delay assures that the ball has traveled as far wide off the court as possible so that you'll be able to completely clear the post. Remember, this shot does not go over the net, but rather around it, so for maximum advantage, try to hit the ball so that it just barely skims the ground. Wicked!

You have a few things to consider when it comes to attempting an ATP. Not every pickleball venue has enough space on the sides of the court to hit the ATP. If you try this shot where there's not enough room, you may find yourself with chain link–shaped "grill marks" on your face and body. Ouch! Also, if you and your friends pile up your pickleball bags, chairs, and water bottles along the side of the court, you may be ruining your chances to hit an ATP. It's always safest to keep these items entirely off the courts, if possible.

To defend against an opponent's ATP down your sideline, shuffle back and get low. This ball is likely to come at you deep and low. Defending the ATP is not easy, but it can be done! The smartest move is to prevent the ATP in the first place by not hitting a ball out too wide. Although sharply angled dinks can be a great tool for moving opponents off the court and creating a hole, if you're playing against someone who is skilled at hitting ATPs, you will need to tread a fine line. Dink wide, but not too wide. At advanced levels, a dink that bounces in bounds but travels out too wide is considered an error because it invites an ATP. As mentioned earlier in this chapter, adding some backspin to your wide-angled dinks will help prevent them from bouncing too far and setting up your opponent for an easy ATP.

Attacking with flicks and rolls

Two more attack shots to add to your toolbox are *flicks* and *rolls.* These are both speedup shots that you typically hit from the kitchen line. The beauty of these two shots is that they can easily be disguised as dinks. Your opponent won't see the attack coming until it's too late!

The flick shot

A *flick* is a forehand or backhand speedup on a dink that may have set up a bit too high (often off the bounce). It's hit from a height slightly below the top of the net. Disguise your flick to look like a regular, straight-ahead dink. Remember, surprise attacks are the best attacks! Drop your paddle head below the height of your wrist, just as you do on your dinks. Then accelerate forward with your wrist and arm. This is one time you're allowed to get wristy, because we want you to quickly generate paddle-head speed by flicking your wrist. Be sure you're still swinging upward and forward to generate the topspin needed to clear the net.

Flicks are typically aimed right at the chest of the opponent standing closest to you, or even better, to their dominant side hip or shoulder. You're counting on the element of surprise and defeating your opponent's reaction time, so watch for moments when an opponent is off-balance or has dropped their paddle down low. Flicking the ball right at an opponent who is standing in good ready position won't be particularly effective.

The roll shot

A *roll* is a heavy topspin shot that you hit farther out in front of your body, just like you hit your dink volleys. Hit plenty of dink volleys in your game so that your opponents won't expect this speedup when you decide to use it. Stay as close to the kitchen line as possible. Bend your knees and bring your paddle down by your toes for the backswing. The follow-through involves essentially driving your paddle upward and forward at an angle of approximately 45 degrees. This motion imparts generous amounts of topspin and some forward momentum on the ball. To get that heavy topspin, it can help to think about brushing up the back of the ball as you push forward.

In case you're wondering what the difference is between the flick and the roll shots, it is essentially that the flick is more of an abrupt, forward paddle motion, whereas the roll uses more of an upward brushing motion, with your paddle face almost parallel with the net.

Your targets for the roll shot are similar to the flick because they are both surprise attacks from the kitchen line. Hit them to the opponent directly in front of you, aiming for their dominant side in the hip-to-shoulder area. You can also aim for spots just out of reach so that your opponent has to stretch. Because the attack is a surprise, the stretch is likely to be awkward for them. Be ready to attack again because even if they do get their paddle on the ball, it's likely to be a pop-up. Nice job!

Roll shots also make great passing shots. If you see an opponent pinching the middle, set up as though you're going to dink to the middle, but instead hit an inside-out roll shot behind them and down the sideline. Or push your opponent wide with a dink and then follow up with a roll shot down the middle. We also love using the roll shot as a fourth shot, when you're up at the line but your opponents are still making their way in. If their third shot wasn't attackable with a volley, you can still make an offensive shot by rolling the ball up and over the net, aiming for their feet. If they allow the ball to bounce, the heavy topspin you added will cause it to kick up into their body, making for a very awkward shot.

Chapter **15**

Strengthening Your Mental Game: Use Your Noggin!

Pickleball is a physically demanding game that can push your body to its limits. You'll obviously play better if your body is prepared for the fast moves and athletic twists and turns that pickleball requires. Equally important to your pickleball success and enjoyment is your mental fitness. As with physical fitness, mental fitness takes focus, training, and maintenance. Do not skip over the development of your mental game. Commit to working on it. It may just be one of the best things you ever do for yourself outside of a therapist's office!

For many players, the biggest obstacle to playing well arises from their mental game. You may have recognized this obstacle in others, or even yourself. A couple unforced errors in a row, a bad line call, tournament nerves — these are all seemingly small things that have the potential to implode your game. Even if you have no issues with your mental game right now, this chapter can help when issues come up in the future. You also learn how to become the World's Greatest Doubles Partner by consistently supporting your partner with positivity. It's one of the best things you can do to increase your team's chances of victory.

Competing under pressure can bring up feelings of insecurity, lack of self-worth, anger, frustration, envy, and many other unpleasant emotions. Think of it as an opportunity to confront these feelings, learn, and grow. Thankfully, many top athletes have recently been sharing their struggles and shedding light on the mental health issues so many people deal with. Leave the stigma in the past and allow your strength of mind to become a great asset to your pickleball game, and your life.

Keeping Patient and Focused

You have probably noticed throughout this book that we encourage patience when playing this great game. Rushing through your shots, or speeding up balls that aren't ripe enough to attack, will almost always work against you. You need to slow down, do the work, build the point, and finish it off when the time is right. Some of us are naturally more patient than others. If you're typically short on patience, here's some good news: Pickleball gives you a great opportunity to cultivate it!

Along with patience, staying focused is also challenging for many players. After a couple hours of hard play, you are likely getting tired, hungry and sore. Instead of focusing on your game, you're busy daydreaming about going home to devour a charcuterie board and drink champagne while soaking in a bubble bath. (We hear pickleball is big with celebrities these days, so we wanted to make sure they feel included in this book.) Sometimes, external distractions like loud music, funky smells, or especially boisterous players can cause you to lose focus.

Fortunately, there are some tricks to staying patient and focused on the pickleball court:

>> **Arrive prepared:** If Serena Williams unexpectedly showed up at your door, you may be totally freaked out and overwhelmed. If you had a chance to prepare for her visit by cleaning your house and hiding all your Serena posters, you would be able to enjoy her visit with a much calmer demeanor. Readiness brings calm, so do everything you can to be ready. Pack your bag carefully, dress for success, eat something nourishing, hydrate, arrive early, stretch, and warm up fully. Then you'll know you're ready to play your best. Bring it on!

>> **Walk, don't run:** Try to walk as much as possible whenever you're on the court. Sure, you should hustle up to the kitchen line as soon as you've hit a serve return. In most other situations, you will find that you're better off walking throughout the court. Make adjustments to get to the ball and then return to being in good court position, and in good balance. (See Chapter 11 for more on staying in your lane on the court) Wild, frantic, anaerobic movements are not going to help you stay in a Zen frame of mind!

>> **Use your time wisely:** If you are not currently hitting the ball, instead of just stopping to admire your partner's pretty forehand or your opponent's cute skort, use that time to improve your court position. This gives you a goal to focus on even when it's not your turn to hit. Getting caught "spectating" is common but easily avoidable. Along with keeping you focused, being in good position means fewer frantic moments trying to scurry for a ball your opponent has wisely hit into the open court.

>> **Paddle track:** In Chapter 11, we talk about *paddle tracking,* which means keeping your paddle and both hands out in front of your body while squaring to the ball. Good paddle tracking helps you maintain focus throughout the point and is an invaluable habit to acquire. Not only is it almost impossible to lose focus while paddle tracking, it also helps to keep you ready at all times. With readiness comes calm. You will be amazed at how much the game seems to slow down!

>> **Remember to have fun:** You most likely took up pickleball because you wanted to add more play to your life. Hold that intention close. Make sure that you are *playing* pickleball. Relax and enjoy your time. If your goal is to get every rally over as quickly as possible, you won't be making smart decisions. Instead, have fun using the different shots in your toolbox and moving your opponents around to create different patterns and plays. You're on a pickleball court with friends. Hopefully, that alone brings you joy, so don't be in a rush to get out of there!

Patience ultimately comes from confidence. If you know you can hang in there indefinitely in a long dinking rally, why get impatient and attack a ball that isn't attackable? Build the point and wait for your moment. It may come early in the rally. That's great! It may come at the end of a long and exhausting exchange, but that's fine, too. The rally may speed up and slow down several times. Just stay calm and stick to your plan. When you get the chance to end the rally with a high-percentage attack, take it. Or, your opponent may be less consistent or less patient than you and hit the ball out or into the net. In that case, your patience just became your greatest weapon! We think that's one of the coolest things about this sport.

Assessing Opponents' Strengths and Weaknesses

One way you can really help your mental game is to know what you're up against. Fewer surprises mean less chaos. Less chaos means calm confidence. So, whenever possible, try to assess your opponents' strengths and weaknesses.

Advanced players know that to get the upper hand in a match, you must prevent your opponents from hitting their best shots while trying to pick on their weaker shots. Simply playing the same game against every team does not work. As a fun bonus, you can employ this strategy quite sneakily. Your opponents may notice they're not playing their best but not recognize why, and frustration sets in. Now you've disarmed both their physical and mental games at the same time! (Winning isn't always pretty.) To use this strategy successfully, you need to figure out your opponents' strengths and weaknesses. You do so through careful observation before or during your own match, or by gathering intelligence from other players.

If you get a chance to watch your opponents play another match before yours, take it! This is an opportunity to glean a ton of valuable information. Here are some things to note while you observe your opponents:

>> Are they left- or right-handed?

>> Do they switch hands when they play (ambidextrous)?

>> Is the team stacking or switching?

>> What types of serves do they use?

>> Which partner has a weaker return or third shot?

>> How mobile are they?

>> How long can they last in a dinking rally before making an error?

>> Do they like to lob, and in which situations?

>> Are they typically the first person to speed up the ball?

>> How well can they handle a body shot?

>> Is the team pinching the middle or backing up off the line?

>> Do they communicate well on middle balls?

Often, you don't get a chance to really study your opponents. You watch them warm up only while you're also trying to warm up, making it tough to concentrate on getting the information you're looking for. At least you can tell whether they're left-handed, tall, short, fast, or slow. You can gain more information after the match starts, so try testing your opponents early on. How do they handle a drive, a lob, a flick? Are they lining up to return your serve in such a way that they won't have to hit a backhand? Hmmm, this probably means they don't have a good backhand, or at the very least that they don't believe in their backhand. Good to know. Hit to their backhand! Adjust your play to take advantage of their weaknesses and minimize their strengths.

TIP

Communicate regularly with your partner to point out what you're noticing. You may each notice different things, so share them and work as a team to adjust your strategies. If things go well for your team when you are playing either diagonally or straight across from a certain opponent, consider stacking or switching (explained in Chapter 12) to be able to set up that situation regularly. If your opponents pinch the middle, hit out wide to the angles they're leaving open, or jam them up by driving it straight to the middle. If they bend forward at the waist, they may be good players to lob over. You have many options if you pay attention to the players and patterns on the other side of the net. Make the adjustments as a team and then watch your step as you ascend the medal podium.

Developing Anticipation Skills

Pickleball is an incredibly fast-moving sport. Without good anticipation skills, you will find yourself always reacting to the ball rather than deliberately acting on it. This means your opponent gets to dictate what happens throughout the point. That's no good! You can't implement any of your smart strategies when you have zero say in what's happening.

Learning to anticipate the next ball before your opponent even strikes it helps to situate you in the right place most of the time. The game slows down for you because of your increased readiness. Shots feel easier because you're in good balance and have more time to think about where to place them. You may wonder whether you've suddenly developed psychic powers. Perhaps so, but it's probably just your enhanced anticipation skills!

Reading your opponents

The previous section delves into assessing your opponents to anticipate what will happen next. Are they hard-hitting bangers? You just fed them a yellow-light ball to their forehand — gird your loins; it's coming back fast! Are they soft-game aficionados? That same yellow-light ball will likely be returned as a well-targeted dink. Knowing what shots your opponents love to hit helps you predict what they'll do next.

TIP

Knowing your opponent's tendencies also helps you anticipate "out" balls. You don't need to be ready for a huge drive at your chest if that particular opponent always hits them out. You know to just get out of the way and be prepared to extend your index finger to indicate that the ball has sailed past the baseline, just as you anticipated. The same goes for lobs — no need to waste energy chasing down every lob if your opponent hits 90 percent of them out. It's smart to play the percentages, even if you lose a few points here and there when your opponent manages to pull off a shot they almost always miss.

In addition to learning your opponent's preferred style of play, you want to develop your ability to read a player's body language. Most players project their intentions much more obviously than they realize. Deception is an advanced skill and is hard to pull off while you're busy executing a finesse shot.

As your opponent sets up to hit, pay attention to the following clues:

>> **Backswing:** If you see your opponent taking a giant windup, they're probably about to drive the ball hard!

>> **Feet position:** On groundstrokes, watch where your opponent plants their feet, and notice which direction their front foot is pointed in; this is where their weight will be transferred, which usually indicates the direction of the shot.

>> **Direction of head and eyes:** Unless they are deliberately trying to deceive you with a "no look" or a "head fake" shot, players tend to look exactly where they are aiming.

>> **Paddle-face angle:** The ball generally goes where the paddle face is pointed at contact. Watch for an open, closed, or flat paddle face, as well as the angle (right or left).

>> **Swing path:** Are they swinging low to high, or high to low? Obviously, these will result in two very different shots. You can also learn to anticipate spin based on an opponent's swing path (see Chapter 14 for much more about spin).

>> **Facial expression:** This one's a little more subtle, but if you play with the same people all the time, you may begin to notice that their face gives their intentions away. Our friend loves to lob, and we swear she gets a "lobbish" look on her face every time she's about to hit one! Like a great poker player, look for these sorts of "tells" to gain the advantage.

WARNING

Reading your opponent's face and body language is an incredibly useful skill, but don't be discouraged if it takes some time to develop. As a beginner or intermediate player, you're mostly focused on what you and your partner are doing. As you acquire experience, you start to notice what's happening across the net more easily. You will eventually gain the ability to track the ball, your partner, and your opponents' subtle movements all at the same time. Just keep playing and practicing, and trust that it will come!

Having a plan

A great way to slow down the game in your brain and improve your ability to anticipate is to have a plan. You can form your initial plan before the point even begins. It feels a bit like cheating, but it's not!

Your plan will vary based on your role:

» **Server:** This is a great position to be in because the server is the first player to dictate how the rally will go. Think through what type of serve you want to hit, and where you want it to land. Your decision should depend largely on what type of serve you think that particular receiver will struggle with the most. Next, think about what to do if the return comes back to you. Where do you want to hit the third shot? That's right — you plan your third shot before the point even begins! It's best to get as many decisions out of the way before all the excitement begins.

» **Server's partner:** As the server's partner, make a plan to stay back behind the baseline (don't creep!) until the ball comes back to your team. You should plan your third shot as well. You don't know which partner will get the return, so you may as well be prepared in case it's you. Have an alternative plan for what to do if your partner ends up hitting the third shot. (See the section in Chapter 12 about going hunting for our favorite option.)

» **Receiver:** We hope you've been paying attention to how your opponent tends to serve. Line up in an optimal position based on whether you think the ball will come short, deep, wide, and so on. Next, make a plan about where to return the ball: to the weaker opponent (who has an inferior third shot), the stronger one (to keep them back), or to the middle (to cause confusion or cut down available angles for their return). This is also a good time to remind yourself that right after you've hit your amazing return, you need to get your booty up to the kitchen line and join your partner.

» **Receiver's partner:** In this position, you strive to perfect your ready position at the line. Be prepared to look over your shoulder to call the serve short or out if necessary, and watch your partner hit their return so that you can collect as much data as possible. You may also make a plan to slide a half step to the middle just before the third shot is struck so that you can intercept it with an offensive volley. (We detail this play in Chapter 14.) Think about what targets to aim for should you get to hit the fourth shot. Your shot selection and target will vary based on whether it's a low or high ball and how close your opponents are to the kitchen line.

All this planning ahead can improve both your game and your mental state. Planning makes you hit the ball mindfully instead of just getting it back over the net. Planning can also increase your confidence. Of course, plans can, and must, change mid-rally based on what your partner or opponents decide to do; you can't, after all, control three other people. If you have to adjust your plan, do it consciously. Try to play your game the way you want to play it instead of reacting unconsciously to your opponents' game.

Be prepared to let your plans evolve throughout the match. Your plan on the first serve of the game will probably not be the same on the tenth, unless you're currently winning 10–0–2, in which case, don't change a thing! When things aren't going your way, do something different. If returning to one player isn't working, return the serve to the other player and see how that goes. If your crosscourt drops are all going into the net today, aim for the middle where the net is slightly lower. Mix up your serves if your opponent has started expertly handling the serves you've been using so far.

REMEMBER

Remember to always share your brilliant plans with your partner. If you are planning to beat a team with your well-honed soft game, but your partner has decided that it will be "all hard, all the time," this match is not going to end well (but it sounds fun to watch)! Keep checking in with your partner throughout the game. In a tournament setting, that's what time-outs are for, so be sure to take advantage of them. Your partner may have noticed something you haven't. If you've realized that every time Bob goes out wide for a backhand dink, he pops it up, share this with your partner. This shared intelligence is gold and can often lead to medals of the same color. See Chapter 11 for more on partner communication.

Adapting to Unfavorable Weather Conditions

When you play pickleball outdoors, you have to consider the weather conditions. Being poorly prepared can really throw off your mental game. It's distracting to constantly think about how cold you are because you underdressed. ("Pants. I should have worn pants.") Becoming overheated or dehydrated will tank your game faster than just about anything ("Why on earth did I wear pants?!") Your authors live in Sacramento, California, where summer temperatures regularly soar over 100 degrees, so we know a thing or two about getting overheated. The more practice you have playing in different environments, the less challenging these problems become, because you can mentally prepare and adapt.

When playing outside, be sure to dress appropriately for the weather, including potentially changing weather. Layers are always your best bet. Your body temperature will almost certainly rise as you get moving. Breathable, moisture-wicking performance fabrics are ideal for keeping you cool and dry. Hats and visors can also help you to deal with sunny or cold conditions. If you tend to sweat quite a bit, a hat, visor, or headband can prevent that wonderful feeling of an ocean of sunscreen pouring into your eyeballs.

Many players like to wear gloves in cold weather to prevent their hands from becoming stiff or numb. For your paddle hand, we recommend a thinner type of glove (such as a racquetball glove) to maintain a good feel on the paddle. You can also try the Tourna Hot Glove, which is a fleece mitt that goes over both your hand and paddle handle, helping your hand to stay warm without losing the feel of the paddle.

On sunny days, beware of players whose lobs make you look directly into the sun. If you come up against a lobber, do your best to prevent the lob (see Chapter 12 for tips on prevention). If they do send a ball up over your head, try blocking the sun with your nondominant hand. Wearing sunglasses is always a smart move because it helps you avoid blindness both from the sun and from getting hit in the eye with the ball. (Chapter 3 has more about protective eyewear.)

When it's hot, safety becomes a real concern. An asphalt pickleball court runs around 10 degrees hotter than the outside temperature. Please be sure to hydrate before, during, and after you play, and supplement with electrolytes. Cooling towels soaked in ice water and personal misters are incredibly helpful. Sunscreen is a must. If no shade is available at your courts, bring your own stuff; you can even buy a folding camping chair with built-in shade! (Just know that everyone else will be jealous and try to sit in it when you're not looking, possibly leaving gross sweat stains on the seat. Ew.)

Windy days make pickleball highly challenging. After all, you're using a lightweight plastic ball that is full of holes. When the wind gusts higher than 12–15 MPH, a pickleball flies around unpredictably. This scenario can lead to a fun time with lots of surprises and giggling, but it can also be frustrating if you were hoping to hit precise shots that day.

Here are some tips to adapting to wind and playing your best:

>> **Get ready to lift the ball:** Keep in mind that the wind not only blows the ball from one side or another but often pushes the ball downward. Remember this tendency when both hitting and chasing after balls. The ball may travel or bounce much lower than you expect.

>> **Check the flag:** Many outdoor pickleball venues have a flag or windsock. Refer to that indicator frequently during your games because the wind direction can change. If you see that the wind is blowing hard in one direction, be sure to adjust your targeting accordingly.

- >> **Choose a bigger target:** When playing in the wind, never aim too close to the lines; allow yourself more wiggle room instead.

- >> **Avoid lobs:** A pickleball is difficult to control in the wind, and even more so when lofted high in the air. A lob must be struck carefully to be effective: not too low, or it will be taken as an overhead smash; and not too high, lest it be easily chased down. Add wind to the equation and a lob is a very low-percentage shot for most players.

- >> **Take a compact backswing:** This type of backswing makes it easier to make the micro adjustments necessary for windy play. If your paddle is way back behind you and the ball bounces either away from you, or into your body, making good contact with the ball will be challenging.

- >> **Don't set your feet too early:** The ball is moving around in the wind, so keep your last few steps quick and small to make the fine-tuned adjustments necessary to compensate for unexpected ball movement.

WARNING

Remember, the pickleball addiction is real, but don't ever play in unsafe conditions. It's just not worth it. Stay home, study this book, watch pickleball videos, and live unharmed to play another day.

Here are our rules for playing in various weather:

- >> **Rain, sleet, snow:** Don't play. It is far too easy to slip and fall on wet or icy courts.

- >> **Hail:** Hail no, don't play!

- >> **Sunny:** PLAY! What on earth would you consider doing instead?

- >> **Windy:** Play, if it's reasonable enough to still be fun. Be careful if you have a bad back because wind can lead to a lot of last-second jerky movements.

- >> **Cold:** Play, but layer up and bring plenty of balls (they crack easily in cold weather).

- >> **Hot:** Play only if it's safe for your body. (Everyone's heat tolerance varies.) Stop if you experience dizziness, nausea, or any other signs of heatstroke.

Maintaining a Positive Attitude: I Dink I Can, I Dink I Can . . .

Coauthors Mo and Reine named their teaching business "Positive Dinking" because they saw how vitally important the power of positivity is in pickleball. They had both taken lessons or clinics that sent them home crying and wanting to quit the game. Ugh! Pickleball is supposed to be fun, right? The moment a game turns into a negative experience, people's minds start to close up. The learning stops and the stress and self-doubt begin. It's the same way in a match. When a player's mind turns really negative, the ability to play well and adapt to changing conditions and strategies shrinks.

Some players find they play better when they adopt a serious, intense, and aggressive mindset. Smashing pickleballs may be their best outlet for relieving stress. That's fine. Harness that intensity and make it work for you, but try not to turn your aggression against yourself. You're doing the best you can. Keep reading for some ways to support a Very Important Person in your world: you!

Developing your on-court presence

Have you ever noticed that most of the top golfers don't show much emotion, at least until the round is over? They need to have steady nerves to deal with the pressure and accuracy required in their sport. This kind of steady calmness is also useful in pickleball. If you can stay calm, cool, and collected, you are much more likely to be a strong and consistent competitor that day.

The image you present on the court through your body language, self-talk, sense of fair play, and overall demeanor is more important than you may realize. Ideally, the qualities you want to project are confidence, power, and positivity. Yes, you project these qualities partially to intimidate your opponents, but mostly you do it for your own state of mind. You may feel as though you're acting or must "fake it till you make it," but that's actually the point. Even when it feels forced, consciously choosing to project strength and positivity helps you channel those feelings into reality.

You may have heard the expression "Look good, feel good." You can start by dressing for success. If a certain style of shirt makes you feel like a suave pro athlete, buy five of them! If a floppy bucket hat helps you to channel your inner chilled-out beach bum who loves the soft game, wear one. Stand up straight as your mother told you. Walk tall, holding your head high and shoulders back. Look confident, even if you're not. Looking confident tends to translate into actually *being* confident. At the very least, you will fool your opponents into thinking you've just figured out how to beat them and are sure you're going to win.

Also important is to display good sporting conduct. Nobody likes playing with or against a player who cheats, uses underhanded tactics, or throws temper tantrums. Such behavior can be distracting or embarrassing for your partner. They may decide (either consciously or unconsciously) that they would prefer to get off the court as quickly as possible, even by losing. Don't be that person! Never be afraid to say "Nice shot" when your opponent does something awesome. You aren't displaying weakness; in fact, you're showing that you aren't buckling under pressure. A competitor who is positive, kind, and plays with integrity will quickly win the crowd over on their side. The boost of energy you get from spectators rooting for you (as opposed to booing) is hard to quantify, but certainly real.

TIP

When you feel frustrated, nervous, or upset, don't reveal these emotions to your opponents. They will mark it as a "win" in their corner, likely only emboldening them to play even better. Experienced players can easily identify when their opponent is starting to emotionally crack. They will exploit your negative state of mind by isolating you or sending more aggressive attacks your way. This tactic will, of course, only cause you to feel more frazzled and upset. Keep projecting your best self and keep your opponents in the dark whenever you're in a less-than-ideal state of mind.

Talking to yourself as though you're talking to a friend

Yes, you are reading a book called *Pickleball For Dummies*, but the somewhat tongue-in-cheek title refers only to your level of expertise on the topic, not intelligence. You are obviously brilliant, or at least superior in your taste of reading material. So now that we have reminded you of how smart you are, please start treating yourself that way.

Self-talk refers to what you say to, and about, yourself, either out loud or silently in your head. We hear players call themselves unkind names, or say cruel things to themselves that they would never say to another person. If another person said those things to them, they would be aghast. We want you to always talk to yourself as you would talk to a dear friend, using only positive, kind, supportive words (both on and off the court). If you aren't already using this kind of self-talk, we have now identified the very first thing you need to do to improve your mental game.

If you tell yourself how stupid or terrible you are, you believe it. Negative self-talk is sometimes tough to identify or stop; you may not even realize you do it. Ask a trusted pickleball friend to help you by calling you out when they hear you say negative things about yourself. Have them ask you to repeat the same thing to them. You will soon clearly see how awful your language about yourself can be. When you are asked to call your doubles partner a "stupid idiot" to their face, you learn to break this habit very quickly.

When your thoughts turn negative and feelings begin to boil over, immediately stop and smile. It sounds silly, but it really works! Conjure up a happy thought of something that brings you instant joy, like your favorite pet or grandchild.

Or maybe it's the delicious turkey and avocado sandwich waiting for you after the match. Try to recall why you came to play pickleball that day in the first place. We're assuming it was to have a good time, not to endure two hours of unnecessary self-flagellation. Whatever may be going wrong on the court, it beats that root canal you keep rescheduling, so keep things in perspective.

Psychologists use the term *negativity bias* to describe how negative events tend to have a greater impact on people than equally positive ones do. People tend to dwell on the bad stuff, instead of remembering the good stuff. This is certainly true for many pickleball players. You may mentally tally your errors and replay them over and over, forgetting all about the great shots you made in between. Try to be conscious of this tendency when you are playing. Sure, you just hit the ball out and lost the point, but five shots earlier, you hit a beautiful reset that kept your team alive. That deserves to be celebrated and tallied on your mental statistics sheet!

TIP

One way to combat negativity bias is to start complimenting your opponents or partners, regardless of the outcome of the rally. Most players say "nice shot" only to the person whose shot just won the rally. If your partner flubs their third shot into the net, you can still say, "That was a great serve you hit!" If your opponent misses their put-away, you could say, "Wow, you had me pulled out really wide. Nice set up!" The more you practice identifying what went right for others, the more you'll recognize the small successes in your own game. This habit will also make you an in-demand player whom everyone wants to partner with!

REMEMBER

If you're not playing all that great today, remember that the very worst thing that can happen is that you lose the game. It's just a game, after all, not a life-or-death situation. Believe it or not, your worth as a human being is not defined by how well you play pickleball. (For those of us who are particularly competitive, it can sometimes feel that way!) Try to enjoy your time on the court. Not everyone gets to have that opportunity. Gratitude can help to keep the stress in check.

Supporting your partner

Doubles is a team sport. Your number-one job is to lift your partner up, period. If you're having a bad day and missing every shot, you can still do that one job. Who knows, with your stellar support, you may just be the "wind beneath their wings" that allows your partner to rise to the occasion and lead you to victory! We call this being the World's Greatest Doubles Partner, and it has nothing to do with your shot-making skills.

We know how easy it is to get down on yourself when playing sports, and the whole "winners and losers" aspect often doesn't help. When the conditions are right, a few unforced errors or missed opportunities can quickly send even the highest-level players hurtling down a shame spiral that can be difficult to climb out from. If you see your partner even *thinking* about getting down on themselves, go over to them, tap paddles, and say something positive. Try supportive words like "We've got this," or "No worries," or "You're so mad when you're cute." That last one will get them thinking and laughing at the same time. Tension broken!

TIP

The paddle tap is a great way to remind your partner that you are connected. Players get down on themselves more easily when they feel alone. Your doubles partner should never feel alone. Pickleball courts are quite small, so that never has to happen! In competitive play, we like to paddle tap and make eye contact with our partner between every point. See Chapter 11 for more tips on partner communication.

If you need more support from your partner than you're currently receiving, tell them that. Not everyone can pick up on little cues like a slight frown, a subtle foot stomp, or a thrown paddle. If necessary, call a time-out so that you and your partner can huddle and talk it out.

REMEMBER

When playing singles, be your own World's Greatest Double Partner. Make it your goal to stay positive and lift yourself up constantly so that you can play your best. The "two of you" are going to beat that lone player on the other side of the net and have a ton of fun doing it (who else laughs at all your jokes?). This is fantastic training for all the moments you must "go it alone" in life and be your own partner, parent, and cheerleader. Adulting is hard, no matter your age!

Comparing yourself to others ("Nothing Compares 2 U")

In pickleball, and life in general, people's feelings of frustration and inadequacy often come from comparing themselves to others. Stop — it's a trap! Comparing yourself to someone else is generally just an attack on your own self-esteem. Consider who is making the comparison: it's you. Are you an objective observer of yourself? No, you are not. People do not see themselves accurately. We tend to judge ourselves in the harshest of lights.

Comparing yourself to other players is a futile exercise. Everyone shows up to pickleball with different experiences, knowledge, aptitudes, and challenges. In Chapter 5, we discuss how your prior athletic experiences (or lack thereof) can greatly influence how you approach the game. If you've never held a paddle or racquet before, you can't expect to play the same as a former tennis pro. That doesn't mean you'll never be as good as them; it just means your journey will look different. It's simply impossible to freeze-frame any singular point in your two journeys and make a valid comparison.

Not many players can be coached to reach the pro level, so don't compare yourself to the pros, either. (We're pretty sure most of them are superhumans from another planet.) Compare yourself only to *you!* Are you improving? Yes? That's great! Reward and praise yourself for your own improvement. Did you struggle this week? That's okay. Just reflect on why you may have struggled. Were you well-rested, fed, and hydrated? Did you arrive at the courts ready to play with a positive mindset? Perhaps your opponents were having a particularly great day. You have many variables to consider, so worry only about the ones you can control.

Realize that a player who started playing at the same time and skill level as you may eventually wind up being better than you. This does not make them a better person, just a better pickleball player. (We heard they like pineapple on pizza, so clearly they're not perfect.) If you're enjoying yourself, let that be enough. Sure, you'll want to try to improve, but do so in a way that is kind to your psyche. For example, if you were missing your serves last week, maybe you will arrive early today and practice serving. If you get most of them in, it's time to celebrate a personal victory (even if you lose every game that day). Who needs a gold medal when there's gold-medal ribbon ice cream waiting at home?

Salty Situations: How to Dill

As with any human endeavor, especially those involving other people, awkward or difficult situations may arise. Pickleball is no exception. No worries! We're here to help you navigate these occasionally rough seas. Know that many of the tough spots you may find yourself in are very common and happen to most of us at one time or another.

Pickleball should be fun and positive, even when you're competing. When you let it be less than fun, tough times ensue. Most of the pressure you feel comes entirely from yourself, not others. Try to stay positive and trust in your abilities. You're not perfect, but neither is anyone else. Practice and court time will help to build confidence that you can deal with just about any pickleball-related situation. Arrive prepared and warm up well so that you are always starting the session in your best frame of mind.

Dealing with nerves

Everyone gets nervous, so don't attach any stigma to it. It doesn't mean you're a weak loser. (You *never* talk like that to yourself, right?) What being nervous does mean is that you care. Caring is a good thing. Let that caring be a positive force. Try not to come from a place of fear. Don't be *afraid* of losing or playing poorly.

Everyone has lost or played poorly and lived through it. Nobody was told to hit the road and never come back to the courts. Regardless of the outcome of a match or tournament, you will be fine. You're still a great person with a fun, healthful hobby, and that means you're winning at life!

Whether it's your first tournament (or your fiftieth), a recreational game with higher-level players, or your first time at a new venue, nerves can rear their ugly heads.

Here are some of our best tips for "dilling" with them:

>> **Be prepared.** If you're playing at a new venue or a tournament, gather as much information ahead of time about what to expect so that you have no last-minute surprises. Be sure to arrive early to avoid unnecessary stress from getting lost or being unable to find parking. Prior to your matches, do everything you can to make yourself ready, including self-care like hydrating, stretching, warming up, applying sunscreen, preventing blisters, and so on. Get that all squared away so that you can focus on the task at hand: playing your best pickleball. You are the player who is ready to go and feeling good!

>> **Get focused.** Tune out the rest of the world and focus on playing smart, aggressive pickleball right out of the gate. Nervous players tend to play tentatively, from a place of fear. You can't take charge of what's happening on the court if you're being tentative. If your mind starts to drift and you feel the nerves creeping in, just remind yourself to keep playing the way you have been practicing. Using the paddle tracking technique that we cover in Chapter 11 can help you to maintain laser-like focus throughout each rally.

>> **Play one point at a time.** Focusing on only the current point helps to make the task at hand feel manageable. You can definitely handle playing one point in pickleball, right? Then, win or lose, it's time to move on to the next point. Keep going, one foot in front of the other, one point at a time. Don't dwell on past mistakes; take a second to grieve the missed shot, consider what you could have done differently, and then put it behind you. Developing a case of short-term amnesia can help you stay in the moment until the match is over. Be a goldfish!

>> **Remember to breathe.** Slow, deep breaths calm your nervous system and lower your racing heartbeat. While you're at it, remember to smile, too!

>> **Stay busy.** You always have something to do when you're in the middle of a pickleball rally. If the ball is coming to you, set your feet, select a target, and hit that ball in the smartest, prettiest way you know how. If you're not the player hitting the ball, you still have the job of getting yourself into a better position. That may mean getting your paddle up and forward, or moving into a better

court position, or both. Keeping up with your current tasks help you tune out the rest of the world, including your nervous thoughts.

>> **Communicate.** Be sure to tell your doubles partner what you need. Do you need a reassuring paddle tap between each point? Your partner should certainly be able to provide that. Tell your partner how you're feeling. A good partner will reassure and support you. Be sure to be that person for your partner, too. Remember, your number-one job as a doubles partner is to lift up your partner.

>> **Use your time-outs**. If you're feeling rattled or need a minute to catch your breath, call a time-out. Come back to the game and focus on playing one point at a time. If you're playing recreationally and need a moment, take your time retrieving the ball or take a few extra breaths before serving. Many recreational players don't mind if you say you want a quick time-out.

>> **Practice playing under pressure.** Joining a ladder at your local club can help you learn to play under some pressure without feeling like you're at the National Championships. Under this more manageable amount of pressure, you can learn to play confident, aggressive pickleball. You can even add some "practice pressure" to your drilling and practicing. Try starting a game down by five points to practice climbing out of a hole. Play some games that start at 7–7 to learn to keep a game from getting away from you when it's tight. Turn drills into competitive games. Whoever hits the target the most, wins. Whoever gets to the kitchen line in balance as a team wins two points, and so on. You can make any drill into a competition.

REMEMBER

There's no skill in pickleball that you can't practice. That includes dealing with nerves. It's just another part of the game that you can work on and master. If needed, you can turn to a sports psychologist for extra help. That is no different than turning to a pickleball coach for help with your technique and strategy. The mind and body have to work together in order to play good, quality pickleball.

Getting over "the yips"

Yips are barks from young puppies. *The yips* refers to when you are not able to perform an athletic skill after doing so successfully many times before. Suddenly you are "in your head" and freaking out because a certain skill you believed you owned has left you entirely and taken a cruise to the South Pacific. *Bali Ha'iiiiiii!*

Because the pickleball serve is the one thing you do all by yourself, it's usually the first thing that breaks down when players get nervous. "OMG! Everyone's watching me! What if I screw up?" This thought process goes on repeat in your head, and the problem before you seems to get bigger and bigger until you simply cannot hit the same serve you've hit a million times before. Yikes!

It's okay. Breathe into a paper bag until you stop seeing stars. You can fix this.

If the yips have infected your serve, here are some ways to help yourself:

>> **Get back to basics.** First, be sure that your serve is as simple and compact as possible. The more moving parts there are, the more ways there are to break down — just ask any car owner. If you normally have a nice compact serve with an extended arm and a great follow-through, make sure you're using the serving style that you have honed. Sometimes nervousness makes your follow-through disappear (or change) for no apparent reason. If you usually use a fully extended arm when serving but now find that you're bending your elbow, your serve will struggle.

>> **Try something totally different.** If the preceding tip doesn't help, try a new approach. If you normally use the traditional "out of the air" forehand serve, experiment with the drop serve or even a backhand serve. Sometimes a fundamental change to your serve helps you build the new serve and make it better than the old one was. The drop serve can make it easier to time the ball, so if nervousness is affecting your timing, that can help. View it as hitting a regular forehand groundstroke instead of a big scary serve.

>> **Ask a friend or coach for help.** An outside observer may easily spot what has suddenly gone funky with your serve. You may even ask them to take a video of your serve so that you can see what's happening from an outside perspective.

>> **Relax your follow-through.** Many serving-mechanic issues come from being too tense and trying to control exactly where the ball goes using your elbow or wrist. This situation only gets worse after you've decided you have the yips! After making contact with the ball, follow through up and over your nondominant shoulder and let your wrist naturally relax.

>> **Watch the ball hit your paddle.** We don't usually advise you to watch the ball hit your paddle, but serving is the exception. At all other times, we recommend keeping your chin up so that you can see what's happening across the net, while also seeing your paddle strike the ball. Watching across the net is less important on the serve because your opponents probably aren't doing much of interest. When you serve, it's okay to drop your head and watch the ball contact the paddle so that you can try to get it right in the sweet spot.

>> **Shrink the problem in your head.** Either before the match, in warm-up, or during a time-out, go up to the kitchen line and hit a serve into the crosscourt service box. That should certainly feel manageable. If your serve goes in, which is likely, take one step back and hit another serve. When that goes in, take another step back and do it again. Repeat until you are back at the baseline where you normally serve. You have just proven to yourself that you can do this!

TIP

If the yips are affecting another shot in your game, you can do a similar exercise to the one we just described by hitting a shot to a bigger or closer target until you regain your confidence. For example, if all your lobs are going long, try aiming two or three feet closer inside the line than your normal target. If your swinging volleys are going in the net, simplify your attacks and use a compact punch volley instead. As we say previously, the more compact and efficient your shots are, the less likely they are to break down under stress.

Playing with unruly opponents: Bad line calls and more

Competitive sports don't always bring out the best in people. You may have seen professional athletes throw racquets, chairs, and even punches on the sports segment of the news. Pickleball rarely gets ugly like that. Etiquette and good sporting conduct are encouraged in this sport. In the rare instances that things turn ugly, we truly hope that you didn't start it or add to it. Keep pickleball civil!

If you wind up facing some unruly opponents, you always have the option to walk away. Don't escalate the situation. Take the high road and move on. If you are in a tournament and your opponents make bad line calls on purpose, or just don't play fairly, ask your referee to intervene. If you don't have a referee, go find the tournament director or head referee. They may decide that your match needs a referee and maybe even line judges. Stay calm and cool, without working up excess emotion. The goal is just to play the game fairly.

How such situations affect your play is up to you. The more upset you become, the more it will interfere with your concentration and execution. At one tournament when coauthors Mo and Reine played doubles together, Mo hit her backhand with a little too much gusto. A player on the other team caught the ball out of the air before the bounce and called the ball out. The ball has to bounce out of bounds to be called out, though. Mo started seeing red. Reine, ever the Zen player, turned to Mo and calmly urged, "Don't get mad." Reine diffused the situation because she knew that if they'd decided to dig in their heels and argue about the call, Mo's game would have suffered. Yes, they had a valid argument, but their team was better off not fighting that particular battle. They realized that the ball certainly would have landed out anyway if it had bounced, so the error had been made. The team stayed calm and moved forward without letting their emotions get the best of them. Smart playing!

Your best approach to pickleball is to play fairly, by the rules. Call the balls in or out, but only when they land on your side of the court. Trust that your opponents are doing their best to make their line calls fairly, too. In most cases, a bad line call is caused by faulty vision rather than faulty morals. Call your own kitchen faults as well as your partner's. Foot faults are difficult to call from the other side of the net. If you feel that your opponents aren't playing fairly, have a calm and reasonable discussion about it. If you can't resolve your issues calmly, don't play together.

If you find that the vibe at one of your local pickleball clubs is too snobby, or not friendly to players of your level, look for another club. You can also lobby the board of directors or other influential folks in the club to change their ways. Suggest a 2.0–2.5 mixer or social event to make everyone feel welcome (see Chapter 18 for some fun ideas). Find positive ways to channel your frustrations. Rather than complain, volunteer to help fix the problem. Clubs function at their best when all levels are well represented and players find ways to work and play together harmoniously.

Ideally, pickleball is about having fun. If some players in your community are making it less fun, you can find other people to play with. There are plenty of pickleball-playing fish in the sea! This is your chance to bring recess and play back into your life. Leave your anger at home, or if you must, burn it off while warming up your overhead smashes. Bringing a spirit of generosity and fair play to the courts will serve you well. It's also infectious. If you show others by your example that salty situations can be diffused with kindness, you and your fellow players will get to play this wonderful game in a more joyful way. That sounds like a winning formula!

Chapter **16**

Improving Your Game: DIY or with an Expert

O ne of the joys of improving your pickleball game is being invited to play more often. When coauthor Diana started to play, she guessed the rest of the players were quietly fighting over who had to play with her. Did she give up and sulk? No! She kept on showing up and working on her game. She listened to coauthors Mo and Reine and started kindly coaching herself, as she would a friend. She took a few lessons and clinics and began to improve. She listened to her playing partners, who encouraged her and showed her tips. Now she gets invited to play on a regular basis, playing five days a week if she can. A personal triumph!

Another joy of improving is taking on a challenge and conquering it. As we mention many times in this book, pickleball is addictive, so you will want to play often and keep getting better. It's best to have a plan that incorporates focused practice. You can practice through a do-it-yourself program by grabbing a buddy and running specific drills, or you can take lessons, attend specialized clinics, or travel to a pickleball camp. In this chapter, we provide ideas for different ways to practice and improve — and wow your opponents.

Practice, Practice, Practice

One of the best aspects of pickleball is its low barrier of entry. Experience with playing other sports can often help but isn't necessary. (See Chapter 5 for more about transitioning from other sports.) Practicing frequently and efficiently creates muscle memory (which technically occurs in the brain) along with confidence and increased skills. These benefits translate into calm, patient pickleball.

Don't concern yourself with perfection. No one will ever be perfect, so constantly looking for perfection is an exercise in frustration. Keep working toward improvement and congratulate yourself when you see positive results.

The first step to improving your game is to assess your strengths and weaknesses. If you aren't sure where to start, ask a friend or coach what areas you need to work on. Sometimes just trying certain drills will show where your weaknesses lie.

REMEMBER

No law proclaims that you must drill to play good pickleball. If practice drills don't bring you joy, don't do them. Pickleball should be about enhancing your life with joyful play, not tedious drudgery. There are other ways to practice besides drilling. If you do enjoy drilling and the improvement that comes with it, then by all means drill! If not, don't feel pressured.

Practicing two-, three-, and four-person drills

Imagine this: You show up early to the court and the rest of your doubles foursome hasn't shown up yet. You can sit on the bench, watching silly cat videos on your phone, or you can start practicing solo. You may be able to recruit another player or two to practice with you. Being at different skill levels doesn't matter; everyone has room to improve. When drilling, we recommend that you

>> **Start in a cooperative way.** The first ball is a "courtesy feed," meaning that if you're practicing volleys, don't start with an untouchable slam at your drilling partner's feet. You may need to make a rule that the first two or three touches must be gentle dinks.

>> **Build increasing difficulty.** The best drills have progressive phases, so as you master one phase, you can move on to a slightly more difficult version. Vary the speed or height of the ball, shrink the target, or require more movement.

>> **Add a competitive element.** Many players need this element to keep interest and focus. Have some way of keeping score or earning bonus points when players successfully perform the desired skills.

>> **Practice from both sides.** Practice all skills from both the right and left side of the court, using both forehands and backhands.

>> **Have plenty of balls.** Don't waste your precious drilling time chasing balls if you can avoid it. A hopper, bucket, or pouch full of balls makes practicing easier.

>> **Be creative!** Make up your own drills, and continue to tweak ones you've learned to make them as fun and challenging as possible.

If you're looking for drill ideas, you'll find plenty of videos and books online. Coming up with your own isn't as hard as you may think, either. Just think about which skills you would like to practice and how they normally fit into gameplay scenarios; then isolate those scenarios. To get you started, here are some of our favorite drills:

>> **Dingles:** You need four players and two balls for this drill. Everyone lines up at the kitchen line, and both players on one team start by dinking a ball cross-court. Keep dinking the two balls crosscourt until one of the balls is hit out or into the net. The player who made the error should yell "Dingles!" Now, all four players play out the point with the remaining ball, and anything goes — not just dinks! Whichever team ultimately wins the rally gets a point. **Note:** If the two balls collide in the air, it's known as a *dingle berry*. If both balls go out or into the net at the exact same time, it's called a *double dingle*. Both result in a replay.

>> **Moving Targets:** Start at the kitchen line, hitting crosscourt dinks to your drilling partner. After each dink, take a side step toward the opposite sideline. For a brief moment, you will be directly across from each other in the center, but mostly you're hitting crosscourt shots. When you get to the other side, reverse direction and keep moving. Focus on keeping the ball in front of your body and dinking with intention toward the other player. This drill helps you incorporate movement and precision. You can perform the same drill using volleys.

>> **Two-Touch:** Two players perform this drill in a dinking format. Let the ball bounce in front of you, but rather than hitting it directly back over, hit it up to yourself, let it bounce again, and then dink it back over. You must touch the ball twice before it goes over the net. This drill helps improve coordination, paddle feel, placement skills, and reaction time. You will quickly find that this drill is successful only if you keep the ball out in front of you. You can make this drill harder by doing it without letting the ball bounce.

>> **Figure Eights:** You need four people for this cooperative drill. The only rule of this drill is that you can't hit it back to the person who hit it to you. So if you receive the ball from the player straight across from you, you need to hit your

shot crosscourt. You can make this drill more fun and focused by counting how many shots your group can accumulate before someone misses. This drill encourages intentional hitting and lets you practice changing the direction of the ball. It works great for dinks, volleys, and groundstrokes.

>> **Double Dutch Volleys:** Two players hit volleys straight across from each other using two balls at one time. Not easy!

>> **Boogers (a.k.a. Dink it or Flick It):** Dink straight across with a partner, but occasionally surprise each other by speeding things up (flicking). Constantly be ready for a speedup or attack. When you least expect it, expect it! (Tip: Always expect the unexpected.)

>> **Target Shoppers:** You can practice and improve any shot by simply throwing down a target and hitting toward it. Challenge your drilling partner to a showdown: The first one to hit the target ten times buys lunch! Targets can be just about anything. Cut up a yard-sale yoga mat, or use dish towels, shopping bags, pool noodles, fitness hoops, bowling pins, or anything brightly colored that you happen to have lying around.

>> **Shout It Out:** Stand at the kitchen line and have your drilling partner hit balls from the baseline. Your goal is to predict whether the ball will be in or out before it crosses the net. Don't actually hit the ball back or you won't know whether your prediction was right. Your partner should vary the shots with height and speed to replicate real gameplay. Players rarely practice this important skill, so you'll be ahead of the curve if you can learn to let more "out" balls actually go out!

>> **Protect the Hoop:** Place painter's tape or cones down to indicate the area around each player's feet that comprises their "hoop" (the radius a player can comfortably reach to play a ball out of the air; see Chapter 8 for more details). Each player should dink offensively and try to land the ball in their drilling partner's hoop while fiercely protecting their own with dink volleys. Keep score to make the action more competitive.

>> **Close-Up Volleys:** Stand across from your partner, just inside the kitchen line. Practice volleying back and forth from this technically illegal position. You won't have much time to react! Next, step back to your normal position behind the line. Volleys will suddenly feel a lot easier! This drill is a great way to improve your reaction time and hand speed. Soon you'll be catching flies with chopsticks.

>> **Deep, Deep, Short:** This drill lets you practice the first three shots of the game, which, as Chapter 7 makes clear, are critical. Your goals are to serve deep, return deep, and then hit a short third-shot drop. You can set up lines or cones to delineate whether a shot is deep. It can be helpful if the closest player calls out to say whether the shot was deep. Your group can keep score

of how many times you managed to execute the perfect sequence of deep, deep, short.

>> **Feet-Sets:** One player stands at the kitchen line while the other player stands at midcourt. The kitchen player aggressively hits balls toward the other player's feet, and the midcourt player attempts to reset the attack with a drop volley or half-volley. Switch roles halfway through.

One is the loneliest number: Doing solo drills and wall drills

Solo and wall drills allow you to practice hand–eye coordination, readiness, and accuracy. Even though these drills may not feel like the most realistic gameplay scenarios, you can still find ways to practice the fundamentals discussed in Chapter 6. For example, when practicing against a wall, focus on good footwork and setting up well to receive the ball. Keep the ball under control and in front of your body (between you and the wall).

Drilling alone takes some of the pressure off. You can feel free to play around with new things, fail, and fail again without judgment. Pickleball is very social, which can be overwhelming sometimes for introverts who need a little more "me" time. Here are some ways you can practice pickleball while enjoying the pleasure of your own company:

>> **Going Solo:** Bring a bucket of balls to the court and work on your technique. Serves are the natural choice, but you can practice any shot. Focus on using compact strokes, striking the ball out in front and within your "V," and using a proper follow-through. No matter what shot you're working on, always have a target in mind, and hit with intention.

>> **Relax That Backhand:** Many players struggle with their backhand because they're too tense, tending to stick out their elbow and jab at the ball instead of swinging from the shoulder. A great solo drill for retraining your backhand is to hit against the fence. Focus on simply striking the ball out in front, leading with your shoulder, and opening up your chest in a pretty Statue of Liberty follow-through. This drill helps you to build muscle memory without worrying about where the ball goes.

>> **Balls to the Wall:** Find a wall that you can hit pickleballs against. It may be the side of your house or a special ball wall at a park. You can also purchase pickleball "rebounders." Mark off (or visualize) a small window, just above net height, to hit the ball through, and see how consistently you can hit that target. Then take it to another level by standing closer and hitting only volleys or by speeding up your shots. This drill improves your accuracy and reaction time.

>> **Bounce Back:** Here's a drill you can do using just a paddle and a ball. Try bouncing the ball on your paddle over and over without letting the ball drop to the ground. Focus on getting into a rhythm and set goals of how many times you can tap the ball on the paddle without stopping. Practice this drill using alternating forehand and backhand (like you're flipping a pancake). Also try tossing the ball up high in the air and "catching" it on your paddle with minimal bounce. You have to soften your grip and lower your arm slightly as the ball contacts the paddle in order to absorb its energy. This drill is great for practicing the "soft hands" required for resets (see the section about controlling the pace in Chapter 14).

>> **Machine Learning:** If you frequently practice alone, a ball machine can provide more realistic drilling scenarios. However, ball machines are expensive and sometimes don't feed balls as reliably as you would hope. A ball machine is particularly good for working on your serve return, swinging volleys, drives, and drop shots. If you're a glutton for punishment, have it lob you repeatedly and work on retrieving those lobs. See Chapter 3 for more details on investing in a ball machine.

Just the two of us: Playing skinny singles

If you're hankering for a game but have fewer than four players, skinny singles may be your best bet. Of course, you can always play regular singles — if you have that kind of energy! Skinny singles can take several forms. You can play straight-ahead, crosscourt, or with three people. Chapter 13 provides detailed explanations and diagrams of these common skinny singles variations.

Regardless of how you play, skinny singles forces you to return the ball to a specific side of the court and really focus on where you place the ball. If you don't place it on the correct side, the ball is called out and you lose the rally. The lack of open court and available angles requires you to use varying depths in front of, and behind, your opponent to win the rally.

Practicing while you play

Each time you play offers an opportunity to work on some aspect of your game! For example, if one of your goals is to hit deeper serves, you may drill a few times and then start integrating those serves into your game. You gain confidence with each success on the court.

Some players don't enjoy drilling at all, and that's perfectly fine. If that's the case for you, use your recreational play as your time to work on your skills. It's all about mindfulness and intention. If you simply go out and play mindlessly, exactly the same way you played last time, you will be slow to improve. Instead, pick one skill a day, week, or month to focus on. Don't try to improve everything simultaneously. Nobody's brain can handle all that!

Here are some skills you may decide to practice while playing:

>> **Serve returns:** Focus on being aggressive and using good forward weight shift. Try to hit your return to the back third of the court. Next, work on hitting to your opponents' weaker sides.

>> **Backhands:** Position yourself for the serve return in a way that forces you to use your backhand. (This may be the exact opposite of what you've been doing, as someone who favors their forehand!)

>> **Dinks:** Instead of dinking simply to get the ball over the net, try working on the Evil Dinking Genius patterns we detail in Chapter 12. Make it your goal to dink more offensively and move your opponents around.

>> **Third shots:** Work on becoming more proficient in analyzing the returns that come your way so that you can quickly decide whether your third shot should be a drop or a drive.

>> **Serves:** Experiment with a variety of targets, spins, and speeds. Note which ones seem to cause the most trouble for your opponents.

>> **Resets:** Try spending some games being the player who is always willing to slow down the ball after the game speeds up. Slowing down the game may feel strange but it will help you become a more well-rounded player. You want to be the player who controls the tempo.

>> **Resist overattacking:** Tell yourself, "Today I will do only what is necessary to win the point." Find another outlet for your anger and instead play smart pickleball. Instead of trying to cream the ball, just punch it through a hole in your opponent's defense, or down at their toes. Using this approach trains you to stop overhitting your attacks.

>> **Targeting:** Challenge yourself to recognize areas of open court and accurately hit your targets.

>> **Lobbing:** Many players are scared to lob because if they don't do it well, they feel like they're just giving the point away. Lobs can be a great offensive weapon, or at least a way to cause a little chaos for your opponents. If you're normally a shy lobber, set a goal to lob at least once per game. Make sure you have a target in mind beyond just "Lob!"

>> **Partner communication:** Work on calling the ball more, yelling "stay" or "switch" as needed, and lifting up your partner when they're feeling down. Try to always call the third shot. That's a great way to create the habit of calling the ball "mine" or "yours."

> » **Strategy:** Spend some games really thinking about what strategy you need to solve the puzzle in front of you. Be mentally nimble and ready to change tactics as the puzzle evolves. Be sure to communicate your ideas to your partner. Practice stacking or switching to complicate the puzzle for your opponents and emphasize your team's strengths.

Improving while playing up or down in skill level

Most people would agree that playing with others of similar skill level leads to the most fun and competitive pickleball. That's perfectly understandable. However, forming a perfect foursome isn't always possible. Maybe you go out of your way to avoid playing with lesser-skilled players or feel too intimidated to play with higher-skilled players. However, mixing skill levels provides more opportunities to improve than you may think.

If you're playing with opponents who are significantly below your own skill level, try playing counterintuitively. Emphasize your weaknesses instead of your strengths. If you're good at driving the ball hard, try playing with slow, soft shots instead. If you normally dominate the line with your amazing dinking skills, engage in more volley battles instead. This is a great opportunity to develop parts of your games that need a little extra attention. Remember to be kind as you play with lesser-skilled players. Keep in mind that they are most likely intimidated by playing with a more advanced player.

Playing with higher-skilled players can induce nerves or feelings of inferiority and cause you to play much worse than you normally do, which only exacerbates your negative emotions. Keep in mind that most players are busy thinking about themselves. More than likely, no one else on the court is keeping track of your mistakes or negatively judging you for supposedly being the weakest player. If you're nervous, try to focus on keeping the ball low and in play. Don't show off or make risky moves — advanced players will be waiting to pounce on any mistakes. A patient, steady partner is appreciated at all levels of play.

TIP

Don't expect higher-level players to give you free coaching during recreational play. They are there to enjoy themselves or work on their own games, not analyze yours. Although many advanced players do enjoy helping others, they are not obligated to play with, or coach, everyone who asks.

Here are some more ways to hone your craft while having fun with players of mixed skill levels:

>> Work on your dinking.

>> Ask the other team to hit the ball hard so that you can practice blocking and resets.

>> Serve to specific targets.

>> Practice adding spin to your shots.

>> Stand on one foot, close one eye, and switch your paddle to your other hand. (Just kidding — don't do that!)

>> Practice slowing down the game with soft shots.

>> Nail those third-shot drops and drives.

Most important, playing with people of different skill levels provides an opportunity to practice compassion. We were all beginners once. It's a beautiful thing to see experienced players enthusiastically help new players learn the ins and outs. Pickleball for all! (We'll work on world peace next.)

Improving when playing the same people all the time

For a variety of reasons, many people tend to play with the same people all the time. Doing so is not ideal for improving your game, but you can still keep your skills moving forward even if your playing group stays the same.

For example, you may decide to focus on deep serves for an entire game. The next game, you focus on deep returns. Or spend a game or two concentrating on your drop shots. It's best to challenge yourself with as many different playing styles as possible. So, try one game as an aggressive, hard-driving beast, and then play the next game as a soft and stealthy ninja. If you know what your opponent's favorite shots are, avoid hitting to their strengths. Many players never venture outside their normal routine and therefore don't really know what they are capable of. If you've never hit a drive in your life but suddenly force yourself to try it against your usual, safe group of players, you may find that you're very good at it.

Another way to get out of your rut — if your group agrees to it — is to change the rules of pickleball. Use your creativity to encourage certain shots and targets while still in a gameplay scenario. It's fun and can get your group to break free from the old familiar routine. Here are some examples of fun "rules" to shake things up:

>> Each server must whisper their serving target (wide, middle, or center) to their partner before serving. If they miss their chosen target, the serve is called

"out" by their own partner. Give the server two tries, if needed, to make this less stressful.

>> Require that all shots after the serve and return are drop shots until all four players are at the kitchen line.

>> If your group feels like practicing the Erne shot (Chapter 14 explains this shot), require that all dinks be hit straight ahead, near the sidelines. This rule should create quite a few opportunities to attempt an Erne.

>> Award bonus points for various achievements, such as hitting a deep return, resetting after an attack, successfully lobbing over an opponent, or hitting an Around the Post (ATP) shot (we explain the ATP in Chapter 14.) Coauthor Mo keeps trying to make a new rule that if you hit the "T" on your return (the spot where the baseline and centerline meet), you have to buy tequila shots.

Practicing through visualization techniques

It turns out that visualizing yourself as the pickleball player you want to be is not only an enjoyable daydream but can actually help you become that player. Scientific studies show that visualization techniques are effective for all kinds of athletes. The swimmer Michael Phelps has spoken often about using visualizations as "mental dress rehearsals" to help lead him to 28 Olympic medals.

Try this: Imagine that it's a cool, clear day. Your bag has brand-new balls and you're wearing your favorite shirt. You are calm, relaxed, and confident. You are light and quick on your feet. You hit your dink, drive, and volley targets and immediately snap back into ready position. Your serves blow your opponents away. You're playing your best match ever!

Imagining your perfect pickleball scenario is just one way to use visualization. You can also use this technique to overcome challenges. For example, if you are about to play opponents who intimidate you, visualize that you play masterfully the whole time, taking advantage of their weaknesses and winning the game. Or visualize that those pesky drop shots you've been struggling with lately are now perfect every time. Take the confidence gained from this visualization onto the court.

Here are some other ways to use visualization to improve:

>> **Watch videos of the pros.** Visualize yourself playing the way they do. If you watch the top pros play and admire their efficient footwork, imagine your feet moving the same way. Emulation can be very effective when trying to improve.

>> **Practice with shadow swings.** Standing in front of a full-length mirror, practice your strokes with perfect technique. Make your strokes look smooth and graceful while building muscle memory. ***Note:*** Be sure to remove your favorite kids and pets from the room when doing this exercise.

>> **Turn your back to the wall.** Stand with your back facing a wall and then step forward about 6 inches or so. Practice imaginary volleys without taking big backswings. The wall will prevent that huge windup.

>> **Do a mental fitness workout.** If you struggle with negative self-talk or other mental challenges, make time to work on those things. That time can be while you're standing in line at the store, or anywhere else you may have a few quiet moments to yourself. Develop a new, positive narrative and come up with a mantra for when your thoughts turn negative. Try one of these: "I am a problem solver" or "I am a strong and smart player" or "I have put in the work. I've got this."

>> **Create mental targets.** Using mental pictures when you are practicing or playing can be very helpful. We often encourage players to keep the ball low by imagining they are hitting the ball through a window that sits just above the net. When trying to get players to hit through the ball rather than poking, jabbing, or carving at the ball, we ask them to visualize hitting through three pickleballs aligned in a row. There are plenty of ways to use your imagination!

Learning from watching live pickleball

There are some great ways to practice pickleball without even playing it. Consider this idea whenever you have a long wait to get on a court at your local pickleball venue: Instead of becoming impatient or annoyed, put this time to good use. Become your own expert pickleball analyst by carefully watching other people's matches.

Start to look at each team or player as a problem to be solved. Look for weaknesses and strengths in their game. How could you exploit their weaknesses and avoid their strengths? Analyzing other players is more difficult when you're busy playing across the net from them.

Practice judging the drop shots of other players. Judging drop shots is just as important as hitting them. Evaluate the drop shots in real time and try to articulate (silently to yourself) whether that drop shot worked. Was it good enough to move in behind? If so, just say "yes." Is it better to hang back because the drop shot carried too high and far? Then say "no." Try to call it as early as possible. You will eventually begin to tell from the hitter's setup and body language whether their drop is likely to be successful. Practicing analysis like this can enhance your ability to quickly judge your own team's drop shots, as well as your opponents'.

TIP

If you're watching a team who's using an unfamiliar strategy, observe closely and try to figure it out. If you can't decode their strategy, ask the players about it after the game is over. Pickleball players are often supportive of players who are trying to improve. If you start your inquiry with a flattering compliment, you'll rarely be turned down!

Learning online (Be careful what you watch)

Hundreds of videos, blogs, newsletters, and websites about pickleball are available online. You can even attend some online pickleball academies through a paid subscription. These videos are typically longer and go into much more detail than the standard free YouTube videos. Some experts also offer analysis of your game if you send them a video of one of your matches.

Anybody with a computer can publish their content online, so use caution when someone professes to be an expert. The real trick is to find the resources that are right for you. Ask your court buddies for recommendations, and read the online reviews. You can also contact your friendly USA Pickleball Ambassador or local coaches for suggestions.

Some of our favorite online content comes from these professional coaches:

>> Sarah Ansboury

>> Mark Renneson

>> Simone Jardim

>> Jordan Briones

>> Deb Harrison

>> Tony Roig

>> Morgan Evans

>> Mike Branon

>> Zane Navratil

Taking Lessons, Clinics, and Camps: The Sweet and the Sour

When you're ready to improve your game but aren't sure how, consider seeking some professional help. As with anything in life, there's no shame in asking for help. You can find many competent coaches who are glad to help you on your journey of pickleball improvement. This section can serve as a guide to choosing a coach who fits your needs.

Choosing the right coach for you

If you're lucky enough to live in a region where pickleball is booming, it's likely to offer multiple pickleball coaches available for hire. Finding the right coach for you will take some thoughtful research. Consider these questions:

>> **How much does the instruction cost?** Clinics and lessons can range from free to several hundred dollars.

>> **Where will the instruction take place?** Find out whether you need to be a resident or club member to take instruction at that venue.

>> **What is the experience or certification of the coach?** Many good coaches are not certified, so you'll have to decide whether that's important to you. See the upcoming section on coaching certifications.

>> **Does the coach teach their own style of play or do they customize instruction based on the student?** The best coaches will assess individual playing style and strengths, and help maximize your abilities.

>> **What can the student expect to learn?** Some coaches love to teach their "greatest hits." These topics may or may not be of value to you. Make sure the coach is comfortable teaching all aspects of pickleball, or at least the ones you're interested in.

>> **Do you feel more comfortable with a coach of a certain age or gender?** Putting yourself in the role of a student can sometimes feel a little scary and vulnerable. You may feel you can relax and open your mind more around someone of a particular gender or age.

>> **Are private or group lessons offered?** Many students learn best when taking lessons with a friend of about the same skill level. They can practice together between lessons. Others feel more comfortable blending in to a group, or taking private lessons for more individual help.

>> **What sort of delivery style does the coach use?** Are they kind and gentle, or more like a drill sergeant? Are they silly and upbeat, or more serious and technical? Different personalities and delivery styles may work better for you than others.

>> **What sort of learning styles do they accommodate?** Some students prefer to learn one concept and spend an hour drilling it. Others prefer to soak in as much information as possible and drill on their own time.

>> **Do you connect well with the coach in regular conversation?** If you struggle to make coherent small talk or schedule a lesson time with this particular coach, they certainly won't communicate in a style that works well for you as a student.

Ask around to get reviews from other local players. USA Pickleball and their Ambassadors are good resources for recommendations. You can also find coaches in your area by searching websites like Professional Pickleball Registry (https://www.PPRPickleball.org) and Pickleball Teachers Network (https://www.PickleballTeachers.com).

If you don't immediately click with your coach, don't feel guilty about trying a different one. You may not know exactly what you're looking for until you find it.

WARNING

We cringe when we hear the suggestion that folks simply take lessons from any 4.5 or 5.0 player. As with any sport, the top players don't necessarily possess great coaching abilities. Many top athletes are unable to communicate clearly to others how they are able to make their spectacular plays.

In contrast, some of the very best coaches may have never played competitively, or can no longer play. To be a great coach, they need to know the game inside and out, and be able to analyze and solve problems well. Look for a coach you personally connect with — someone who explains what to do in a straightforward and approachable way. Find a coach who is encouraging but also honest about your strengths and weaknesses. Be wary of coaches who seem more interested in touting their own abilities or accomplishments than focusing on you.

TIP

If you take a lesson with a coach and leave with only frustration (or worse, in tears!), look for another coach. You should leave feeling positive and focused on the tasks at hand. You should know what to work on before your next lesson. Unless you are happy paying for the same lesson over and over, be sure to put the work in and practice what you learned. Not only will this provide you with the best value and biggest jumps in your game, it will make your coach feel proud and motivated, too!

Coaching certifications

Understanding pickleball coaching certifications can be confusing. Ask the prospective coach about what those acronyms and organizations they tout on their bio mean. (LOL is not a certification, BTW.) Certified coaches have been trained and evaluated to prove they can do the job. Coaches can be certified to teach pickleball from a few different organizations:

» **Professional Pickleball Registry (PPR):** PPR is currently the official certification and education partner of USA Pickleball. Becoming PPR certified involves attending an in-person workshop and then completing written, skills, and demonstration tests. There are two levels of PPR certification: Coach and Pro.

» **International Pickleball Teaching Professional Association (IPTPA):** The IPTPA has three levels of certification available. Candidates are evaluated through a written exam, skills test, and teaching demonstration. To maintain their certification, instructors must complete continuing education credits each year.

» **Pickleball Coaching International (PCI):** PCI is the official coach education provider of the U.S. Open. It is a certification program and online education resource developed by Mark Renneson, a world-renowned professional player, coach, and commentator. Coaches participate in either an online or in-person workshop and must pass a written test, skills test, and teaching evaluation. Two levels of certification are currently offered.

» **US Professional Tennis Association (USPTA):** The USPTA partnered with the IFP (International Federation of Pickleball) to create a pickleball certification program for certified tennis professionals. Coaches may obtain a certification from one of several USPTA Pickleball Testers or an IFP training center.

Getting the most out of instruction

Remember that getting the most out of instruction is your responsibility. Be a sponge, ready to absorb what the coach is telling you. Listen closely and ask questions if you need clarification. Don't just smile and nod if what you're hearing doesn't make sense! Try not to derail the topic at hand with unrelated stories or tangents. Here are some additional tips for getting the most out of any pickleball lesson:

» **Show up on time.** Figure out where your lesson is and arrive at least a few minutes early. If possible, warm up on another court ahead of time so that your instructor doesn't have to get you warmed up. You can then jump right into your lesson and use your valuable time learning.

>> **Prepare your questions in advance.** Some questions will also invariably come up during the lesson, too, but wait until the right time to ask. If you have one or two things you'd really like to concentrate on, let your coach know up front. You will be disappointed if you expect your coach to navigate through 30 topics in an hour. A good coach welcomes questions and will make you feel safe in asking them.

>> **Focus.** Being a good listener means not whispering to your friend or daydreaming about the hot date you have planned for after the lesson. Show respect for your coach by giving them your undivided attention.

>> **Have a good attitude.** You're learning. Don't expect to get it right every time. Stay positive, laugh together, and keep trying.

>> **Don't be afraid to fail; you're in learning mode.** Make mistakes, keep focused, smile, and try again. No one will spend the rest of the day thinking about how bad you were, so don't worry about what others think of your performance. Just try your best and know that is enough.

>> **Make notes afterward.** As you leave your lesson, hopefully your head is swimming with pearls of wisdom and your heart is brimming with excitement. As soon as you possibly can, write down a list of the ideas that resonated for you. Next time you go to play or practice, choose one item from your list to work on.

Dealing gracefully with unsolicited advice

When another player starts to coach you in the middle of play, it can be awkward and frustrating. Most of the time, the person is just an overly enthusiastic player who wants to share their knowledge. Too often, the advice given is wrong, conflicting, or presented poorly. Almost all of us were told at one time to "get up to the kitchen line as fast as possible." This incorrect advice will cost you many points. (See Chapter 11 for our take on this topic.)

If someone is bothering you with unsolicited advice, tell them their comments are a distraction and to please save them for another time. Mid-game is typically not the best time to contemplate advice, especially if it comes out of nowhere. A mid-game mini-lesson also interferes with the flow of play and is inconsiderate to your opponents. You can always say, "Thanks for your input, but I'm currently working with a coach." That usually ends the conversation. If it doesn't, just be respectful and walk away, or choose not to partner with that person again.

Some players will ask you first if you would like their advice. As a learning player, be open to hearing their suggestions. Listen respectfully to everyone, try things, and then integrate the tips that work for you. Don't take advice as a personal criticism; we all have a lot to learn.

Your Own Point of View: Using Self-Assessment Tools

Learning how to analyze your own play can be informative for your ongoing improvement. Identifying a baseline of your current skills will help you understand what your next steps should be. Identify specific skills to work on so that you can focus on them during drill sessions, lessons, or play. Here are some questions to help you evaluate the current state of your game:

>> **Serve:** Can you get your serve in bounds and deep? Can you serve to a variety of different targets, such as to the opponent's backhand or out wide? Have you incorporated different types of spin?

>> **Return of serve:** Do you sometimes or often miss the return against better players? Do you return serves deep most of the time? Can you return almost all types of serves?

>> **Forehand:** How often do you pop the ball up? Do you hit into the net or out of bounds often? Do you miss the hard and fast ones?

>> **Backhand:** Is your backhand weak? Do you avoid it at all costs? Can you hit a backhand slice?

>> **Drops:** Do you use the drop shot effectively and move in behind it? Are your drops mostly unattackable?

>> **Dinking:** Are you dinking consistently, both straight across and crosscourt? Do you move your opponents around and force errors?

>> **Lobbing:** Do most of your lobs land in bounds and near your intended target? Do you understand when it's a good time to use the lob?

>> **Footwork:** Are you light on your feet like a stalking cheetah, anticipating where the ball is going? Are you always in good balance? Do you maintain a good ready position most of the time?

- » **Communication**: Do you communicate well with your partner throughout the game? Are you keeping in touch throughout every rally? ("Yours! Mine! Switch!")

- » **Strategic thinking:** Do you use a variety of shots? Do you have a plan going into each rally? Can you solve the puzzle in front of you?

Doing your own video analysis

You may be a little shocked the first time you see yourself playing on video. Coauthor Reine was quite certain she possessed the intimidating court presence of pro player Jessie Irvine until she saw footage of herself. Oops. Maybe not so much. That's okay; it gave her something to work toward! We are all our own worst critics, so before you get into panning your own performance, be sure to read our advice on positive self-talk in Chapter 15.

You can buy a tripod to use with your phone or camera, or ask a buddy to hold it. Mix up the camera angles when possible. If you have access to a drone (fancy!), overhead footage can be a great tool for evaluating court movement and positioning. Don't worry if your practice videos aren't primetime worthy; for this purpose, all you need is to be able to see how you are hitting and moving on the court. (How's that paddle tracking, by the way? See Chapter 11 if you're not sure what paddle tracking is.)

Document the areas to work on and track your progress. Just think: You can even determine your shot selection percentages. Are you hitting mostly drops or drives? Which is working better for you? Notice areas you need to work on. Be sure to pat yourself on the back when you notice improvement and overcome each challenge.

TIP

Some coaches offer video analysis for their students. You may wind up sending your video to a top coach who lives across the country for expert analysis. Ain't modern life grand?

Using match-charting tools

It takes discipline, but charting matches is a great way to analyze your play and progress. You can do match charting with just a plain old piece of paper and pencil, or you can get fancy and create a spreadsheet. Free charts are available online for you to print, or you can purchase a copy of *The Pickleball Workbook* (https://www.pickleballworkbook.com) — a spiral-bound journal, planner, and charting tool. You can chart your own matches from video footage or have a friend do it for you in real time. Some different options for charting include:

» Creating a grid of all possible types of shots (dinks, returns, third shots, and others) and tracking how many of each type you hit and how many attempts resulted in an unforced error.

» Tracking each player's impact on the match by counting their total number of touches, unforced errors, and winners.

» Charting third-shot types of shots (drop versus drive) and their effectiveness. Were you able to get to the line after the drop? Did you get a pop-up off your drive?

» Tracking your various types of serves (location, speed, spin) and how well your opponents returned.

» Looking at how the score of the match progressed over time. Are you slow to start and always end up behind, only to make a big comeback? Did you get to 9–0 and fall asleep? Did you manage to earn 19 sideouts but never score a single point on serve?

» Charting your dinking patterns, total dinks, and dinking errors.

Evaluating your own data can be eye-opening! Match charting also helps you log a history of selected matches in case you play against certain opponents again. Many competitive players keep detailed notes on various opponents so that they don't have to start from scratch every time they face them.

Chapter 17

Playing Tournaments

Coauthor Mo had been playing pickleball for only a few months before she decided to try her hand at tournament play. She grabbed her sister, Lisa, and headed to the tournament venue on the other side of town. They played pretty well despite their nerves. Then they came up against some familiar faces: coauthor Reine and her friend Pat. The match was close, and the lead kept changing back and forth. Then Mo hit a shot that ticked the top of the net and dribbled over, well out of reach of Reine and Pat, who were clearly not pleased at this "cheap shot." Oopsy. It was now 14–13. Match point!

A long, intense rally ensued. The players ran all over the court, trying to finish the point. Lisa hit an amazing lob that sailed over the heads of Reine and Pat, landing just inside the baseline for a winner. End of match. Nobody likes to get lobbed, but a perfect lob to end the match, especially right after a dribbler on the previous point? *Grrrr!* The only thing that could possibly have ruffled Reine and Pat's feathers more would be to have to read about it in a book one day.

Tournament tales, like the one above, are great fun. So are the friendships and adventures that come with hanging out with friends between matches, cheering each other on, taking goofy medal-stand photos, and celebrating with food and drinks after a long day of competition. Court time is only a small fraction of your time at most tournaments. Embrace the camaraderie of the "campsite" where everyone plops down their chairs, sunshades, coolers, and bags. Sit back, relax, and get to know your fellow players better. Invite newer tournament players to join you. We all want to feel like we belong.

If tournaments sound like fun to you, read this chapter to understand the various formats, player ratings, what to expect, and how to cope with competitive play. Tournaments can be an enjoyable way to test your skills, travel, meet new people, and take your hobby to the next level.

Understanding Different Tournament Formats and Types

Pickleball tournaments come in a variety of competitive formats. You'll need to put some thought into what you are looking for in terms of the event type, competition level, and distance you're willing to travel. If you aren't sure at first, just pick a tournament, hold your breath, and dive in! (Oops, scratch that — we don't recommend holding your breath when playing pickleball.) Competition can bring new excitement to your game. It can provide added motivation and a deadline to train for. It can usher in new friendships and experiences that you didn't expect.

Don't dismiss the idea of tournaments because you feel you're too young or old, or not skilled enough to compete. Tournaments always have divisions based on skill and gender. The larger tournaments are divided based on skill, gender, *and* age. So you may find that the 80+ 3.0 Men's Doubles division is perfect for you. There are also the Pro and Senior Pro (50+) divisions, so stay inspired to keep working on your game, no matter what your current age is.

Because tournament play can seem a little scary at first, we recommend that you start off with a small, local tournament. The stakes are low and you'll be among familiar faces, so it's a fantastic way to dip your toe into the tournament pond without a lot of stress.

Pickleball tournaments, large or small, have the following characteristics in common:

>> **Event categories:** Most tournaments offer Women's Doubles, Men's Doubles, and Mixed Doubles (in which one partner must be female and one male). Some also offer Women's Singles and Men's Singles, as well as wheelchair divisions.

>> **Skill divisions:** Tournaments offer skill divisions, typically based on the rating scale range of 2.0–5.0 (see "Knowing Where You Stand: Player Ratings," later in this chapter, for more on ratings). Larger tournaments may offer pro divisions, usually with prize money attached. Smaller tournaments may use more casual

labels such as "Beginner," "Intermediate," and "Advanced." Your team's skill division is determined by the highest-rated player.

>> **Age divisions:** Depending on the size of the tournament, skill divisions may be further divided by age. Your team's age division is determined by the youngest player on your team, so if you're planning to team up with your grandson, be ready to play in a much younger division!

>> **Medals:** Pickleball tournaments traditionally award gold, silver, and bronze medals to the top three players or teams.

>> **Souvenirs:** Most tournaments provide a swag bag for all participants as well as some sort of tournament souvenir, such as a t-shirt, hat, or towel.

Pickleball tournaments are run using a number of different formats. Familiarizing yourself with the three most common, described in the following sections, will help you feel more comfortable on game day.

Round robins: We all get a turn

A popular format in competitive pickleball is the *round robin*. In this format, every player or team plays all the other players or teams in their division or pool. This standard round-robin format works well if each division has around six to eight teams. If you have six teams, each participant is guaranteed five matches (obviously, they can't play against themselves). Matches typically consist of either two out of three games to 11, or one game to 15 or 21. If the division has fewer than five teams, you may even play each team twice in what's known as a *double round robin*. Get the Epsom salts ready — that's a good long day of highly competitive pickleball!

After all the matches are complete, the winner of the round robin is the team who won the most matches. If two or more teams are tied, the match is decided by "head-to-head," which means that when the two teams played each other, the winner of that match is considered the overall victor. The rule book details additional tie-breakers to be used if needed. The tournament director has the final say on how the outcome is decided, unless it is a tournament sanctioned by a governing body, in which case their official rule book dictates how the winners are decided.

Double elimination: The "Two and Out Club"

Another common format in pickleball tournaments is a standard "knock out" or elimination type of bracket called *double elimination*. If you lose two matches, you're knocked out of the tournament. Time to pack up your paddle, swap your sneakers for the "Sandals of Shame," and head home. No, wait — don't do that! You may be done playing for the day, but you can still continue to have a great time. You're off the hook and can just relax, have a margarita, and enjoy watching some great matches. Figure 17-1 shows an example of a double-elimination bracket chart.

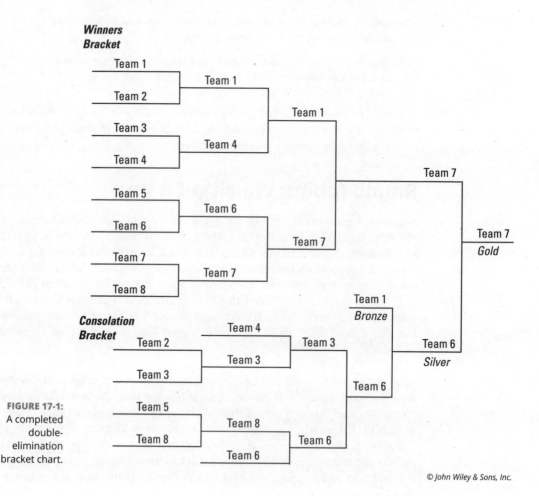

FIGURE 17-1: A completed double-elimination bracket chart.

For a double-elimination tournament, tournament staff post a bracket showing the matches arranged for the first round. Depending on the number of teams in the division, some participants may receive a "bye" in the first round.

As you win matches (typically two out of three games played to 11 points), you move on in the bracket. If you lose, you drop down into what's known as the "back," "consolation," or "losers" bracket (that last one seems harsh). In this bracket, matches are typically one game played to 15 points. If you lose a second match, you are out of the tournament.

As players keep winning and progressing, eventually the remaining team in the consolation bracket meets up with the remaining team in the "top" or "winners" bracket to play the gold-medal match. The winner of that match gets gold; the loser, silver. Bronze goes to the team who lost the final match in the consolation bracket.

Remember that you must lose twice to be out of the tournament, so the team coming up from the consolation bracket will have to beat the team from the winners bracket twice if they want that gold medal. *Say what?* Remember, the team in the consolation bracket already has one loss. The team in the winners bracket doesn't have any losses. The team in the winners bracket has to lose *twice* in order to be eliminated. So if the consolation bracket team beats the winners bracket team in a two-out-of-three match played to 11 points, they must then turn around and beat them *again* in a single game played to 15.

TIP

If you ever find yourself in a tournament in Bend, Oregon, at the Pickleball Zone, don't be dismayed if you lose your first two matches. You will be invited to join the not-so-exclusive "Two and Out Club." The perks of this club are many! They include a discount on a new paddle in their pro shop (because of course you lost as a result of an inadequate paddle) as well as a sticker that shows your proud membership. You'll also receive a discount at their bar (for obvious reasons), where the bartender promises to listen to you complain about your partner and slip you a confidential list of potential new partners. The best part is, club membership is free! All you have to do is lose your first two matches. It's great when pickleball players don't take themselves too seriously.

Single elimination with consolation

A third possible tournament format is the *single elimination with consolation*. This one is nearly identical to the double elimination format described in the previous section. The difference is that after you lose a match and are knocked down into the consolation bracket, the best you can hope to place is bronze. A team in the consolation bracket has no opportunity to work their way back up to the gold-medal match. The gold and silver will go to the final two teams who reach the end of the winners bracket.

Sanctioned versus non-sanctioned tournaments

When signing up for a tournament, you need to know whether it's a sanctioned tournament. A *sanctioned tournament* must meet specific requirements and guidelines established by USA Pickleball. The goal of sanctioning is to provide a consistent and fair playing environment. Here are some important things to know about playing in a sanctioned tournament:

>> You must be a USA Pickleball member to participate.

>> You must use a USA Pickleball–approved paddle and ball. (See Chapter 3 for more on equipment standards.)

>> Your results will count toward your UTPR (USA Pickleball Tournament Player Rating). We discuss ratings more in the next section.

>> It will likely be more expensive to enter because of the additional referee, software, and sanctioning fees.

>> The level of play is typically higher because sanctioned tournaments attract players from a wider region.

A non-sanctioned pickleball tournament may follow the same guidelines, or it may stray from the guidelines for any reason. It is entirely up to the tournament committee. To be clear, non-sanctioned tournaments are not necessarily poorly run. Tournament committees can have many good reasons not to pursue sanctioning. In fact, a number of major tournaments are not sanctioned, yet are professionally run and attract thousands of participants. If you're looking for fun and competitive play, you will find it at all types of events, from a non-sanctioned tournament at your local park all the way to the officially sanctioned National Championships.

Knowing Where You Stand: Player Ratings

Most people who choose to compete in something don't want to be in way over their heads, or have to play far below their skill level. Imagine entering a slam-dunk contest and your opponent was either LeBron James or a four-year old kid. Neither situation sounds like much fun!

Pickleball has numerical rating systems in place that indicate players' skill levels. Each player may have a different rating for singles, mixed doubles, and gender doubles. The intent of rating systems is to level the playing field so that you have the opportunity to compete against similarly skilled players, making for the most competitive games.

Rating systems are not perfect by any means. You may find that your official rating doesn't accurately reflect your level of play. If that's the case, we encourage you to play at the higher level. It's always better to challenge yourself against better players than to play beneath your skill level and be accused of *sandbagging*, or knowingly playing at a lower level just to ensure that you win. Sandbagging is for flood control, not pickleball!

Defining the digits: Official skill-rating definitions

USA Pickleball has defined a skill-level rating system that ranges from 1.0–5.5+. For general purposes, such as club or league play, your rating will be a two-digit number, such as 3.0 or 4.5. For tournament purposes, it can be as precise as a four-digit number, such as 3.899. Your skill rating is determined by your ability to understand the game and perform various shots.

Table 17-1 provides summarized descriptions of each skill level. For the complete, official descriptions of each skill level, check out the USA Pickleball website (http://www.usapickleball.org).

TABLE 17-1   Skill-Level Rating System

Level	What It Means
1.0–2.0	This player is just starting to play pickleball and has a basic understanding of the rules of the game.
2.5	This player has limited experience. They can sustain short rallies and know how to keep score.
3.0	This player can hit medium-paced shots. Shots lack depth, directional intent, and consistency. The player understands fundamental strategy and is learning proper court positioning.
3.5	This player has improved stroke development with a moderate level of shot control. They are developing their soft game of dinks and drops. They move toward the kitchen when the opportunity is there.
4.0	This player consistently hits with depth and control. They are still perfecting shot selection. They selectively mix soft and power shots to create an advantage, but with inconsistent results. They're aware of their partner's position on the court and move as a team. They're learning to identify opponents' weaknesses and formulate game plans to attack them.
4.5	This player has a high level of consistency. They use pace and depth to generate opponents' errors. They understand strategy and can adjust style of play according to the opponent's strengths and weaknesses. They make a limited number of unforced errors.
5.0	This player hits all shot types at a high level of ability and rarely makes unforced errors. They have mastered pickleball strategy.
5.5+	This player is a top-caliber player. Performance and tournament wins speak for this player's ability to consistently perform at a high level.

Reading the descriptions in Table 17-1, you may notice that they sound quite subjective. The USAP skill-rating definitions aren't without controversy. Some players feel they are outdated, inaccurate, or don't reflect regional or individual differences in playing styles and abilities. Don't worry if you're still a bit hazy about your own rating after reading these descriptions. We offer more tips for self-rating later in this chapter, in the "Self-Rating for Your First Tournament" sidebar.

Tuning in to tournament rating systems

Competitive pickleball uses a few different rating systems. The difference between these systems and the skill-level definitions in the previous section is that they are objectively based on match results, rather than on the more subjective system of how well you perform various skills. The following subsections describe the main rating systems to become familiar with for tournament play. When you register for a tournament, the website should tell you which system (if any) is used.

USAP Tournament Player Rating (UTPR)

UTPR is the rating system developed by USA Pickleball. It is a calculated rating based on sanctioned tournament results. You must be a USA Pickleball member and play in sanctioned tournaments to earn a UTPR.

Your UTPR can range from 0.000 to 6.999 and is displayed as a four-digit number. Players have separate ratings for gender doubles, mixed doubles, and singles. Age is not accounted for in UTPR.

Your four-digit UTPR is updated weekly based on any sanctioned tournaments you played that week. Your two-digit UTPR is updated quarterly. Every win or loss affects your UTPR — but only by a tiny amount (no more than 0.1 per match). The degree of change will depend on several factors that include your rating, your partner's rating, and your opponents' ratings.

TIP

Don't be surprised if you don't see much movement in your UTPR after your first few tournaments. If you and your opponents were pretty evenly matched, earning enough fractions of a point to get up to the next level will take time.

World Pickleball Ratings (WPR)

PickleballTournaments.com created its own rating system known as World Pickleball Ratings (WPR). Their system calculates your WPR based on your results from any tournaments utilizing their software. Similarly to UTPR, your WPR consists of separate four-digit ratings for gender doubles, mixed doubles, and singles.

The goal behind WPR was to incorporate the greatest number of match results and therefore eliminate the hazards of self-rating and "sandbagging." Many players had been finding that because they rarely played sanctioned tournaments, their UTPR was not accurately reflecting their current skill level. As with most technology these days, the accuracy of the rating comes down to the various algorithms used. We leave that debate to the more mathematically inclined!

WARNING

SELF-RATING FOR YOUR FIRST TOURNAMENT

If you've never played in a tournament before, you won't have a UTPR or WPR rating yet. You will enter your first tournament by reporting a self-assessed rating. We have seen this requirement cause a lot of stress for new tournament players because it's difficult to be objective about your own skill level.

Here are some tips on determining where to begin:

- **Ask more experienced players' opinions.** Preferably, consult players who attend similar-sized tournaments to the one you are planning to enter.

- **Ask a coach's opinion.** If you've been working with a coach, they probably have a good idea of your skill level.

- **Attend a rating clinic.** If the timing is right, you may be able to get evaluated prior to the tournament at a rating session offered by a coach or IPTPA Certified Rating Specialist.

- **Check out the tournament roster.** Most tournament registration sites show you who has already signed up. See whether you recognize any other players. If you see players you normally match up with pretty evenly, consider playing in their division.

Please do not just automatically put yourself in the lowest skill level because it's your first tournament. If you're beating 4.5 level players on a regular basis in recreational games, don't enter the 3.0 division in the tournament. You will probably feel a bit sheepish collecting your medal. Pickleball is more fun when you challenge yourself against true peers.

After the tournament, reevaluate your self-rating. If you easily cruised to the gold medal, you should probably move up a level in your next tournament. Another sign that you may have entered too low is when your opponents' primary strategy was to hit every ball to your noticeably weaker partner. If you never scored more than a few points in any of your matches, you may be better served by moving down a skill level. Or stay at the same level but concentrate on improving through coaching, training, and more court time. Things can only get better from here!

Dynamic Universal Pickleball Ratings (DUPR)

DUPR (rhymes with "super") was developed by Steve Kuhn, founder of Major League Pickleball (MLP). It's also the official rating system of the Professional Pickleball Association (PPA). Your DUPR rating is a four-digit number that ranges from 2.000 to 8.000. With DUPR, you have only two ratings: one for singles and one for doubles.

Interestingly, DUPR accounts for *all* matches you play, including recreational play (though tournaments and other official DUPR events do count more). In addition, your exact scores are also factored into the calculation, so every point counts, not just wins and losses.

To get a DUPR rating, simply sign up for a free account on the app and start playing matches with other users. As soon as you log the match results, you'll see your ratings change. Many players enjoy participating in DUPR because it adds higher stakes to recreational play. It also makes your rating more dynamic because it can change with every match you play — not just after a big tournament.

Walking the Line: Tournament Roles and Expectations

If you intend to play tournaments, it's helpful to know what to expect and what will be expected of you. We're here to guide you through the mountains, valleys, lakes, and streams of the competitive landscape (yodeling optional).

Expectations for players

As a tournament participant, your choices and behavior can greatly affect not only your own experience but everyone's around you as well. Tournaments are complex events requiring quite a bit of "cat herding" on the part of organizers. They must stick to a schedule, making sure all matches are played fairly and results are recorded accurately. Be mindful of doing your part to ensure an enjoyable, successful tournament for all. As a player, you are expected to

>> **Enter the appropriate division.** Don't sign up for a division that is clearly below your skill level. It's always better to play "up" than to play "down" if your desired division is full.

>> **Register and pay your fees early.** Be sure that both you and your partner register and pay your fees before the deadline. Tournament directors have enough to do without dealing with last-minute registrations.

>> **Carefully read all emails.** Be aware of any notices, changes, prematch briefings, and other information. Don't cause yourself unnecessary stress on tournament day by ignoring important instructions regarding parking, start times, or check-in requirements.

>> **Listen carefully at the player briefing.** Nerves are riding high, but as best you can, listen carefully as the tournament staff explain the format and procedures for the day. You'll be able to relax more if you know exactly what's expected of you and how the event is being run.

>> **Keep your phone nearby.** Many tournaments notify players of court assignments by text, so keep your cellphone charged and close by so that you don't miss your match.

>> **Be ready to play.** When you're called to your court, get right down to the business of warming up. Not only is it rude to keep your opponents and referee waiting, but taking too long to arrive may result in a forfeit.

>> **Respect your referee.** If you have a referee, you may get another short prematch briefing. Listen closely and treat your referee with respect. Most referees are either volunteers or are being paid very little. Referees deserve our appreciation, not grief!

>> **Play your match with integrity.** Play to win, but maintain good sporting conduct. Call the lines and foot faults as fairly as you can on your side of the court. Your honesty is good for the sport.

>> **Turn in your scorecard promptly.** At the end of your match, you may be expected to take the scorecard back to the tournament desk. Report the results of your match promptly to avoid delays in getting your court turned over for another match.

Cooperation is essential. Players should be ready, respectful, and reasonable. Tournaments are difficult to run, so do your best to be a help rather than a hindrance. This approach is great for the tournament and the sport as a whole.

Calling 'em as they see 'em: Referees and line judges

Some tournaments have no referees, some provide them only for medal matches, and some have referees for all matches. A referee's role is to help your matches run smoothly. The referee is there to help, not hinder, the flow of play. Referees keep track of the score and time-outs, both to keep the play fair and so that players don't need to waste their own precious brain power. Referees also constantly monitor players' starting positions, ensuring that the correct person serves and receives from the correct side. They watch closely for kitchen and service faults, but they don't call the other lines. That responsibility falls on either the players or line judges. The ref has authority to overrule a line call, but they will do so only if the call is challenged and they were able to see it clearly.

Stepping out on the court with a ref for the first time ("Who is this extra person on my court? Security!") can be a bit intimidating. It helps to know how this experience will differ from your average, everyday pickleball match. Here are some things to expect from your referee:

>> **Prematch briefing:** The referee introduces themselves, confirms that the correct teams are present, and explains the match format. They will remind you that they watch for service and kitchen faults but that calling the other lines is your responsibility. They may also warn you of any potential safety hazards specific to that court or venue.

>> **Paddle inspection:** In a sanctioned event, the referee quickly inspects each player's paddle to make sure it conforms to USAP equipment regulations. If you've coated your paddle in super glue and sandpaper, your ref will definitely notice!

>> **Determining first serve:** The rule book states that referees may use "any fair method" to determine who gets the first choice of serve, receive, or end (meaning which side of the net they'll start on). Typically, they write "1" or 2" on the back of the scorecard and ask one of the teams to guess the number. Your ref will provide some sort of wearable identification, such as a wristband, to mark the first server on each team.

>> **Calling the score:** After players are in position, the referee starts each point by calling the score. It can feel strange to not call the score yourself, but be sure to wait for the referee to call the score before you serve; otherwise, it's a service fault! After each rally concludes, the referee verbally acknowledges the result by calling "point" (if the serving team won the rally), or "second serve" or "sideout" (if the serving team lost the rally). As a player, keeping an ear out for these calls to make sure they are correct is a good idea. Sometimes even our most brilliant, beloved refs can make mistakes. They are human.

>> **Line calls and foot faults:** The referee's primary job during a rally is watching for service faults and kitchen faults. Don't assume the ref will acknowledge that a ball was out, even if it clearly sailed way out of bounds. The referee will wait for you to make the line call on your side of the court, either verbally or both verbally and with a hand signal. (An index finger pointed straight into the air is the signal for "out.") Be "loud and proud" when you call "out!" Your ref will thank you.

- >> **End changes and time-outs:** The referee lets players know when the time has come to change ends (in the middle of a game or between games). The rules ensure that teams play on both ends during a match in case of issues with sun, wind, or other factors. You have one minute to relocate, get a drink, towel off, and strategize with your partner. When a time-out is called mid-game by a player, the referee will pull out their trusty stopwatch and start the one-minute countdown. You get a 15-second verbal warning before the ref calls "time in." (If you've been looking for a good excuse to carry around a stopwatch and a tiny clipboard, become a pickleball referee!)

- >> **Overruling calls:** If you feel strongly that your opponent has made a poor line call, you can ask the referee whether they saw things differently. In most cases, the ref will respond, "I didn't see it well enough to overrule." The call stands. The ref was probably busy watching the kitchen line or didn't have a clear line of sight. However, be aware that a referee does have the authority to overrule a line call, but only when challenged by the team who lost the rally.

- >> **Monitoring player behavior:** One of the ref's most important duties is to make sure players are behaving fairly and acting appropriately. Profanity, excessive arguing, delays of game, ball abuse, throwing paddles, or other dangerous and unsporting behavior can result in a verbal warning, a technical warning, or a technical foul.

Referees often volunteer their time for free or are paid only a nominal fee, so please treat these wonderful rule-book experts with kindness and respect. Trust that they are doing their best. They certainly did not become referees to get rich! Pickleball is growing incredibly fast, and nearly every tournament is faced with a shortage of referees. If you think refereeing might be an enjoyable way to get more involved, consider training for it. See Chapter 19 to find out how referees begin as tiny seedlings and mature into the cherished chestnuts of a pickleball community.

Some of the very biggest events also provide line judges for their medal matches. Line judges call the lines and service-line foot faults. Line judges go through training and certification, but it's a much shorter and less rigorous process than the one required to become a certified referee. There is, thankfully, a vision test involved!

TIP

You can make tournament life much easier for yourself, your partner, your opponents, and your referees by reading the entire rule book before competing. The middle of a tournament match is not the time to quiz your referee with rules questions or start unnecessary disputes because of your own ignorance. You can purchase an official rule book or download the PDF version from USA Pickleball's website at https://www.usapickleball.org.

Cheering appropriately: Coaches and spectators

Pickleball is an exciting sport to watch! If you haven't had the chance to watch high-level tournament play, especially at the pro level, we strongly encourage you to do so. It's extremely intense and fun. Coauthor Mo is well-known for her loud cheering and ability to drown out any public address system. She also carries great signs, so you definitely want her in your corner (unless such exuberance embarrasses you, in which case it's best to sit elsewhere and pretend you don't know her).

WARNING

It's great to cheer on your favorite players, but be aware that some cheering can be considered coaching. Coaching is allowed only during time-outs and between games. *Coaching* is defined as any communication that a player can act on to gain an advantage. You don't want to accidentally cost your favorite player a point. During a game, as a spectator, you *cannot* yell things like

>> "Let it go!" (When a ball is headed out)

>> "Be aggressive!"

>> "Hold the line!"

>> "Hit it to his backhand!"

>> "Wrong server — switch sides!"

Do not participate in line calls or scorekeeping if you are a spectator. You may in fact have the best view of anyone in the stadium to see that a ball called out was in fact in. Keep this knowledge to yourself and let the officials do their jobs. There is absolutely no scenario in which a call will be overruled thanks to your "helpful" interjection. Spectators are disruptive when they give their two cents on line calls, and players violate the rules if they consult a spectator regarding a line call.

You can yell things like "Here we go!" and "You've got this!" and "Go team!" or other generally encouraging things. Be a good spectator by bringing positivity not only to your favorite player or team but the experience as a whole. Stay out of any drama. Certainly never insult a referee or line judge. Please don't ever show disrespect for anyone with your cheerleading. Cheer *for* people, never *against* anyone. If your favorite team's opponent makes a great shot, you can still applaud their thrilling display of athleticism. They are putting on a great show for you!

If you are a player's chosen coach, feel free to offer words of wisdom during time-outs and between games. Great coaching can be an invaluable tool and turn around the momentum of a match on a dime. Be sure to coach your player or team privately if you don't want their opponents to know what you said. Friends, family, and fans of a given player are more than happy to share the coaching they overheard you dishing out, so keep it hushed and private. Sneaky! Don't be so sneaky that you break the rules, though. Coaching violations can be called because of verbal, nonverbal (meaning hand signals), or electronic communication.

REMEMBER

Coaching between doubles partners can occur at any time and is considered to be partner communication. No time-out needed.

Putting Yourself Out There: Tips for Your First Tournament

So you've decided that you want to try your hand at formal competition. Good for you! For some players, this is the natural choice because competition sounds fun and intriguing. For others, it's an extremely brave choice. Either way, we commend you. Competition can really enhance your enjoyment of the game and lead to wonderful new friendships and adventures. This section offers some tips to make your first tournament the best experience it can be.

Choosing a doubles partner

Coauthor Mo's mother gave her two of the best pieces of advice ever uttered in the world of competitive sports:

>> Choose a great doubles partner.

>> Win the last point.

Are there any arguments against those two golden nuggets of wisdom? Nope. Thanks, Mom! To get started, you need to find a great doubles partner.

First consider what you need in a partner. Think about people you play well with *and* enjoy spending time with. Doubles partners often hang out and travel to tournaments together. If you don't have good "off court" chemistry, you're not likely to have good "on court" chemistry. As a team, you want to be a well-oiled machine, working together toward a common goal — not two individuals working at cross-purposes. Here are some aspects to consider when looking for a partner:

>> **Dominant hand:** Are they right or left-handed? Pairing a right-handed player with a left-handed player can give the team a significant advantage. If such a

team stacks or switches (explained in Chapter 12), they can play with both of their forehands in the middle. Watch out!

>> **Time and commitment:** Are there days and times when you're both available to practice together? Getting in sync with a partner you've barely played with before is hard. How committed is your partner to practicing with you? Any amount is okay, as long as you both agree.

>> **Skill level:** Try to partner with someone who is close to your skill level to enable simplicity and fairness when choosing what division to enter. It also allows both partners to contribute to the team instead of one player dominating or the weaker player being picked on.

>> **Age:** You may also want to choose a partner who is near your own age. If you are 83 years old and decide to partner with a 24-year-old, you will wind up having to enter the 19+ age division. (We're not implying you can't hang; it's just something to consider.)

>> **Communication skills:** Before, during, and after the match, you need to communicate well with each other.

>> **Attitude:** As we say elsewhere in the book, the number one job of a doubles partner is to lift their partner up. Look for someone who is good at supporting you in the particular ways that help you, and who brings positive energy to the court.

The best way to find your next doubles partner is to simply start asking. We know this idea can be daunting, like finding a date to prom! You might get a few no's before you get a yes. Don't take the no's too personally. Someone may simply have other plans in mind.

TIP

If the deadline is looming and you're still having problems securing a partner, most tournaments maintain a list of "Players Needing Partners" on the registration site. As with any blind date, it's a bit of a gamble. You might end up having a wonderful time, or it might turn out to be a horrible match, but at least you'll get a funny story out of it. (As much as she loves a funny story, coauthor Mo has had a few too many "hilarious" blind dates for her taste.)

Knowing what to bring

Nothing is worse than arriving at a tournament and realizing you don't have what you need. Attending a tournament with nothing but a small water bottle and a granola bar is a bold choice indeed, but not the smartest. Here are some essential items you definitely want to pack in your bag:

- » Your favorite paddle, plus a spare, if you have one
- » At least two balls that are the same brand the tournament is using
- » Court shoes
- » Towel
- » Water and electrolytes
- » Meals and snacks
- » Chair, possibly with a shade umbrella
- » Medications and a small first aid kit
- » Sunglasses or other eye protection
- » Sunscreen and headwear
- » Money and ID
- » Change of clothes if you sweat a lot
- » Comfy sandals or shoes for after your matches

TIP

Always bring plenty of food! Too often, players start to crash mid-tournament because they aren't eating enough between games. To sustain your mental and physical energy, you'll want to graze on healthy snacks throughout the day. Don't count on finding food available for purchase. Even if you do, it may not be suitable in the middle of an athletic competition. (Chili dogs, anyone?)

Setting expectations for tournament day

When you arrive at a tournament, you'll walk into an event that is charged with energy. Players will be staking out areas to park their chairs and gear. Shady spots will be snapped up quickly. You may see endless rows of shade canopies spread out before you, and even some elaborate tailgating setups with misters, ice chests, and massage chairs.

As your first task, stop at the check-in desk. (Feel free to stride up to the desk and confidently declare, "I've arrived!") Next, find your partner and make sure they're ready to play. Locate and use the restroom to avoid doing some suspicious dancing during your match. It's always best to show up early and allow plenty of time to set up your "campsite" and get stretched out, warmed up, and hydrated. If you're feeling nervous, you can try techniques like deep breathing, meditating, jogging laps, listening to music, or sharing laughs with friends before it's time to get down to business.

When you are called to your first match, you typically have ten minutes at most to warm up, so get there quickly! If you're playing doubles, warm up on the opposite side of the net from your partner who, if you've planned ahead, knows your preferred warm-up routine. Check out where the wind sock or flag is so that you can monitor the wind conditions. For safety reasons, you won't be allowed to carry anything but a towel and your water bottle onto the court.

If you have a referee, they will give you a short prematch briefing and randomly pick which team gets to select "serve or side." If you don't have a ref, the players determine who gets to choose, usually by having one write a "1" or a "2" on the back of the scorecard (or holding up one or two fingers behind their paddle), and asking a player on the other team to guess the number. If they guess correctly, they get to choose either which team serves first or which side of the net (end) they want to start on. Whichever one they don't pick is decided by their opponents.

In a match of two out of three games played to 11 points, the teams switch ends of the court after each game. If the match goes to a third game, the teams switch ends again after one team reaches 6 points. If you're playing only one game to 15 points, the teams will switch ends as soon as one team reaches 8 points.

At the conclusion of each game, players should come to the net, gently tap paddles, and say, "Good game." At the end of the match, the winning team makes sure the scorecard is filled out properly and initials it. Be sure to return the scorecard to the tournament desk expeditiously to help keep the tournament moving.

For a variety of reasons, tournaments commonly run late. You may have long waits between matches. It's best to go with the flow and not let unexpected delays upset you. If you're lucky enough to keep progressing in the tournament or are playing in a round robin, you can expect your event to last around 4–8 hours.

If you manage to win a medal (congrats!), you will be called to the medal stand to collect your gold, silver, or bronze and take photos with your fellow medalists. It is customary to bring your paddle with you and display your medal hanging around your neck, resting on your paddle face (see Figure 17-2). Many photos are usually taken on the medal stand with multiple cameras and phones, so be patient and smile pretty.

Maintaining your mental focus

Tournament days can sometimes feel very long. You may find your attention wandering as you think about the pizza and beer you'll be sharing with friends later to celebrate (or commiserate). Or maybe it's 90 degrees out, and all you can think about is jumping in a kiddie pool full of ice cubes. Wait — hold up! Get your mind back to the current task at hand: playing your very best pickleball.

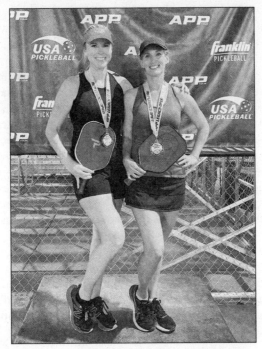

FIGURE 17-2:
Nothing is quite like perching atop the medal stand after a long day of hard-fought matches.

Arrive at each match ready to play and in a positive mental state regardless of how intimidating your opponents may look. Connect with your partner and make sure you're on the same page as far as strategy. Get yourselves pumped up! After all, you're a team, and you're counting on the other to give it their all. Nobody likes to feel that they have let their partner down. Use that partnership as motivation to keep battling hard until the very end.

It's important to clear your head of anything that's not currently happening on your court. Now is not the time to mentally compile your list of tomorrow's errands. Don't worry about who's playing on the court next to you (OMG, is that Anna Leigh Waters?). You also need to let go of whatever happened in your last match. Try to imagine your court as an island in the middle of the ocean. It's just you, your partner, your opponents, and the ball.

During the match, stay well-hydrated and toweled off. Cooling towels doused in ice water can quickly offer relief and ward off a heat-related injury. Use your paddle-tracking technique from Chapter 11 to help you stay focused and squared to the ball. Stalk that ball like a cougar stalking its prey. It's almost impossible to let your mind drift over to the food trucks (gosh, something smells good!) when you're busy paddle tracking. Stay hungry for the ball instead! One of coauthor Reine's tricks to maintain intensity through a long tournament day is to think to herself repeatedly,

"Gimme the ball! Gimme the ball!" It sounds a little crazy, but it works much better than thinking, "Please don't hit it to me, I am so, so, so, so tired . . ."

REMEMBER

Between points, please use only positive self-talk. Dwelling on your mistakes certainly won't undo them and will only distract you going forward. One error can suddenly multiply into three before you even realize what's happening. If you notice your partner getting flustered or dwelling on their own errors, call a time-out and have a pep talk. Don't wait until the match slips away from you to step up and be the supportive partner they need.

Some people find that repetitive physical actions between points, like tapping, wiggling their fingers, hopping back and forth, spinning their paddle, or performing certain breathing patterns, helps them stay present and focused. You've probably seen tennis or pickleball players with some pretty elaborate pre-serving routines: bounce the ball 19 times, pull up their sleeve, adjust their hat, bounce the ball 19 more times, rock back and forth, grimace, and then finally serve. No matter what habits work for you, be sure to check in with your body regularly. Are you clenching your teeth, squeezing your paddle too hard, or holding your breath? Nerves can do that to you. Make a conscious effort to relax, breathe, and find your Zen between each point.

TIP

Every match is a puzzle to be solved, and the puzzle may keep changing as your opponents try new strategies. Never get complacent, even if you're winning 10–0. Most tournament players have at least one sad story of "the match that got away." Try to forget about the score and focus on one point at a time. Keep after it with full intensity until the very end.

Using time-outs wisely

In games played to 11 or 15 points, each team gets two one-minute timeouts. Use them both! You can use time-outs just to give yourself a break if you're feeling winded or mentally overwhelmed. More commonly, players use time-outs strategically. If one team is on a roll and seems to have too much momentum in the match, the other team wisely calls a time-out, which can often swing the momentum the other way.

Detailed changes in strategy may be suggested during a time-out, or partners may just pump each other up and change the energy dynamic. Coaching is allowed during time-outs, so your supporters may be able to offer advice. Sometimes an outside perspective can really help!

TIP

If your opponents get to game point or match point and you have time-outs left, this is a good time to hit pause and try to find a way to turn things around. It certainly can't hurt! Never give up until the match is over.

Reflecting after the tournament

If you took home a gold medal, you're probably pretty happy about having played in a tournament. If you lost your first two matches, donned the "Sandals of Shame," and cried all the way home, perhaps you're having regrets. Either way, take a few days and let the dust settle. After you've taken a few long Epsom salt baths and plenty of ibuprofen, you can reflect on the experience and decide whether tournament play is right for you.

Deciding whether tournaments are for you

Tournament play is not a good fit for every player. That's okay. Your desire, or lack thereof, to play in organized competitions is no reflection on who you are as a person. Tournaments can bring out the worst in some players. If they transform you from a happy-go-lucky recreational player into a nasty, temper-tantrum-throwing player, please decline the next opportunity to sign up for a tournament. On the other hand, if tournaments light a fire of challenge and enthusiasm in your soul, by all means, play in them!

You may have other barriers to enjoying tournaments, such as health conditions, financial priorities, discomfort with large crowds, or a dislike of traveling. Some players hate waiting around for matches and are happier playing rapid-fire pickup games at their local park. Just remember that there is no shame in it either way. Never feel pressured to play in tournaments just to prove you're a great pickleball player. Your abilities speak for themselves, no matter the stage. Make sure that pickleball remains fun for you! It is a game, after all.

WARNING

Use caution if you're considering throwing in the towel after one bad tournament experience. Most tournament players have had very good *and* very bad tournaments. Different events can have different vibes. If your first one was a disaster, perhaps your next one will be great! Getting back on the horse takes courage and can be a good mental and emotional challenge for you to tackle. No matter the outcome of the next one, you can still be proud you gave it another go.

Determining what to do differently

After a tournament, it's a good idea to take some time to think about what you might do differently should you decide to dip your toes back into the competitive pool. You probably found that certain aspects of your game need some work. You can turn to a coach for help or just focus practice sessions on turning your weaknesses into strengths. Some players thrive on the extra bit of motivation that tournaments give them.

You might consider a smaller or larger tournament, or one that uses a different format. If double elimination feels like too much pressure, try a round robin next time. You'll be guaranteed to keep playing even if you lose your first two matches. There are indoor and outdoor tournaments, so if the sun and heat were your downfall in the last tournament, you might want to try an indoor competition next time. If you didn't particularly enjoy getting beaten by your own grandmother (dang it, Nana!), try a tournament with separate age divisions next time.

Maybe you and your partner didn't quite jibe, or you found that you overpacked. Perhaps your breakfast of prunes and coffee was ill-advised, or you failed to bring enough snacks. We hope you didn't skip our advice in Chapter 15 about dressing in layers and try to play in a fleece onesie in the middle of summer. Try to reflect on everything that went right or wrong for you that day. After just a few tournaments, you'll probably be totally dialed in to what you need to be comfortable, play your best, and have a great time.

Breaking Up Is Hard to Do: Changing Partners

This might be the most delicate topic in this book (gulp!). Please have a seat, because it's time for some real talk about doubles partnerships.

Doubles partners usually start out as friends who enjoy playing with each other recreationally. When you create a doubles partnership, having a conversation about the permanence of this relationship is worthwhile. Doubles partnerships are *not* marriages! (This is true even if your current doubles partner also happens to be your spouse.) If either of you decides to switch to a different partner in the future, be sure the friendship stays intact.

If you decide to change to a different doubles partner, be forthright with your soon-to-be ex-partner. Give them enough notice so that they are not in a tough spot trying to find a new partner for the next tournament. Lead the conversation with kindness. Tell them that you've enjoyed playing with them, but you'd like to branch out to broaden your experiences. Be honest. Don't take the coward's way out by suddenly ghosting your partner or concocting an elaborate lie. By doing so, you are being disrespectful and endangering a friendship that could have a lot more to give.

If you're on the receiving end of a doubles partnership "break up," please don't take it too personally. Very few humans are great at handling rejection (or what we perceive as such). Your feelings will probably be a bit hurt, or maybe you're just disappointed, which is natural. Keep things in perspective: Very few doubles partnerships last forever because individual players don't stay the same forever.

Your individual games might not always change in the same exact way, or at the same rate, affecting your team dynamic. Switching things up might spark an exciting opportunity for you both. If you can put your hurt feelings aside, you can still maintain a supportive friendship with your ex-partner. Keep cheering each other on!

You might consider a change in partners if your partner does not enhance your tournament experience. Playing as a team should be a fun and uniting experience that builds over time. If your dynamic is fraught with strife and conflict, it is definitely time to look for a new partner. Yes, even if you are married! Not all couples pair well together as doubles partners. The pickleball court shared by couples is often referred to as the "divorce court"! It's almost as bad as getting in a two-person kayak together. ("Are you even paddling? Why am I the only one paddling?") If competing together is harming, rather than enhancing, your relationship, try to put the relationship first.

Another reason to change partners is when your skill levels are no longer comparable. It's not good for anyone if a 3.0 player is forced to compete at their partner's 5.0 level. They will get picked on, and that's a tough place to be. It's also not much fun for their more skilled partner because they won't get to hit many balls. We all want to feel like we are positively contributing to our team.

If you and your partner don't communicate well, have very different ideas about strategy, or just don't mesh well for any reason, give yourself permission to move on. There are plenty of fish in the pickleball sea. Try to find someone who will add to your joy of the game in addition to helping you play your best pickleball. A well-oiled doubles team is built from communication, mutual respect, and balance. A truly great doubles partnership can become a unique and treasured relationship.

5
Enjoying the Wider World of Pickleball

Chapter **18**

So Social: Jumping into the Pickleball Scene

When you were a little kid, you'd probably meet another kid at the playground, say your name, and within a minute or two ask, "Want to be friends?" And that was it. You had a new friend.

As an adult, making new friends gets a little harder. Careers, families, and the daily grind can make it difficult to connect. But there is an easy way to make friends again. Just step onto a court, paddle in hand, and say, "Want to play pickleball?" You just made at least three new friends!

Pickleball tends to be a more social sport than most, for a variety of reasons. The court is smaller than a tennis court, so talking with the other players is easier. Players often show up individually rather than as a prearranged foursome. A large portion of the pickleball population picked up the game in their forties, fifties and sixties. They show up to get exercise and often to meet new people. If you get nothing else from pickleball, we hope you make many wonderful friends. We did!

The pickleball social scene is everywhere, from public courts operated by city recreation departments, community developments, and private clubs to homemade courts on the streets, driveways, and inside garages or basements to fancy custom courts in backyards. There's little barrier to diving right in and meeting lots of like-minded folks!

Joining a Pickleball Club

As you play more pickleball, you may find yourself wanting more: more time to play, more players to play with, more fun. All these outcomes may await you through a local pickleball club. If you're thinking about joining a club, here are some factors to consider:

>> **Cost:** Are you willing to pay monthly or annual fees, and if so, how much?

>> **Location:** How far are you willing to drive to play, potentially several times a week?

>> **Size:** What size club are you interested in? Are you looking to meet a few hundred players, or are you more comfortable with smaller sized groups? If it's a large club, how do they manage court usage and crowds?

>> **Culture:** Do you want to join an informal group at the local park or one at an upscale country club? Try to get the feel of the club. Do they offer events for players of your skill level?

>> **Activities:** Are you interested in lots of organized play like ladders, leagues, tournaments, and social gatherings or do you prefer more casual play? Does the club offer the kind of competition you enjoy?

In the next section, we outline the benefits of joining a club, or forming a club yourself if you don't find one near you. Starting a club may seem daunting at first, but folks all over the world are starting pickleball clubs with no prior experience — just passion for the game and some plucky DIY spirit. Pickleballers are unstoppable!

Enjoying the benefits of a club

Whether you join an informal club at the local park or pay for a membership to an athletic or country club, you can experience some definite advantages of being a "joiner." Benefits vary, but you may get to

>> **Drop in.** Most clubs have several drop-in times a week. No hassle of finding partners and organizing a court. You simply drop in and play with whomever is there, which is a nice way to meet new people. You can also learn more about pickleball and hone your skills by playing with people of different styles and skill levels.

>> **Reserve a court.** You don't have the hassle in waiting for others to finish. Some (but not all) clubs have reservation systems, so you're guaranteed a court time.

>> **Learn from a pro.** Most larger clubs have teaching pros who offer clinics and private lessons.

>> **Party on.** Clubs are primarily social and make parties a priority because they add to the fun. It can be a perfect way to get to know the people you play with a little better.

>> **Play tournaments.** Club-run tournaments are often low-key compared to large, sanctioned tournaments, so they're an easy way to get your feet wet before entering any major events.

>> **Get discounts.** Who doesn't love a deal? Often, clubs offer discount pricing for members on court time, lessons, and tournaments. Many clubs also negotiate discounts from equipment retailers.

>> **Volunteer.** If you enjoy sharing your talents and giving back to the community, joining a club provides many opportunities for you to get involved and make a difference.

To gain maximum enjoyment from the club experience, we recommend finding your tribe. You will instantly meet a lot of people who may have similar interests. From your new pickleball club friends, you can learn how to play better, what equipment to buy, where to get lessons, and where to find the best tacos in the neighborhood after you've won all your matches. (Tacos are for winners.)

Forming a new club

Anyone can start a club, including you! Most pickleball clubs begin as grassroot efforts, and their organizers are just regular people who see an opportunity to unite the players in their community. Sometimes the impetus comes from seeing a problem and wanting to collectively improve the local pickleball experience. Players organize into clubs for several reasons:

>> **Scheduling:** Clubs offer a way to organize drop-in play, ladders, and leagues. Organizing not only helps players mix and mingle but can also help ease overcrowding by redirecting court traffic to less busy times.

>> **Communication:** Forming a club is one way to gather contact information and efficiently communicate with players in your area. Some important topics to communicate on include court closures or openings; local tournaments and events; advocacy opportunities; lost-and-found items; and club rules and regulations.

>> **Advocacy:** Organizing local players into a club allows you to advocate collectively for additional courts, more gym time, and facility improvements, among other issues. In some cases, it may be necessary to represent the

interest of pickleballers when cities or neighborhood associations want to limit the use of courts.

>> **Rules:** Sometimes forming a club is necessary so that someone has the authority to set rules and regulations. When courts get overcrowded, bad behavior can occur. Rules about court rotation, sharing, and etiquette can go a long way toward keeping the peace and making sure everything runs smoothly during crowded play times.

Starting a new pickleball club may seem daunting at first, but you are also becoming a trailblazer, which can be fun and rewarding. It's an opportunity to bring your community together and play more pickleball at the same time (a win-win.) Although forming a new club entails a lot of work, you can recruit volunteers to bring their unique talents to the table and you may well end up with lifelong friendships in the process. Here are some tips for setting up your own club:

>> **Decide where to play.** Make sure the times you want to play are accessible and enough courts exist. Also confirm that you have the blessing of the venue owner, city, or park district before formally organizing a club at their courts.

>> **Give your club a name.** Go with something that is easily identifiable and indicates the venue, town, or region your club plans to serve. Potential members need to easily be able to find you on Google and social media.

>> **Recruit members.** Go to local events or other clubs and ask around to see who's interested, or just start with a few friends and spread the word. Distribute flyers and post on social media. One of the best ways to attract new members is to offer some sort of free weekly clinics for beginners. See Chapter 19 for tips on holding an introductory clinic.

>> **Identify the decision-maker(s).** The organizer may be just you for a while, but be on the lookout for people to delegate tasks to. Fortunately, many people are passionate about pickleball, so finding others who want to get involved won't be that hard.

>> **Determine dues.** Determine monthly or annual dues (if any) and what benefits you can offer members in exchange for paying them.

>> **Have ongoing communications.** Keep your peeps connected! Create a Facebook group, email list, website, or a simple newsletter to keep people up to date.

>> **If you have enough players, form committees to help with the club.** You are only one person and can't do everything. Pickleballers love to help! It never hurts to ask.

>> **Don't get discouraged.** It's important to realize going in that pleasing everyone all the time is impossible. Focus on the positive outcomes you're achieving, and be sure to take time to step back and enjoy actually playing, too! After all, the love of the game is what motivated you to step up in the first place.

It's really cool to see a newly formed group gather to organize fundraisers and social events, or convince the park district to convert unused tennis or basketball courts into thriving pickleball courts. We see this positive energy for change happening all over the world. Imagine all the picklebilities — er, possibilities!

Playing in Ladders and Leagues

All clubs that host pickleball engage a wide variety of levels of players and competitiveness. Offering ladders and leagues is a good way to keep your club programs fresh and courts full. Organized play is a nice alternative to casual drop-in play, which can be a bit of a hit-or-miss proposition for competitive players. Organized play can also help new players feel included.

A ladder league is designed to help players get a chance to play with others of a similar skill level. The rungs on the ladder represent each player's ranking over a certain period of time. During ladder play dates, typically held weekly, a foursome meets and plays three games. Each player teams with a different partner each game. Players track their total points for these three games. Based on the points earned for that day, you move up or down the rungs of the ladder. The more weeks that everyone plays, the more closely players become grouped by skill. Every time the ladder meets, you play with the three players closest to your current ranking.

Another type of league you can run is a team-based league. Teams may consist of two, four, or more players depending on the format. Each week, two players from each team play a match against another team and record their scores. After every team has had a chance to play each other over the course of the season, the top teams go into a playoff round to determine the league champions. Team-based leagues build camaraderie. You can run them from within your own club or between nearby clubs and cities.

Leagues are extremely popular. To run one, you need a system for tracking everyone's scores and rankings. You can use good old-fashioned pen and paper or a spreadsheet. Easy-to-use software is also available to help you keep track of everything, such as ClubExpress, R2 Sports, Global Pickleball Network, TopDog Sports, and others.

Organizing Fun Events

Because pickleball is such a social sport, organizing events is a natural next step. Don't do it alone! Recruit fellow players to help you and come up with a plan using your combined creativity. Social media is an abundant source of ideas from other clubs and players around the world.

Running round robins, mixers, and scrambles

Round robins, mixers, and scramble events are a fun way to mix up a group. Events like these also provide opportunities for club members to play with new partners and opponents. They take some work to set up, but the rewards are many, and with luck, you'll have some friends to help you. You can also use apps like Round Robin Assistant, Scoreholio, Pickleball Scoreboard, and others to help you track the progress.

In a nutshell, here's how these formats generally work:

>> **Round robin:** Typically, a round robin is a team event in which doubles teams play against all the other teams in their pool. Winners are determined by total wins followed by total points.

>> **Mixer:** For each game, players are randomly paired up, but they individually track their total wins and points. You'll get to play both with and against a lot of different people in one day.

>> **Scramble:** A scramble is similar to a mixer, but rather than completing games to 11 or 15, players engage in timed rounds (typically 10–12 minutes). Players track their total points over the course of the event. Scrambles are an efficient and lively way to squeeze a lot of pickleball play into a short time because no one is waiting around between matches.

>> **King/queen of the court:** In this format, courts are ranked from highest to lowest. When you win a game, you move "up" a court. When you lose a game, you move "down" a court. You may play as either a team or an individual (changing partners each time). After a few rounds, the more skilled players are grouped toward the top court and the lesser-skilled players are on the bottom courts.

Follow these steps to successfully organize these types of events:

1. **Determine the location.**

   You need to make sure there are enough courts, parking spaces, bathrooms, shade, and seating.

2. **Set a registration fee.**

   Clearly define what players get in exchange for their fee.

3. **Create an easy way for players to sign up, and post a registration deadline.**

   You can even have early-bird deadlines with a discounted fee to drum up early interest.

4. **Decide whether you want to have event t-shirts made and order medals or other prizes.**

   Instead of ordering t-shirts, you may consider hats, towels, or water bottles because you don't have to worry about sizes so much. Be sure to plan ahead for ordering.

5. **Provide refreshments, especially water.**

   Look for sponsors for giveaways like lip balm, water bottles, snacks, and so on. Sometimes sponsors donate pickleball equipment for prizes, too.

6. **The day of the event, be sure to have someone checking people in.**

   Make sure the check-in person can explain the format and direct people where they need to go.

7. **Have fun.**

   Even though you're running the event, don't forget to join the excitement. You may not be able to compete in the event if you have too much cat-herding to do, but you can still have a fantastic time.

Camaraderie is vital for any club. Continually find ways to help people feel welcomed and have positive experiences. It's the pickleball way.

Letting your creativity run wild: other fun event ideas

Just playing pickleball is a blast, but coming up with new ways to enjoy the sport is even better. You can plan fundraisers, competitive events, or a social event like a potluck or happy hour. In addition to the obvious holiday-themed events, here are some other creative ideas:

>> Costume Contest

>> Crazy Socks or Hat Day

>> Dinks and Drinks, or Pizza and Pickleballs

>> Poker Pickleball (collect a playing card for every win; try to make a winning hand)

>> Pickleball Bingo (mark off a square for every person you play with)

>> Glow-in-the-dark pickleball

>> Dinking-only tournaments

>> Age-split tournaments (one partner under 30 and one over 60)

>> Skills and drills events

>> Pickleball carnivals with skill games and prizes

>> Bring a Newbie Day

>> Blind Date/Luck of the Draw tournament (partners are randomly paired up)

>> Wacky Rules Day (three bounces? overhand serves? no forehands allowed?)

The only limit to new pickleball event ideas is your own creativity. Besides offering events from within your own club, consider networking with other clubs for some interclub play and social mixers. We warned you that you may end up with *a lot* of new friends.

Traveling and Pickleball: *Always* pack a paddle!

Avid pickleball players often keep a spare paddle, shoes, and a ball with them at all times to be prepared in case an impromptu pickleball game breaks out anywhere. (It has never happened to us, but we keep hoping.) The beauty of a pickleball paddle is that it fits in almost any suitcase, keeping you ready to play pickleball on vacation, too! You find instant friends in a different town, plus you get to see how other clubs play. Pickleball players always seem to help each other find the best restaurants and attractions in any given location. You can even find or provide housing for another pickleball player through Picklebilly Hosted Housing (https://Picklebilly.com). There are also Airbnb and Vrbo vacation rentals that have pickleball courts right on the property! What could be better?

Meeting up with the locals for casual play

We've taken our paddles with us on vacation and found that each club or park has its own way of doing things. To learn the etiquette of each club, review its information online beforehand, if possible. Find out about its drop-in times and protocol, time limits for court usage, and how to get in the queue to play. After you arrive at the courts, players are typically happy to explain their way of doing things. No need to be shy! Most groups are thrilled to welcome visiting players.

Enjoying pickleball entertainment venues

If you're looking for a super-sized day of pickleball with food and drinks in a fun atmosphere either locally or while on vacation, check out the pickleball entertainment centers that are popping up all around the country. Franchises like Chicken N Pickle have opened to rave reviews, offering pickleball courts, beverages and fried chicken — three of our favorite things! They have indoor and outdoor pickleball courts along with tasty food and specialty drinks, plus shuffleboard and bocce ball.

Another enjoyable venue, Pickle & Social, sports a rooftop bar and cornhole in Atlanta, Georgia. There's a House of Pickleball in Leland, North Carolina; Pickleball Zone in Bend, Oregon; and Smash Park in Des Moines, Iowa. Several locations of Electric Pickle, by Eureka Restaurant Group, are opening around the country. Pickleball entertainment venues are growing faster than you can say "Great minds dink alike!" Figures 18-1 and 18-2 show entertainment venues featuring pickleball courts.

FIGURE 18-1: Pickleball (left) and great eats (right) is a winning combo at Chicken N Pickle.

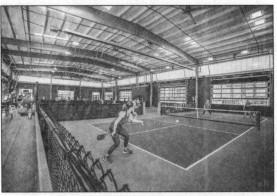
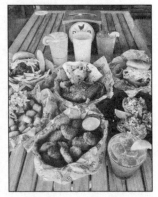

© John Wiley & Sons, Inc./Photo Credit: Kacy Meinecke/Chicken N Pickle

© John Wiley & Sons, Inc./Photo Credit: Amanda Spencer/Chicken N Pickle

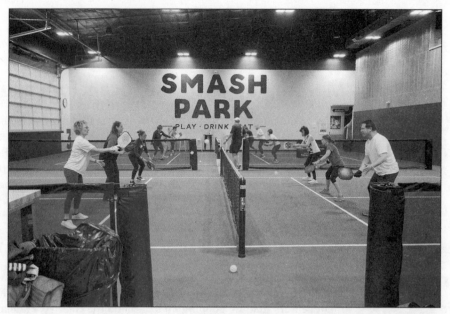

FIGURE 18-2:
Pickleball entertainment venues like Smash Park are popping up all over.

Probably the most ambitious pickleball-related venue is Dreamland, in Dripping Springs, Texas, which is owned by Steve Kuhn, a former hedge-fund manager turned pickleball fanatic. He has built a Disneyland-style venue for adults on 64 acres, with room to have next-level mini golfing, craft breweries, art sculptures, live music, delicious food, and tons of pickleball courts. Kuhn had a dream, built the venue, and in no time, the players came.

We've covered just the tip of the pickleball entertainment scene. Next time you plan a trip, Google the city you're visiting to find the best venues. USA Pickleball's Places2Play website and app (https://Places2Play.org) and the PlayTime Scheduler website (https://PlaytimeScheduler.com) list open courts and play times all over the world. (You can find more details on these sites in Chapter 4.)

Joining organized pickleball getaways

Some players enjoy pickleball destination camps for getting away from their daily routines. There are travel companies that specialize in pickleball trips and do all the planning for you. Destination camps offer an opportunity to experience amazing sites domestically and internationally — in Mexico, Portugal, Croatia, Costa Rica, Thailand, Italy, and Japan, to name a few. You can meet cool people and play lots of pickleball. Here are some resources to get you started on your dream pickleball vacation:

>> **Pickleball Getaways** (https://www.pickleballgetaways.com/): Run by two professional pickleball players, this group creates destination pickleball getaways, camps, and clinics at exciting places all over the world.

>> **Pickleball Trips** (https://pickleballtrips.com/): Through this group, you can sign up for intensive training with a certified instructor at camps and clinics in the U.S. and all over the world.

>> **Pickleball World Tours** (https://www.pickleballworldtours.com): Along with providing all-inclusive authentic and cultural travel experiences, this group provides an opportunity to compete as a representative of the USA in international competitions.

Training clinics and camps

Many organizations offer various types of single-day clinics and multiday camps. Players can work on everything from stroke techniques to advanced strategies, all while expanding their pickleball world view at the same time. Here are some of the major pickleball clinics and camps to check out:

>> **Rise Pickleball Camps:** https://www.risepickleball.com/

>> **Engage Pickleball Camps:** https://www.engagepickleball.com/

>> **Boost Pickleball Training Camps:** https://www.pickleballcentral.com/ Pickleball_Training_Camps

>> **LevelUp Pickleball:** https://www.leveluppickleballcamps.com/

>> **Nike Sports Camps:** https://www.ussportscamps.com/pickleball

>> **Never Stop Playing Pickleball Camps:** https://www.neverstop playingpbcamps.com/

These companies offer improvement opportunities for all skill levels, including camps where you can learn from your favorite pro. Follow your favorites on social media to see where they may be teaching next. Figure 18-3 shows Wayne Dollard, founder of LevelUp Pickleball Camps and publisher of *Pickleball Magazine*, running drills at a camp.

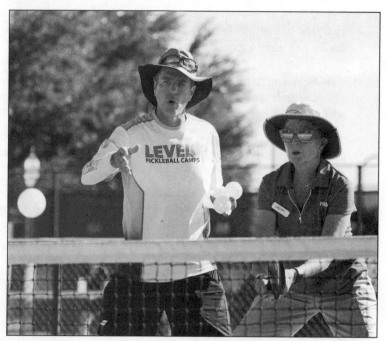

FIGURE 18-3:
Wayne Dollard at
a LevelUp
Pickleball camp.

Getting to the Net: Keeping Up Online

The internet can be a useful tool for finding tips and advice from famous coaches, keeping up with your local scene, or even arguing over rules interpretations with players 3,000 miles away. Spending time online researching or discussing pickleball can be a pleasure, or it may make you want to slam your laptop shut and go hit some balls really hard. You can decide how deeply you want to wade into that pool.

Magazines, newsletters, and blogs

In your search for pickleball enlightenment, you can find dozens of pickleball magazines, newsletters and blogs, but these are some of the best:

>> **Pickleball Magazine** (http://pickleballmagazine.com): The official publication for USA Pickleball Association, *Pickleball Magazine* offers readers the opportunity to learn more about the sport and the people involved with it, including instruction, tournament information, player profiles, destinations and more.

>> ***InPickleball Magazine*** (`http://inpickleball.com`): *InPickleball* readers will find useful information to improve their on-court skills, including curated gear guides, fitness and nutrition tips, and advice from professional players and sports medicine doctors.

>> **Third Shot Sports** (`http://thirdshotsports.com`): World-renowned coach and commentator Mark Renneson offers a wealth of content via multiple e-newsletters (*Third Shot Sports, Pickleball Coaching International, and The Pickleball Lab*) as well as videos, e-books, podcasts, and more.

>> ***Pickler*** (`http://thepickler.com`): Subscribe to the free bi-weekly newsletter or catch up on the "Tips & Stories" blog for tips, strategies, news, and more.

>> **Pickleball Central** (`http://pickleballcentral.com`): Not only is it a top online pickleball retailer, Pickleball Central also offers a weekly blog. Get insights on the newest paddles and gear as well as playing tips, interviews with industry insiders, instructional videos, and more.

>> **PickleballMax** (`http://pickleballmax.com`): This site provides a blog and free e-newsletter featuring topics like playing strategies, news, and equipment reviews.

Social media

You can also find Facebook groups devoted to playing pickleball in your local area. There are also many national and international pickleball Facebook groups. Here are some of the most popular:

>> **Pickleball Forum by Aspen Kern:** One of the oldest and largest pickleball forums on the internet, this group is incredibly active, with lively discussions occurring on everything from rules debates to pickleball humor.

>> **The Kitchen:** In case you're overwhelmed by the sheer volume of daily posts on Pickleball Forum, this group features curated, high-quality content but still leaves room for open discussion and banter.

>> **The Dink Pickleball:** This group keeps you up to date with pickleball news and media, with a focus on professional players and tournament highlights.

>> **Pickleball Forum for Women:** An international group of passionate, empowered, fearless women pickleball fanatics.

>> **Pickleball Instructor's Forum:** This forum serves as a place for coaches to share ideas and opinions on teaching pickleball.

>> **Pickleball Buy, Sell, Swap:** Looking to sell or buy gear? Join the internet's largest pickleball rummage sale.

>> **USA Pickleball Seniors:** This is a discussion forum just for senior players. Swap stories, ask questions, and share some laughs.

>> **Pickleball Players Seeking Tourney Partners:** It's like online dating, but for tournament doubles partners.

>> **The Pickleball Clinic:** Here you can ask advice about technique, strategy, rules, and anything else while chatting with fellow pickleball lovers.

You can find social media groups for juniors, women, LGBTQ+ pickleball players, and many others — probably any subset you belong to. Are you a left-handed Air Force veteran and former lacrosse goalie with dyslexia and a love of crosscourt dinking? There's probably a group for you.

We are always encouraging players to "find their tribe." One of the avenues to find players you can really connect with is online forums. It's wonderful to go to a tournament somewhere and finally meet someone you've enjoyed chatting with online. Pickleball players love to connect with one another, usually in an upbeat and positive way. We all love the sport of pickleball! That's a solid starting point for any type of relationship.

Apps and websites

The pickleball universe also has a plethora of apps and websites dedicated to helping you connect with other players, finding places to play, and making your playing experience better. Fortunately, we've done some of the homework for you. Here are some of the best apps and websites out there:

>> **PlayTime Scheduler** (http://playtimescheduler.com): This free, web-based app helps you locate or arrange play sessions in your local area. Well over a hundred thousand players are already using it. Log in and view the weekly calendar to find the action in your hometown or anywhere in the world you plan to visit. (Full, proud disclosure: Coauthor Reine created this website!)

>> **Pickleball Buddy:** Pickleball Buddy is an app that allows users to find pickleball players in their area. You can add friends and chat with other players to set up matches or discuss strategies. After you've recruited some buddies to play with and set up a game, you can record your game on your phone via the app.

>> **PickleConnect:** This is a helpful app that was built by pickleball players for pickleball players. This app features an extensive list of courts, tournaments, coaches, and clinics. You can save your favorite courts and chat back and forth with your new friends. Game on!

>> **PicklePlay:** This app helps you find courts, players, events, and club information. You can review courts, invite friends to play, chat, earn badges, and more.

>> **Selkirk TV:** The world's first free pickleball TV app! It features livestream matches as well as past tournaments, video lessons from the pros, podcasts, and other on-demand video and audio content.

>> **Pickleball Tournaments:** Wondering when and where your next tournament will be? You'll likely find it on PickleballTournaments.com (http://pickleballtournaments.com), the official tournament software provider for USA Pickleball. Search by location and date and register to play, all in one place.

>> **Pickleball Brackets:** This website is another primary source for finding and registering for tournaments. If a tournament is not listed on PickleballTournaments.com, it's probably on Pickleball Brackets (http://pickleballbrackets.com). You'll want to bookmark both and check them regularly.

>> **DUPR:** This app allows you to record the results of your matches with other users and develop a calculated rating over time.

Podcasts

Currently, a few dozen podcasts are devoted to discussing pickleball. We're a little biased because coauthor Carl produces the "I Used to be Somebody" show (https://pickleballmediahq.com/). It's a podcast for people aged 50+ who don't want to retire but want to do something new, fun, and meaningful. And the best part of the show is, drum roll, please . . . "Pickleball Life Lessons with Mo," featuring our pickleball instructor extraordinaire and coauthor, Mo Nard.

Some other top pickleball podcasts include:

>> Pickleball Therapy by In2Pickle

>> Pickleball Fire Podcast

>> The Profound Pickleball Podcast

>> Pickleball Kitchen Podcast

>> Pickleball Problems

>> The Eddie and Webby Podcast

>> The Pickleball Guru's Podcast

Videos

You can spend hours every day watching pickleball videos (we suspect some people secretly do) and still never see them all! The videos are instructional, funny, motivational, or all the above. Some of our favorite YouTube channels include:

>> Sarah Ansboury

>> In2Pickle

>> PrimeTime Pickleball

>> Pickleball Librarian

>> RooSportz

>> Pickleball Channel

>> Pickleball Kitchen

>> Selkirk TV

>> Deb Harrison

>> Simone Jardim Pickleball

>> Shea Underwood – Pickleball Road to Pro

Following the Pro Tours

Forget boring office watercooler talk; the hot topics at your local courts likely revolve around the latest pro tournament upsets and controversies. Even if spectator sports aren't really your thing, we encourage you to give watching pro pickleball a try. It's more exciting than you may think!

Pickleball certainly has a colorful cast of characters, with every major tournament bringing together well-decorated veterans along with the next generation of up-and-comers. The pro tour is brimming with innovation as these amazing athletes look for something new to give them an edge — new shots, strategies, and partnerships. If you're into tracking stats, you can even participate in a fantasy pickleball league.

Nothing is like being there, watching a live pickleball tournament. The excitement of the crowd reacting to amazing efforts by professionals and amateurs alike gives you a sense of what the pickleball community is all about. You're with hundreds or even thousands of people who are immersed in this wonderful sport they love. Most pickleball spectators are players, too, so the awe and appreciation for what the pros do on the court is palpable. At most of these tournaments, you'll be able to sit right in the front row to cheer on your favorite pros. Try that at an NBA game without getting kicked out.

In contrast to those of many other sports, pickleball pros are usually low key and approachable. It's not unusual for them to stop and chat, answer questions, and pose for photos with fans. They are happy to do it. Heck, they even carry their own bag. Pickleball is the people's sport!

The two largest tournaments that include both pros and amateurs are the Minto US Open Pickleball Championships and the Margaritaville USA Pickleball National Championships. These mega-tournaments each have more than 2,000 participants. Whether you're a player or a spectator, these tournaments are extremely fun — you can cheer on your friends, watch the pros play, sip a margarita, and meet fellow pickleball enthusiasts from far and wide. If you get a chance to attend, do it!

Currently, three associations conduct professional pickleball tournaments, as described in the following sections.

Association of Pickleball Professionals (APP)

The APP Tour (https://apptour.org/), headquartered in Chicago, Illinois, was launched in 2019. This tour's format consists of a series of men's, women's, mixed doubles, and singles divisions in which players compete against peers in a sanctioned tournament environment. (See Chapter 17 to find out more about tournament sanctioning.)

The APP Tour currently schedules 32 tournaments a year in various cities. The APP has no exclusive contracts, and the prize pool is about $2 million. It will most likely go even higher due to the increasing popularity of the sport.

Pro Pickleball Association (PPA)

The PPA (https://ppatour.com) is headquartered in Dallas, Texas, and features men's, women's, mixed doubles, and singles divisions. Its tour consists of top professionals competing for some of the largest payouts in pickleball. They also welcome amateurs of all skill levels to come and play at tournaments with the slogan "Play Where the Pros Play." The PPA Tour's nationwide tournaments feature professional play, beautiful venues, and unique experiences. The tour currently holds 20 events a year and has instituted exclusive contracts for the top 30 players. The prize pool is about $3 million.

Major League Pickleball (MLP)

Launched in 2021, MLP (`https://majorleaguepickleball.net/`) is headquartered in Austin, Texas, and its format is mixed-gender team tournaments. It has a "Team Competition Draft Format," with team names drawn randomly to determine the order in which team owners will select players for a dual (but directionally opposite) women's and men's snake draft format. This draft format, the first of its kind in pickleball, ensures that doubles pairings are novel and interesting, and also creates evenly-matched games full of drama and excitement. This new team format is exciting to watch and has creatively mixed formats and partnerships to make for great viewing.

Chapter **19**

Becoming More Involved

As you begin to play pickleball more often, all the while honing your skills (because you're reading this book), you may want to take it to the next level and get more involved as a member of the pickleball community. Or you may be injured or unable to play for some reason but don't want to lose touch with your pickleball tribe. This chapter outlines the various ways to get involved beyond just playing, whether locally, regionally or at the national level. The only downside is that sometimes your new responsibilities may cut into your court time!

You can become active in your local club, get training to become a referee, work on behalf of USA Pickleball as an Ambassador, volunteer on a committee, and so much more. Read on to learn more about ways you can fully relish your pickleball experience.

Training to Be a Referee or Line Judge

The rapid growth of pickleball means an increasing number of tournaments going on all the time. And they need officials! Fortunately for the pickleball world, the USA Pickleball website (http://www.usapickleball.org) is chock-full of information on how to become a referee or line judge. You'll find a comprehensive section devoted to officiating (with resources for reference), training, and testing materials for all the different programs available, as well as the process required to become a referee or line judge.

Becoming an official offers many perks. Often you get to travel, sometimes get paid, and have the best viewing position during the games. At larger tournaments, you may get to meet and interact with pro players. If you're dealing with injuries or health problems, refereeing allows you to stay involved even when you can't necessarily play. Plus, you are giving back to the greater pickleball community.

To become a referee, you obviously need to know the rule book backward and forward. You receive training on specific procedures for running and officiating matches. During a match, you're responsible for tracking the correct server, receiver, and score at all times. You also watch for illegal serves and kitchen faults during play. You must ensure that time-outs are legally called and time limits observed. Occasionally, you may need to settle disputes between players. It's a lot to keep track of!

You may have noticed that the referee's job is not so much about making line calls. Unless the tournament provides line judges, the players make the line calls of in or out. The referee stands up at the net on one side of the court (see Figure 19-1). This position is perfect for calling kitchen foot faults, but it's not the best for calling the ball in or out. If a player disagrees with their opponent's line calls, they may appeal to the referee. If the referee was able to observe the bounce of the ball and make a determination, they will either confirm or overturn the line call.

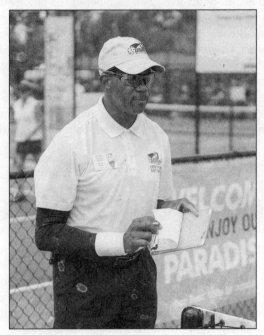

FIGURE 19-1: A tournament referee working hard on behalf of his sport.

© *John Wiley & Sons, Inc./Photo Credit: Steve Taylor/Digital Spatula*

Many pickleballers find refereeing to be a fun and rewarding challenge, and it does get easier with practice. Depending on your experience and comfort levels, USAP offers different levels of referee credentials. The highest level is that of Certified Referee, who is qualified to officiate all types of matches, including those for professional players. Becoming a Certified Referee is a challenging and rigorous process that involves significant study and practice. Please give the folks who attain this level your utmost respect. In fact, give all referees your respect! If you find that officiating is your thing, you can also become a Certified Referee Trainer and teach the next wave of newcomers. Talk about leaving your mark.

Volunteering as a USA Pickleball Ambassador

Ambassadors are volunteer representatives who are also unofficial spokespersons for USA Pickleball, the governing body for the game of pickleball in the United States. If you don't live in the U.S., your country may have its own governing body. If not, maybe starting one is your calling!

An Ambassador's responsibility is to promote and grow the sport in their local and regional areas. As mentioned in the previous section, if you're interested in becoming a USA Pickleball Ambassador, that organization's website is the place to start. It provides excellent resources on codes of conduct, responsibilities, and how to apply. Haven't you always wanted to be called "Ambassador"? Sorry, there's no embassy for you to work from.

Ambassadors can be a force for positive change in your pickleball community. They often help with programs that spread the joy of pickleball to others. Ambassadors have helped to bring pickleball to schools, after-school programs, prisons, parks, churches, senior centers, and other facilities. They can help at local government meetings when players are trying to get more courts built at their community parks. Ambassadors often encourage players to take referee training by coordinating training events at their local clubs or parks. It is not necessarily a glamorous job, but it can be quite rewarding. What's not to love about spreading the joy of pickleball?

Becoming an Ambassador is a great way to feel connected to the larger pickleball community, but it's not a role to take lightly. As an Ambassador, you represent something larger than yourself. You should approach the job with a giving heart rather than a desire for power or authority. You'll be expected to meet high standards of behavior whenever you're on the court or participating in any pickleball-related activities. This means no foul language or unsporting behavior.

Fairness, honesty, and respect are all part of the USA Pickleball Ambassador Code of Conduct. (We hope you're already following that code.) There are also strict rules about flaunting your title or using it for self-promotional purposes. An Ambassador's duty is to serve their community and be a positive role model. (See Figure 19-2.)

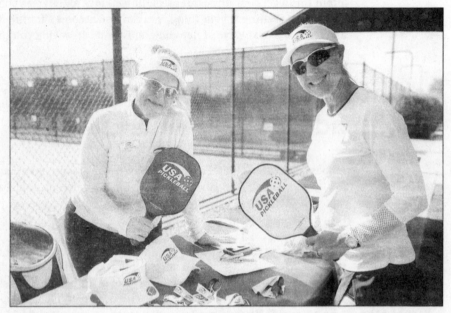

FIGURE 19-2:
USA Pickleball Ambassadors are the heart and soul of it all!

© John Wiley & Sons, Inc./Photo Credit: Bruce Yeung; IG: @yeungphotography

Joining Committees

If you are interested in joining a committee, we commend you! Not surprisingly, many pickleball players are retired or working part-time, so they have the energy, time, and interest to volunteer. All too often, volunteer organizations suffer from a condition called "same ten people (STP)". This means that all the goals and work of the committee fall on the same ten or so people. You can help out by being the eleventh person to volunteer! Grab a friend to join you and keep those numbers going up. Many committee or volunteer positions are easy and fun, so get in there and share your skills with your pickleball community. If your skill is to make holiday decorations out of broken pickleballs, that's great! Offer them as a fundraiser item. Others in the club will appreciate whatever you can do to help. If you have great organizational and leadership skills, consider serving as an officer on the board of directors of your club. These positions are sometimes hard to fill. Pickleball Grand Poobah may be your calling.

Much committee work revolves around tournaments at the regional and national level. The number of tournaments keeps increasing, and these events need all kinds of committee volunteers to make them run smoothly. Besides those for tournaments, other USAP committees include the Executive, Rules, Equipment Evaluation, Recreation, Youth, and Ratings committees.

Many committees are devoted to fundraising. Around the world, pickleball clubs and groups host events, exhibitions, round robins, and tournaments to raise money for specific causes and charities — often for maintenance and improvement of local pickleball courts. Looking for courts to play in your area? A portable net is easy to find at less than two hundred dollars, and a net along with a measuring tape and some painter's tape are all you need to turn a flat surface into a pickleball court. You can organize a group to play at a local school gym or church hall, charge a small fee to play, and then donate the money raised back to the facility. It's a win–win.

Potlucks, mixers, groovy gatherings, oh my! These are just a few fundraising events to consider. You may also volunteer to form a social committee at your local club. There are as many kinds of pickleball social events as there are creative, fun pickleball players. An Earth Day Pickleball Play Day and Park Clean Up? Yep! A glow-in-the-dark pickleball party? You bet! Dink-o de Mayo Taco Night? Early Birdie Donuts and Dinks? The creative possibilities are endless, and the smiles, photos, and memories are likely to be worth the effort.

Growing Pickleball in Your Community

One of the best ways to grow the sport in your community is by creating an informal, DIY-type of club or group at your favorite park or venue. These local groups typically focus on fundraising, networking, and advocacy for new courts and improvements.

Here are some ways your group can further develop the sport and help to organize the players in your community:

>> Establish a newsletter, email list, or social media group for communication among local players.

>> Recruit new players by inviting people to free, introductory clinics on the courts.

>> Post drop-in play times and the information for any websites or tools used for organizing play in your area. Make sure to keep the schedule current. Nothing is worse than showing up to what you thought was an organized drop-in time,

only to find out the time was changed and nobody posted about it. (Why am I in a Zumba class right now?)

Connect with the USA Pickleball Ambassador for your area. They likely already have access to many helpful resources and historical knowledge of what's been happening with pickleball in your area over the past few years.

We've seen many neighborhoods enjoy success in creating their own groups as a force for change (which means more pickleball opportunities for all). Keep in mind that focusing on more courts is only half the battle. You also need to recruit new players to come out and play. Another way to grow your group is to contact other nearby clubs about holding interclub tournaments and events. It's all about connecting, mixing, and mingling with like-minded players. When everyone pitches in, everyone benefits!

Advocating for courts: Working with local government

The sudden explosion of pickleball's popularity has created unique challenges and opportunities for many cities and park departments. On one hand, they see the benefits to the community and are thrilled that so many folks are getting outside and recreating, forming bonds and improving their health. On the other hand, the majority of cities are finding it difficult to keep up with the demand for pickleball courts. Lack of space and funding to convert or build courts are typically the main issues. Other times, city officials are simply slow to recognize that pickleball is not just a passing trend or niche sport. They may be hearing pushback from tennis players who don't want to see their courts converted or shared with pickleballers. In other cases, neighbors and HOAs are upset about the potential crowds, parking issues, or noise associated with pickleball courts.

If you want to grow pickleball in your community, it's important to develop good relationships with local government and park district officials. Recognize that their concerns surrounding costs, crowds, and noise are all valid. Their job is to balance the needs of all their constituents, not just pickleballers. (Beware that our enthusiasm for the sport can sometimes make us a bit shortsighted.) Working together to solve these potential issues will ultimately be the key to growing pickleball with the full backing and support of your local officials. This approach puts you on a much easier road than taking an adversarial stance and having to fight them every step of the way!

Here are some steps you can take to make your efforts go smoothly:

>> **Get organized.** Form a group with a unified goal. Immediately start networking to see whether you can get potential sponsors for the project. Identify your key way to communicate with each other (whether through meetings, emails, or some other way).

>> **Educate your local governmental officials and community leaders about pickleball.** Talk up pickleball's positive influence. Focus on how adults, teens, and kids can all play together and that it's a very inclusive sport. The health benefits of pickleball are also undeniable. Anyone interested in promoting fitness, mental health, or longevity in the community should be on your side!

>> **Offer a free lesson and get community leaders out to play.** Maybe they'll get hooked! Friendly persistence really helps.

>> **Contact your local Parks & Recreation department.** Ask department representatives about future development plans and any possible roadblocks to your project from their perspective. Start the conversation sooner rather than later. Getting early buy-in from them by making sure they feel included and heard can be invaluable.

>> **Spin it to win it!**

Make a professional, thorough presentation. Emphasize that holding tournaments may bring visitors (and tourism dollars) to your community. Another benefit is that pickleballers' presence has also been shown to reduce crime in neighborhood parks.

>> **Offer to help with fundraising.** Pickleball courts can cost hundreds of thousands of dollars, and most park districts aren't exactly sitting on piles of cash with nowhere to spend it. You may need to raise some or all of the money yourself through events and campaigns, or by forming a club and charging dues. Your efforts should help to convince officials that you're serious and willing to work with them to do what is required.

>> **Be good citizens and neighbors.** Whenever resources are scarce, (in this case, too many players and not enough courts), conflicts and drama can occur. Encourage the players in your circle to practice good etiquette (see Chapter 4 for more on pickleball etiquette). Figure out a fair system to rotate when courts are full. Observe all posted park or facility rules. Park district staff don't want to receive angry calls all day from neighbors about your "pickleball drama" or with complaints about parking, littering, or excess noise. Problems like these create a very bad impression with park staff and will not help your cause!

Need more inspiration? Imagine a city council meeting with 45 pickleball players in attendance. High attendance at such meetings has been happening all over the country and leading to positive results. It's true that the squeaky wheel gets the grease, but stay polite and positive and do your best to represent the sport with integrity. It can be frustrating at times, but hang in there. We are optimistic that even the most stubborn local officials will eventually see that pickleball is here to stay!

The kids are all right: Junior pickleball

The popular saying, "Adulting can wait, we want to play pickleball" resonates with a great many players. Pickleball brings out our inner kid, so it's no wonder that pickleball is exploding among young people as well as older people. All you have to do is play once with a 14-year-old to realize that kids are naturals for pickleball, and those whippersnappers can dart around the court faster than you can say "You're grounded!"

Here are some reasons pickleball is the perfect activity for kids:

>> It helps them get away from their various screens and out onto the courts for exercise.

>> The court is already "mini" sized! The smaller court size is perfect for kids who don't have a ton of arm strength to whack a ball all the way across a tennis court, for example.

>> It's a great way for kids (or anyone) to work on their social skills and etiquette.

>> Pickleball is the great equalizer — it's unique in that all generations, sizes, and skill levels can play together and have a blast.

>> For parents always searching for family-bonding activities, we can't think of a better one than pickleball.

>> Score! The matches are relatively quick, which is perfect for children's attention spans.

>> The sport has a low cost associated with it. All you need are a paddle, shoes, balls, and eyewear. Done. No expensive league fees, equipment, or uniforms.

Middle and high schools are realizing the fitness and socialization benefits of the sport and are adding pickleball to their physical education classes. As a low-contact sport, pickleball doesn't require special protective gear or clothing. It also doesn't require a lot of space because you can fit numerous courts and players in a relatively small area. The nature of pickleball is to have fun and be encouraging to others. (We may have mentioned the fun part a few times already.)

Taking it to the next level, USA Pickleball is on a mission to promote and develop the sport to younger generations. USA Pickleball has created a junior membership program that provides assistance to physical education teachers, youth program leaders, coaches, and recreation professionals to develop their own junior pickleball programs. USAP's Ambassadors also offer training and program resources to introduce pickleball to youth.

If a junior player wants to build on their skill set and learn more, traveling to tournaments exposes them to new strategies, new opponents, and different styles of play. Advancing up the ladder or winning a medal is a big boost for self-esteem (no matter how old you are). Many kids are naturally little information sponges, so with some training or study, junior players can develop into pickleball ninjas in no time at all. Even if ninja level isn't in their future, they can be healthy and active and have a great time playing pickleball. (Winning is great for self-esteem! Check out Figure 19-3.)

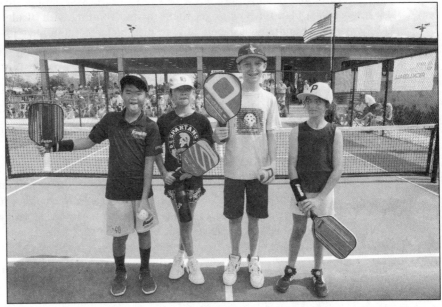

FIGURE 19-3:
Big wins and bigger smiles!

© *John Wiley & Sons, Inc./Photo Credit: Bruce Yeung; IG: @yeungphotography*

Introducing pickleball to others (The gift that keeps on giving!)

After you've caught the pickleball bug, it's only a matter of time before you'll want to introduce the game to your family, friends, neighbors, coworkers, mail carrier, hair stylist, fourth-grade teacher, bowling team, and just about everyone else within a 10-mile radius. They've been giving you grief for constantly talking about pickleball, but it's only because they haven't tried it yet! Introducing friends to pickleball is a win-win. They get to learn a fun new activity, and you have more people to play (and talk) pickleball with. There's also nothing sweeter than hearing those three little words, "You were right."

Coauthors Reine and Mo are now professional coaches, but before their business Positive Dinking was born, they were just two best buds who wanted to teach everyone they knew how to play pickleball. Discovering the game and its community had benefited them both so much that they wanted to shout from the rooftops. After gathering friends for a few informal clinics, they discovered they enjoyed teaching pickleball almost as much as playing it. You don't need to become a professional instructor, but introducing new players to pickleball can be highly enjoyable and rewarding.

After you've convinced a few newbies to meet you out on the courts, it helps to have a plan for how to get them up and running with pickleball. We've taught many hundreds of people how to play pickleball and have found the technique we explain shortly to be fantastic for getting players started in about 60 to 90 minutes. By the end of this lesson, your friends will be playing real games of pickleball and know everything needed to jump into their new favorite hobby/ passion/addiction!

You can do this! Here are some tips for teaching a beginners clinic:

1. **Go over the safety rules.**

    Nothing ruins a fun time like an injury. Be sure that all players are dressed appropriately, especially with proper footwear (no flip-flops or cowboy boots) and eye protection. Caution them to avoid running backward and to call "ball on!" when balls are rolling near anyone's feet. Don't scare them; just help them to play safely. For more important safety tips, see Chapter 2.

2. **Show players the continental grip and have them hit some balls.**

    Great teachers know not to talk too much without letting students actively try what they're learning. At this point, your newbies don't need to worry about any rules — they can just knock the ball around and get a feel for it. We would bet the smiles and giggles have already begun!

3. **Give a tour of the court.**

    Briefly introduce your students to some of the basic terminology used in the game. To understand the rules as you explain them, they will need to know the names of the lines and areas of the court (baseline, sideline, centerline, kitchen, service box). If you need to review, check out the section about the layout of the court in Chapter 2.

4. **Teach scoring in miniature.** As a former newbie yourself, you are well aware that learning to keep score can be tricky. We've found that it's best to isolate scoring as its own mini lesson. Have four students stand up at the kitchen line and play a mini (dinking) game of pickleball; all they need to worry about is scoring and swapping sides (right and left) with their partner. Forget about the Two-Bounce Rule, serving rules, or kitchen violations for the moment. Shrinking the court means less shouting and less pressure to try to hit the ball really well.

5. **Tell a little white lie about the game's starting score at first.**

   Learning (and teaching) the scoring can sometimes be frustrating. ("Why is the score three numbers, and what's this one or two business? I give up!") One trick to help new players is to start your mini game at 0–0–1. We realize that the actual starting score of a pickleball game is 0–0–2, but for a player who has not yet learned about ones and twos, this makes no sense at all. After the basic scorekeeping makes sense, you can confess your fib and tell the players about the starting score exception. It helps to explain the reasoning behind the rule, which is that the initial serving team, who gets to serve first because of luck, can't rack up a ton of points before the other team even gets a chance to serve.

6. **Have the players move to the baseline and practice serving.**

   After all that mental work of figuring out how to keep score, it's time for more doing! Go over the basic rules of serving (see Chapter 2) and show players both the traditional (out-of-the-air) serve and the drop serve. Everyone can now practice serving back and forth. We find that most people, if given a few minutes, will find a serve that works for them. If you see any illegal serves developing, gently correct them (better now than later). Make sure players get a chance to practice from both the right and left sides of the court. They don't need to perfect their serve, just get the general idea and, with luck, get some serves in.

7. **Introduce the kitchen.**

   New players are often curious about this mysterious part of the court and its culinary implications. When we first introduce this area, we like to refer to it by its more informative technical name, the non-volley zone, before switching to its more commonly used name, "the kitchen." Try not to overcomplicate your explanations. Although there are a few funky rules regarding the kitchen (which we outline in Chapter 2), the main point is that you can't contact the ball out of the air (volley) in that zone.

8. **Explain the Two-Bounce Rule, players' starting positions, and how to make line calls.**

   The last three topics to cover are the Two-Bounce Rule, player starting positions, and calling the ball in or out. The Two-Bounce Rule is what informs the typical starting positions of three players back and one player up, so those topics pair nicely together. It always helps to explain the "why" behind a strategy. Practice a few points while directing players where to stand based on who is serving. Point out that everyone starts behind the baseline except for the one player who is looking directly at the server. Their job is to stand up at the kitchen line, staring down the server while looking big and scary. Players often embrace this role with gusto!

9. **Start playing!**

   Congratulations, your friends now know enough to start playing pickleball! Make sure to include enough time at the end of your session to play a few games. Otherwise, it's a bit like sharing one French fry and then taking away the rest of the bag. (That's just cruel.). You'll likely need to help new players with scoring, avoiding kitchen faults, and the Two-Bounce Rule. By now, we bet you are beaming with pride for your newly created pickleball stars. You did a good thing today!

TIP

Be sure to add some humor! People want to have fun, so laugh and enjoy your time together. Don't make your students the butt of the jokes, but you can always laugh at yourself or the game in general. Trying something new (especially something physical) can make folks feel a little vulnerable, so be careful to only laugh with them, not at them. People typically take up pickleball to add fun and friendship to their lives, so help them relax and not take anything too seriously. In addition to teaching them safety and rules, you'll be teaching them how to be a good sport and have a great attitude!

6

The Part of Tens

Understanding what not to do!

Avoiding common mistakes

Chapter **20**

Ten Pickleball Pet Peeves

"Did you see that guy?" or "Can you believe she did that?" Although courtesy, patience, and inclusiveness are part of pickleball culture, it's human nature to have a pet peeve (or ten) that really grinds your gears when you're on the courts.

Pickleball players come from all walks of life. Our shared love for the game brings us together. We urge you to embrace these colorful medleys of pickleball-lovin' folks — but as with any trail mix, you're bound to encounter a few nuts! Every player has a story about another player who got on their nerves, and sometimes rightfully so. Following the rules (explained Chapter 2) and understanding the proper etiquette (see Chapter 4) are important when you play. You want to be invited back, don't you?

Although pickleball is a highly social activity that promotes laughter, smiles, and friendship, it can also be highly competitive — which can often bring out the worst in people. It can be tough to balance your desire to win and perform at your best against the desire to be well-liked by your pickleball peers. We strongly believe that with a little self-awareness and a commitment to kindness, you can easily achieve both!

In this chapter, we reveal the ten pet peeves shared by most players, along with some tips on how not to be that one annoying player whom everyone avoids.

Ignoring Other Players' Goals and Skill Levels

When players tell you that they are purely recreational and not tournament-bound, respect that! Please don't get mad and frustrated at the rest of the group because you have higher goals. Your partner may not feel comfortable diving for the ball or chasing down lobs. That's their choice! Sure, it may cost you a few points, but more important is that everyone can feel safe and enjoy their time on the court. Reserve your ultra-intense competitiveness for when you are actually in the tournament or playing with others who share a similar mindset. You can still spend this recreational time productively by working on various aspects of your game. Chapter 16 offers ideas on how to practice while playing with players of different skill levels.

On the other side of the coin, you may be a recreational player who encounters serious competitive players who are preparing for a tournament. They may request to stay together as partners rather than mixing in. Or they may want to challenge certain opponents so that they can work on specific aspects of their game. Please don't be offended if they turn down your offer to play. We can all work harder at recognizing and supporting each other's goals and unique circumstances rather than taking everything so personally.

Being Rude

Common courtesy and the golden rule should be your guide when interacting with others on a pickleball court. Treat others as you would like to be treated. Rudeness has no place in a game designed to be fun. There are a few pickleball-specific situations in which you'll definitely want to "check yourself before you wreck yourself." Avoid committing the following *faux pas*:

>> **Not tapping paddles.** In pickleball, players meet at the net, *gently* tap paddles between players, and say "Good game!" at the end of each game. It takes less than a minute. Please don't just walk off the court with your back facing the people you just played with. Yikes!

>> **Constantly questioning line calls.** If you are in a tournament and feel strongly that your opponent has made a bad line call, by all means challenge it. In recreational play, be a little more lenient. The stakes are much lower. It's your opponents' prerogative to call the lines as they see them on their side of the court. Constantly stopping play to argue about line calls is just obnoxious and tiresome.

>> **Not politely passing the ball.** After each rally, someone will need to pick up the ball and pass it to the next server. If you're the person closest to the ball, that's you. Wait until the server has turned around and is facing you, and then gently throw or hit it to them. Please do not just carelessly bat it under the net in their general direction, or whack it at them while their back is turned.

>> **Excessive celebrating.** It's totally fine to celebrate when your team wins a point with a joyous exclamation, fist pump, or paddle tap. Keep it positive by saying things to your partner like "Great shot!" "Nice work!" or "Yeah, baby!" Do *not* direct negativity to your opponents by saying things like "In your face!" or "Ha! Take that!" or "Boomshakalaka!" (unless your friends all know you're only joking). Over-the-top celebrations and grandstanding are in poor taste.

>> **Not apologizing for hitting someone.** Getting hit with the pickleball is part of the game. Hopefully, no one intentionally aims for people's faces. It's a much better strategy to hit toward the ground, anyway. If you do hit someone, immediately apologize. It doesn't have to be dramatic, such as falling to your knees and begging forgiveness. Just say something like "Sorry! Are you okay?" and then move on. Failing to extend this simple courtesy will earn you a poor reputation that is hard to shake.

>> **Playing loud music.** Ask around and see whether all the players within earshot want to hear your music. Many players find music to be a distraction and do not enjoy it while trying to play pickleball. It can make hearing the score or communicating between partners difficult. It's also never safe to assume that everyone has the same taste in music. People came to play pickleball, not get down to DJ Steve's smooth jazz playlist.

Being Too Hard on Yourself

Berating your partner or the opposing players is definitely not allowed, and most players would never dream of doing that. But it is also unacceptable to berate yourself! Who wants to hear that? Talk to yourself as you would a good friend (see Chapter 15 for more on supportive self-talk). Please don't slap your leg with your paddle so hard that you startle players three courts away. When you get frustrated, take a deep breath and smile. This technique works! Now you can relax and play on.

REMEMBER

Stop apologizing for every error. You may think your partner wants to hear you take responsibility for losing the point, but we can assure you, they don't! Every rally in pickleball ends because one of four people made a mistake. It's a fair bet that it's going to be you sometimes. Other times, it's going to be your partner. Who cares? Nobody is perfect. (If your partner expects you to be perfect, find a new partner!) Apologies carry an implication that you are requesting forgiveness.

It puts an extra burden on your partner to constantly reassure you with "It's okay" or "No worries." That burden is exhausting for them and doesn't help your team get focused for the next point.

Delaying the Game

It's no fun for other players when you stop the game to change paddles for the fifth time, or to respond to several "important" messages on your phone. C'mon! Also, although it's easy to chat a bit during play, don't become a distraction or hold things up. Your fellow players don't need to hear your movie critiques of the week while they're trying to get their pickleball on. Catching up with friends is great, but please save it for between games.

REMEMBER

Because recreational play doesn't have formal time-outs, there can be a fine line between acceptable partner communication and annoying delays of game. Between points, keep your strategizing and pep talks short. Stopping play for five minutes to hash out a new 12-point strategy with your partner mid-game isn't fair to your opponents.

If you're helping a new player, or your partner asks for some coaching, the polite approach is to check with your opponents first — or better yet, give quick tips only between points while players are getting into position. Again, keep any interruptions brief. Always respect your fellow players' time and the natural flow of play.

Being Ignorant of Rules and Scoring

We know that the rules and scoring of pickleball seem kind of quirky at first. Pickleballers are typically very patient with new players, and everyone forgets details sometimes. But if you've been playing for months and still don't understand the basic rules, it's time to learn them. You can study Chapter 2 and be up to speed on virtually everything you need to know to play recreational games.

TIP

To get a bit more in depth, purchase a rule book from USA Pickleball (or simply download the free PDF version from its website), make yourself a cup of hot cocoa, and curl up for an evening of light reading. (We're just guessing here, but we suspect you may be a book person.) The rule book isn't that long, and you'll be glad you made the effort to better understand the game.

If you don't always know the score, that's okay. It's a running joke in pickleball that nobody can ever remember the score. At least make it a goal to get it right most of the time. Relying on others to keep score while putting in zero effort yourself isn't good pickleball etiquette. Give it your best effort (even if you're wrong a lot), and your fellow players will appreciate it.

Calling the Ball on Both Sides of the Net

If the ball bounces on your side of the net, your team gets to call the ball in or out. If the ball bounces on your opponents' side of the net, they get to call it. You don't get to call your own shots in. Yes, this rule is in the rule book and applies to play at every level, even pro matches.

REMEMBER

Calling the lines on your side of the court is both a right and a responsibility. It's part of your job as a player. Don't be shy about calling the ball out if you're sure about what you saw. If neither you nor your partner is sure, the ball is considered in. Failing to do your job of calling the lines on your side of the court just needlessly delays the game and causes confusion.

Each team should call the ball honestly. Don't try to win points by cheating. For more on making fair and accurate line calls, see Chapter 2.

Losing Your Temper

Don't be a "Mean Matt" who gets so angry during play that you berate other players or throw your paddle in disgust. Such behavior is not only totally unacceptable, it will most likely keep you from having people to play with and may get you kicked out of the club.

Pickleball can be a great stress reliever, but it's never fair to take your anger out on others — anywhere! If you can't control your temper, please stay away from the courts. Find another outlet for your aggression, or seek counseling. Pickleball will be happy to welcome you back with open arms when you are ready to display good sporting conduct.

Not Taking Turns on the Courts

Most pickleball venues have some sort of court rotation system. Just as laws regulate the flow of traffic, pickleball players rely on systems designed to ensure that everyone has access to the courts. You may see a paddle rack, whiteboard, or other method for waiting players to queue for a court. Wherever you go to play, take the time to understand the court rotation rules. If you aren't sure, ask other players around you. They will be more than happy to explain them to you!

WARNING

If many people are waiting and games are going quickly, with players rotating in and out, please don't be that clueless player who never sits out a game. Also, if everyone else is playing games to 11 points, don't try to cheat the system by playing to 15, or sneakily restarting your score halfway through. (Yes, we've actually seen players do this. *For shame!*) Some advanced players seem to think their abilities earn them the right to more court time than beginners. We don't understand this noodle-headed way of thinking, but it's surprisingly common. Everyone wants to play. Strive to be the person that Mr. Rogers always believed you to be. Sharing is caring!

Hanging Back from the Kitchen Line

Most pickleball points are won from the kitchen line. That is the offensive position from which you can hit down on the ball. Try to move forward toward that line whenever possible. If your partner comes up to the line but you don't, you're leaving a huge opening for your opponents to hit through.

You may struggle to find doubles partners if you're the player who hangs back deep in the court all the time, because your team can't play in sync that way. (See Chapter 11 to learn more about proper court movement and positioning.) Your partner is left wondering where you are and what you're doing (unless they are the rare player with eyes on the back of their head). They may feel pressured to cover the entire line by themselves. So much for teamwork. When you get a chance to move forward safely, take it!

Not Bringing Any Balls

Did the ball you were just playing with fly over the fence and tumble off a cliff into the ocean? (We're a bit envious you're playing seaside, but hey, good for you.) Although everyone else runs to their bag to offer up a new ball, are you that one player who never, ever has a ball? You may be saving a few bucks with this scheme, but you can bet that others are beginning to notice! Pickleball is a relatively cheap sport, so pony up and purchase a sleeve of your group's favorite brand of balls once in a while.

TIP

Please don't ruin the parks department's lawn mowers by tossing your broken pickleballs out onto the grass. Throw your garbage in a garbage can, ya filthy animal. Or give your broken balls to your club's resident crafting wizard, who can transform them into something magical, like a holiday wreath or life-sized statue of professional pickleballer Tyson McGuffin.

Chapter 21

Ten Common Pickleball Mistakes and How to Fix Them

Not surprisingly, many pickleball players struggle with the same problems. Some of them are habits picked up from other sports (those giant backswings are fabulous for tennis but don't work so well in pickleball) and others may stem from bad advice. The good news is that they are all fixable!

Before you can correct any mistakes you're making, you first need to know what they are. Sometimes it can be hard to recognize what you're doing, especially when you're focused on winning a point. If you're not sure, ask someone to observe you or record a video. This can be a fun and enlightening exercise to do with your friend or doubles partner. Watch your videos together and help each other look for ways to improve.

It will take practice to train yourself out of these habits. Pick one item to work on for a week (or month). If you try to fix everything at one time, you become overwhelmed and start to feel like you can't do anything right. Be patient with yourself, and celebrate small victories along the way.

Creeping

Players on the serving team often get caught "creeping" into the court following the serve. The problem is that if you receive a deep return, you'll have to retreat quickly. The Two-Bounce Rule requires you to let the return bounce before you can hit it. Clever opponents will see that you've moved up and intentionally hit the ball behind you.

WARNING

Creeping leads to backpedaling, which is something you should never do on a pickleball court. Nothing ruins a fun play session like broken wrists!

Make stepping back a part of your service routine — you're not finished until you've moved into a great position for the next shot. Just keep thinking, "Serve and step back. Serve and step back."

For both the server and server's partner, it's difficult to hit an effective third-shot drop (or drive) if your weight is moving backward. To hit a clean shot, you need to get behind the ball and use both forward weight shift and a forward follow-through. Be ready to launch forward if the return is short, or stay back if the return is deep.

Using the Windshield Wiper Backhand

The *windshield wiper backhand* refers to hitting a volley on your nondominant side with your palm facing the ball — technically a forehand — instead of with the back of your hand facing the ball. It makes your paddle look like a windshield wiper moving in front of your face.

We have a few reasons for you to avoid this shot. Flipping your paddle all the way around to the forehand side (from a backhand-default ready position) takes too long. It's difficult to get the paddle face pointed toward your intended target in time. This shot just doesn't work well once the ball drops below waist height. The awkward twisting motion of the windshield wiper also causes a lot of strain on your shoulder, elbow, and wrist.

TIP

Using this type of backhand can be a tough habit to break. While in ready position, rest your nondominant hand's fingertips on the back of your paddle face. If the ball comes toward your body or nondominant side ("through the doorway" — as explained in Chapter 9), focus on pushing your paddle away from your fingertips, with the back of your paddle hand facing your target.

Hitting with "Wristiness"

"Wristiness" may not be in the dictionary, but we needed a word to describe the overuse of the wrist in pickleball. Your shots are less accurate if you allow your wrist to get overly involved. In general, when hitting softly (dinks and drops), you want a firm but slightly supple wrist. When hitting hard (drives and volleys), you want your wrist to be a bit looser, but it should still follow the natural momentum of your swing rather than try to redirect the ball at the last moment.

Always striking the ball out in front of your body will help solve this issue. After you let the ball get even with or behind your body, you're forced to use your wrist to make the shot work. If you can avoid letting your paddle tip point down toward the ground, that can also help limit the amount of wristiness in your shots. Hinge from your waist and shoulder. See Chapter 6 for more details on good stroke fundamentals.

Sprinting to the Kitchen Line after the Third Shot

Sprinting to the kitchen line is one of the most common mistakes players make, and it's usually due to bad advice. We bet that when you started playing, someone told you, "Get to the line as fast as you can!" It's true that the kitchen line is the offensive position, and ideally, we want to play up there as much as possible. However, blindly running forward as fast as you can is a terrible strategy.

We suspect that this misguided advice stems from confusion between how the serving and the receiving teams should approach the line. If you are the receiver, by all means hustle up to the kitchen line after you've executed your return. However, the serving team does not have the luxury of automatically coming in after the serve. They must hang back and wait for the return to bounce. To get themselves to the kitchen line safely, the serving team first needs to hit a drop or drive that their opponents can't slam back.

REMEMBER

You are far better off if you get to the line carefully and in good balance. The receiving team can easily just hit a ball that bounces between two players who are running. Earn your way to the line by hitting unattackable shots. If your shot was attackable, don't panic; just stay back and try, try again. See Chapter 7 for more on these all-important third shots.

Popping the Ball Up

Chapter 14 details our six "scientifically" proven reasons for pop-ups, but here's a brief rundown on how to prevent them:

>> **Start in and maintain a good ready position.** Keep both arms up and your paddle out in front of you. Playing with your paddle too low will require you to quickly jerk it upward if a ball comes at your body.

>> **Don't point the tip of your paddle toward the ground.** Avoid scooping *under* the ball rather than hitting *through* the ball. You can't get topspin if your paddle head is completely vertical.

>> **Hit the ball in front of your body.** If you're contacting the ball while it's even with, or behind, your body, you're already late. Your wrist will likely get involved to try to make the shot work, leading to inaccuracy.

>> **When it's low, swing slowly.** A low ball requires you to swing from low to high, lifting it back over the net. The faster you swing, the more lift you apply to the ball. Swing slowly to reduce the amount of energy on the ball so that it drops low after crossing the net.

>> **Don't run through your shots.** Keep in mind that there's no shot like the present. When you run through your shot, you're adding too much momentum behind the ball, which can cause it to zing high in the air.

>> **Don't point your paddle face toward the sky.** Using too open of a paddle face directs the ball upward instead of forward.

Using the Bowling Serve

The *bowling serve* refers to pointing the tip of your paddle straight down to the ground as you serve. Your swing motion resembles rolling a bowling ball. Beginners sometimes use this serve to make sure their serve is legal; they run no risk of contacting the ball above the waist or swinging high to low. So this serve is legal, but maybe it's a little bit *too* legal!

This is not a serve that is going to take you places. Earlier in the chapter, we explain how dropping the paddle head leads to "wristiness," but it can also lead to your shots spraying out wide. Even the slightest horizontal angle applied to a dropped paddle head will cause problems. The other issue with this serve is that it allows you to use only the dominant side of your body. You can't get much power or topspin using only your arm, as opposed to swinging through with your hips and core.

To transform your bowling serve into a more effective serve, simply bring the tip of your paddle up a bit so that you are holding your paddle at more of a 45° angle. Hit *through* rather than *under* the ball. Essentially, you're just hitting a regular forehand. You will be delighted to find that you can now hit a much crisper, more aggressive serve using just this minor adjustment in technique. See Chapter 7 for more details on the mechanics involved.

Failing to Get to the Line (Or Hold It)

Many players shy away from playing toward the front of the court. They believe that staying back gives them more time to react. Although staying back does give you a few extra milliseconds, it also makes your shots more difficult. More balls will wind up near your feet rather than above your waist. You will be forced to dig them out of the ground rather than hitting an easy volley. Here are additional reasons to get all the way to the kitchen line:

>> The net can do some of the work of protecting your feet from attacks.

>> You can take balls at their highest point and hit down on them.

>> You take time away from your opponents by hitting the ball earlier.

>> You shrink the court for your opponent and cut off angles.

>> You can consistently play and practice from the exact same position, instead of varying your position every time you are forward in the court.

Think about it: If you could stand all the way up at the net and slam the ball, wouldn't you? You want to be the player who can hit down on the ball. You can't do that if you're deep in the court.

So get up to the kitchen line when you can, and try to stay there. Sure, you may want to back off the line if you're getting attacked, but make it your goal to reset and get back up there.

Relying on the Elbow Hinge Backhand

Backhands often break down when players hinge from the elbow. Some people become increasingly tentative about their backhands. They start to think, "My backhand is terrible. I better just try to get it over the net." They approach the ball by sticking out their elbow and poking at it. This may get the ball over the net but not accomplish much else.

Relax and try hitting your backhand just as you would throw a flying disc. Hinge from your waist and shoulder, opening up your chest as you follow through. You can try this by initially hitting the ball against a fence to remove the big scary net from the equation and help you build confidence. This practice will remind you to lead with your shoulder, not your elbow. Follow through until you find yourself standing in a pretty Statue of Liberty pose, admiring the results of your beautiful backhand (and New York Harbor).

Pinching the Middle

If you and your partner are both playing right next to each other near the center-line (known as *pinching the middle*), that's a problem. If the ball is hit to the middle, neither of you has enough space to work. It's also not immediately clear who should take that middle ball, which can cause the hitter to be late — or the ball may even sail past! Remember, if you've both got the middle, no one's got the middle.

The other problem with pinching the middle is that you've left the sidelines of the court open. Clever opponents will notice this and easily burn you with a passing shot. By covering only the middle, you've effectively abandoned your post and neglected your responsibility to cover your sideline.

After each rally, stop and look to see where you and your partner ended up. Doing so can really help to inform you about what happened. Try to "stay in your lane" as best you can (see Chapter 11). Yes, you sometimes need to leave your lane to hit the ball, but after you've made the shot, return to your lane as quickly as possible.

TIP

Assuming that no one else on your court minds, you can put a small, brightly colored object under the net (such as a piece of painter's tape), one on each side (left and right) of the court, about halfway between the sideline and the centerline. These objects identify where your lane is located.

Attacking Unattackable Balls

If you are trying to attack balls that are well below net height, you are probably a very frustrated pickleball player. Speeding up a low ball usually causes it to go in the net, or pop up. If the ball is low, you should hit a defensive or neutral ball. Swing slowly and gently lift the ball over the net so that it dies as it reaches your opponent, thereby ensuring that they'll be dealing with a low, unattackable ball, too.

Be sure to review the upside-down traffic signal visualization detailed in Chapter 11. "Red light" balls are the ones below your knees — and those mean stop, don't attack! "Yellow light" balls are knee-to-rib-cage height. Use caution if you decide to "run the yellow" and attack. "Green light" balls are chest high or above. Green means go! Attack, attack, attack.

Trying to speeding up a low ball is a very low-percentage shot. Occasionally, you may choose to randomly speed up the "wrong" ball to surprise your opponents. This tactic can sometimes work as long as your shot lands in or is directed right at an opponent's body such that they can't duck out of the way. For the vast majority of the time, though, we encourage you to play the odds: be patient and wait for your moment.

Glossary

This glossary is extensive because there are a lot of pickleball terms (and even slang) you need to know — and we had to have fun with it, too, of course. Read on, learn, and smile. Repeat.

Addiction to pickleball: You can't stop thinking about pickleball. You are always trying to find ways to play and watch pickleball. You have a personalized pickleball license plate or frame. You have more paddles than silverware. You wake yourself up hitting punch volleys in your sleep. You read the glossary of pickleball books.

Altitude sickness: An affliction that affects players who are always on top of the medal stand.

Ambassador: A volunteer who works for the support and growth of the game. They work on behalf of the pickleball governing body of their home country.

Around the Post (ATP): A legal shot that you hit around the net post, as opposed to over the net, and that lands in the court on the opposite side.

Attack: Any shot you hit to capitalize on a weak shot from the opponent. It's a shot hit from high to low, but not always. Sometimes it is just a little "medium speed through the hole" shot.

Attackable ball: A ball that you can attack. A ball that a player does not have to lift up in order to clear the net. A ball that makes a player drool if they're on the receiving end of it. Also known as a "green light" ball.

Backcourt: The deepest area of the court, near the baseline.

Backhand: A shot hit on your nondominant side or in front of you with the back of your hand facing forward.

Backspin: Occurs when the ball is rotating backward on its axis.

Backswing: The action of taking back the paddle just prior to the forward swing and contact with the ball.

Banger: A player who hits every ball hard and does not embrace the soft game. The term often carries a negative connotation, but it just means a player who likes this style of play.

Baseline: The line at the back of the court. The serve must be struck from behind this line.

Behind the Back shot: A trick shot in which the player wraps their paddle arm around and behind their own back to hit on their nondominant side.

Bert: An Erne executed in front of your partner. It occurs when one partner jumps over the kitchen and hits the ball out of the air in front of their partner.

Block/block volley: A volley you perform by putting the paddle up in the path of the ball and deflecting or blocking the ball back to the opponent's side of the court.

Body shot: A shot that is hit right at the body of the opponent.

Bye: A tournament round you sit out because you do not have a scheduled opponent. This occurs when a round robin has an odd number of teams, or a team is not paired to play against another competitor in the first round of an elimination bracket.

Carry: Occurs when a player does not hit the ball so that it immediately bounces away from their paddle, but instead carries it on their paddle surface for a moment or two. May involve the sensation of a double hit. To be legal, a carry must be unintentional and one continuous motion.

Centerline: The line that divides the right and left service boxes.

Chainsaw serve: A serve in which the server spins the ball off their paddle or paddle hand before striking the ball. The ball bounces and jumps either to the right or the left. This was all anyone talked about in 2021 before it was made illegal in 2022.

Composite: Something made up of separate parts or elements. Many paddles and paddle surfaces are composite. Composite paddles usually incorporate an open-celled honeycomb core covered with one or more face materials.

Continental: A neutral grip on the paddle, or a cheap hotel breakfast.

Crosscourt: Hitting to the opponent's court that is diagonal from you.

Cut serve: A serve hit with sidespin.

Cutthroat: A three-person game of pickleball.

Dead ball: A ball that is no longer in play, such as one that has hit the net or bounced out of bounds.

Dedicated court: A court built only for pickleball, as opposed to a multiuser court. This court has painted lines and a net that are specifically for pickleball.

Dig: When a player must field a ball hit low and hard, usually at their feet.

Dink: A shot struck from in or near the non-volley zone (kitchen) that lands in or near the opponent's kitchen.

Dink volley: A dink that a player strikes out of the air before the ball has bounced.

Divorce Court: When married or committed couples play doubles together.

Double bounce: When a ball bounces twice on one side of the net before the player hits it. If you are using a wheelchair, you must hit it prior to the *third* bounce.

Double elimination: A competition format in which a player is out of the competition after they have lost two matches.

Double hit: A ball that hits the paddle twice on the same stroke (*see* Carry).

Doubles: Pickleball played between two teams with two players each.

Doubles partner: Someone who has paired up with another person to play doubles.

Drill: A practice scenario. The act of practicing a particular shot or play. This is both a noun and a verb. ("I know a good drill. Want to drill with me?")

Drive: A faster shot that you hit in an effort to either pass the opponent or put them in a defensive state.

Drop of Doom (DOD): A drop shot that is so good, the opponent hits it into the net.

Drop-in play: A format in which people gather to play pickleball, kinda casual-like. Rather than arranging a foursome, players can drop in as individuals or teams and mingle with other players.

Drop serve: A serve struck off a ball that has bounced. To be legal, the ball must be released from the hand as a dead drop, without any upward or downward force applied.

Drop shot: A low-energy ball that is dropping as it reaches the opponent and is too low for them to attack it. You typically hit it with the intention of moving forward in the court behind the shot.

Edge guard: The material (typically plastic) that wraps around the perimeter of the paddle, protecting it from scrapes or bumps.

Edgeless paddle: A paddle that does not have an edge guard. These paddles tend to offer larger hitting surfaces but can suffer from durability issues.

Erne: A shot hit by a player who has stepped or leapt over the edge of the kitchen to hit a volley very close to the net.

Even court: The right side of the court as you face the net.

Fartner: A doubles partner who is having some gastrointestinal wind.

Fault: Oopsie, you lost the rally. Okay, seriously, a fault is any violation of the rules that results in the loss of the rally. It can be anything from hitting the ball into the net to finishing your volley in the kitchen.

First server: The first player to serve after a sideout or at the opening of the game. This is the player currently standing on the right or even side of the court.

First-server band: A band worn by the first server (usually on the wrist) on each team during tournament play. The band assists the referee and the opponents in tracking the correct server and server's position.

Flob: A failed lob (which usually ends up slammed back at your partner).

Follow-through: The finishing portion of a stroke after the ball has been struck by the paddle.

Foot fault: A baseline serve violation or a kitchen violation. The server's foot may not touch the baseline or the court until after the ball has been struck. At the kitchen, foot faults occur when one touches any part of the kitchen during the act of hitting a volley.

Footwork: The player's movement of their feet in an effort to be in good balance and well-prepared to hit and receive shots.

Forehand: A shot hit on your dominant side with your palm facing forward.

Game: A pickleball game typically ends when the first player or team reaches 11 points, winning by a margin of at least two points. In some instances, a game may be played to 15 or 21 points.

Game point: Occurs when the serving team has the chance to finish the game on the next point (such as when the score is 10–8). You must win the game by two points.

Gender doubles: Women's or men's doubles in which women play against women and men play against men.

Graphite: A lightweight but hard surface used on paddle faces. It spreads out the impact of the ball striking the paddle, giving it more "feel."

Green-light ball: A high ball (chest and above) that you should definitely attack as long as you are in balance and in good position.

Grip: The covering of the handle of the paddle; also, the way the player holds the handle of the paddle.

Groundstroke: A shot that occurs after the ball has bounced on the ground.

Half stack: 1. Stacking only when your team is serving. 2. A more sensible pancake order.

Half-volley: A shot hit right after the ball bounces. Technically not a true volley, but is rather a ball hit just after the bounce. Also called a "short hop."

Handle: 1. The lower end of the paddle. 2. Your pickleball nickname.

Hoop: The area around your feet. It is the area that delineates what a pickleball player can comfortably reach out of the air.

Hydration break: A brief break in competitive play for the purpose of keeping players hydrated on hot days. Usually a 15- to 30-second break with no coaching or strategy talk allowed. Get a drink and return to play.

Inside foot: The foot closest to the centerline on the court.

Kitchen: 1. Slang term for the non-volley zone, the 7-x-20 foot area near the net where a player is not allowed to volley the ball. 2. The area in coauthor Mo's house where she goes to burn food.

Kitchen fault/violation: Occurs when any part of a player has stepped on or touched the kitchen, including the kitchen line, while in the act of volleying.

Kitchen line: The line that separates the kitchen from the service boxes behind it.

Ladder: A format of play, typically held weekly, where players compete and move up or down the ladder based on their individual points earned. Players rotate partners but maintain their individual score.

League: A format of play, usually between local clubs or teams, wherein the players represent their club or team rather than themselves as individuals.

Left/odd service box: As you face the net, this is the rectangle on your left side. The serve coming diagonally from your opponent must land in this box.

Line call: A verbal or physical indication of whether a ball landed in or out of bounds.

Line judge: A tournament official whose job is to call the ball out when it lands outside the boundary lines of the court. They also call serving foot faults.

Lob: A shot hit over a player's head to an area deep in the court.

Lobber: A player who likes to hit the ball over the heads of others.

Lobster: 1. A crustacean often enjoyed with butter. 2. A player who lobs excessively, making people crabby.

Loser's bracket: A term that is too harsh for our taste, but refers to the lower bracket played out by the teams and players who have lost a match in an elimination type of tournament format. Also known as the "opportunity" or "consolation" bracket.

Match point: When the serving team is one point away from winning the final game in the match.

Midcourt: The area from a few feet behind the kitchen that extends to a few feet inside the baseline.

Mixed doubles: Each team is composed of one man and one woman.

Multiuse court: A court with multiple line markings that is used for multiple sports. Many pickleball courts are courts that have pickleball lines taped or painted alongside lines for tennis, badminton, volleyball, basketball, and others.

Nasty Nelson: When the serve strikes the receiver's partner before it bounces, thereby scoring a point for the server.

Nomex: An aramid polymer that is a close cousin to nylon. It is used in paddle cores. Compared to polymer cores, a Nomex core tends to be stiffer, allowing a player to impart more power on a shot.

Non-volley line: The line that is 7 feet away from the net and delineates the non-volley zone (kitchen). This line is considered part of the non-volley zone.

Non-volley zone: The 7-by-20-foot area near the net where a player is not allowed to volley the ball. Commonly known as the kitchen.

Non-volley zone fault/violation: *See* kitchen fault/violation.

Odd court: The left side of the court as you face the net.

Open paddle face: The face of the paddle when it is laid back, causing the ball to rebound upward.

Opportunity bracket: *See* loser's bracket.

Outside foot: The foot that is closest to the sideline.

Overgrip: A covering of the regular grip, usually to absorb sweat and maintain tackiness.

Overhead/overhead smash: An overhand attack struck from high to low on a ball above the player's head.

Paddle: The implement used to strike the pickleball.

Paddle face: The surface of the paddle used to strike the ball.

Paddle tap: The gentle touching (sexy!) of paddles between two or more players. Always done at the net upon the conclusion of a match, but frequently done between doubles partners as a show of connection and support (a pickleball high five).

Poach: A shot hit by a player who has crossed over in front of their partner. Surprise!

Polymer core: A type of paddle core made from a certain class of polymers (such as polyethylene or polystyrene). The polymers tend to be a little flexible, meaning that the core compresses a tiny bit during impact with the ball.

Pool play: A tournament format in which teams or players in a larger bracket are grouped together in subgroups called pools. Typically, each team in the pool plays a round robin with all the others in their pool; then the top finishers in each pool compete against each other to determine the overall winners. Also, *Marco! Polo!*

Punch volley: A ball hit out of the air that the player extends through in a forward direction, as if they are throwing a punch.

Put-away: An attack shot (typically a clean winner) that ends the rally.

Rally: When players hit the ball back and forth. Often confused with the term *volley,* it refers to continuous play that occurs after the serve and before a fault.

Receiver: The player receiving the serve.

Red-light ball: A low ball (near or below the knees) that ideally should not be attacked, but rather lifted up to clear the net.

Ready position: A stance or posture and paddle position that a player assumes in order to be ready for their opponent's shot.

Referee: The boss on the court in tournament play. The referee calls the score, foot faults, language violations (dagnammit), and other violations.

Right/even service box: As you face the net, this is the rectangle on your right side. The serve that is coming diagonally from your opponent must land in this box.

Round robin: A competition format wherein the players or teams each play all the others in their division.

Sandals of Shame (a.k.a. Flip-Flops of Failure): The footwear you put on after you have been knocked out of a tournament. No actual shame is involved! We lose sometimes and that's okay. Now we can get comfortable and cheer on our friends.

Score: 1. The numbers that track the progress of the game. 2. The act of winning a point.

Second server: The player who serves after the serving team has lost their first rally on that particular sideout. The score will end in a "2," indicating that this person is the second server.

Serve: The shot that initiates the point.

Server: The player who is serving.

Server number: The third number in the score, which indicates whether the player serving is the first or second server. If the score is 0–10–2, that server is the second server, and their team is way behind so they'd better get going.

Service box: The rectangular area where the serve must land. It is diagonal from the server on the opposite side of the net.

Shake 'N' Bake: Slang for when a player hits a hard drive that is popped up by their opponent and then put away.

Sideline: The line that runs all the way down the side of the court.

Sideout: Occurs when the serving team or player has lost their serve(s) and has to reluctantly give the ball to their opponents, who now get to serve.

Sidespin: Occurs when the ball is rotating sideways on its axis, like a spinning top.

Singles: Pickleball that is played between two players, with each player being responsible for their entire side of the court.

Sitter: 1. Someone who watches your kids or pets while you play pickleball. 2. A ball that has been popped up high and will be easy to put away.

Skinny singles: A type of singles that is played using only half of the court, either straight on or diagonally.

Slice: 1. Spin applied to the ball, usually in reference to sidespin. 2. A helping of pizza or cake.

Smash (a.k.a. overhead smash): An overhand shot hit from a high ball as an attack.

Split step: A short little hop that gently finishes with the player on the balls of their feet. It balances a player, allowing them to move in any direction.

Stacking: When two players line up on the same side of the court, rather than in the traditional starting positions. Think of it as both players being "stacked" up next to each other. You use stacking to let the players consistently play on a particular side of the court for a strategic advantage.

Starting server: The server who starts the game at the score of 0–0–2.

Stroke: The mechanics of the swing that result in hitting a pickleball.

Swinging volley: A volley that the player takes a swing at. This is an offensive shot with some juice behind it.

Third shot: The third shot in every rally, always hit by the serving team or player (serve, return, third shot). It's typically either a drop shot or a drive and is critical in helping the serving team transition to the front of the court.

Three-quarters stack: Stacking when your team is serving and when only one of the two partners receives serve.

Time-out: A break in the action in organized competition. Called by either team or by the referee, it is usually a one-minute break.

Topspin: Occurs when the ball is rotating forward on its axis.

Tournament: An organized competition between players.

Tournament Director (TD): The Big Kahuna of any tournament. They are in charge of running the tournament. They get the tournament committee working together and do their best to put on a good event.

Traditional/standard/volley serve: A serve that is hit out of the air rather than off the bounce.

Transition zone: The area of the court between the kitchen and the baseline. It's sometimes erroneously called "No Man's Land" (which is a tennis term, not a pickleball term).

Trash talk: Lighthearted banter between opponents, wherein they speak ill of each other's abilities and skills. ("You called that out?! Out of your reach, maybe!") Please make sure your opponent shares that type of sense of humor before engaging in trash talk. Rudeness is not what pickleball is about.

Tweener: A ball hit from between the player's legs.

Two and out: Losing your first two matches in a double elimination tournament. This gives you the opportunity to don the "Sandals of Shame" and relax while cheering on your friends (possibly with a margarita in hand).

Two-Bounce Rule: The rule that both the serve and the return must bounce before being struck. After the first two shots, the ball may be struck as a volley out of the air.

Unattackable ball: A ball that a player must strike from low to high, lifting it over the net. It is usually a drop shot or a dink. Also known as a "red light" ball.

Unforced error: An error a player makes when a player is not under stress from their opponent. The opponent did not "force" the error. For example, it's a routine and easy shot that the player hits out or into the net.

Volley: A shot hit before the ball has bounced.

Volleyball: A completely different sport.

Yellow-light ball: A ball hit from the middle of the hitting player's body (knees to rib cage). This is a ball that requires a decision to be made: whether to attack, or yield and wait for a better chance to attack.

Z Best People: People who play pickleball (and read glossaries all the way to the letter Z.)

Index

defined, 406

dinking, 142–145

effectiveness of, 116

self-assessing, 325

tennis compared with pickleball, 83

force, as a skill transferred from martial arts to pickleball, 94

forehand, 325, 406

forehand groundstroke, 130–131

forehand has middle, 206

forward pressure, 214

four on, four off rotational system, 78

four-person drills, 310–313

frame construction, of portable nets, 57

full stack, 233

fundamentals

about, 99

grip, 100–102

lower-body mechanics, 114–117

ready position, 103–110

upper-body mechanics, 110–114

funneling, 201–202

G

gadgets, 54–60

game point, 406

games, 390, 406

gender doubles, 406

glasses, 16, 54, 182

gloves, 55–56, 297

goals, ignoring of other players, 388

Going Solo drill, 313

graphite surface, for paddles, 40–41, 406

greed, poaching for, 279

green-light ball, 406

grips

about, 55–56, 100

change in size and shape of, for tennis (pickleball) elbow, 185

continental grip, 100–101

defined, 42, 406

eastern forehand grip, 101–102

for paddles, 41–43

pressure for, 102

groundstroke, 85, 130–133, 406

growth, of pickleball, 76, 377–384

H

half stack, 233, 406

half-volley, 406

hamstring injuries, 183

hand injuries, 183

hand signals, 236–238

hand-eye coordination, soccer compared with pickleball, 93

handle, 406

hard pickleballs, 48–49

Harrison, Deb, 370

head direction, of opponents, 294

headwear, 52–53

heat, for tennis (pickleball) elbow, 184

heavyweight paddles, 44

higher-stakes returns, 236

high-percentage pickleball, 215–217

hitting

lob recovery shots, 226

to opponent's weaker side, 252

through windows, 266

with "wristiness," 397

hitting behind, 85, 262

holes, in pickleballs, 48

home position, 143

honesty, etiquette and, 72–74

hoop, 406

House of Pickleball, 363

hydration, 17, 182, 297

hydration break, 406

I

"I Used to be Somebody" podcast, 369

ice, for tennis (pickleball) elbow, 184

icons, explained, 3

In2Pickle, 370

indoor courts, outdoor courts vs., 62–65

indoor pickleballs, 47–48

injury prevention

about, 177

common, 181–186

moving safely and efficiently, 180–181

tennis elbow, 184–185

warming up, 177–180

T

table tennis, transitioning from, 86–87

tap dancing, 143–144

tapping paddles, 388

Target Shoppers drill, 312

targets, 128, 315

team-based leagues, 359

teamwork, as a skill transferred from basketball to pickleball, 90

technologies, for paddles, 39–41

temper, losing your, 391

tennis, transitioning from, 82–84

tennis elbow, 102, 184–185

thickness, standards for paddles, 39

thinking, before dinking, 152–155

third shot, 135–140, 315, 397, 410

Third Shot Sports, 367

three-person "cutthroat," 256

three-person drills, 310–313

three-quarters stack, 233, 410

throwing motion, soccer compared with pickleball, 93

time-outs
  about, 305, 341
  calling, 210–211
  choosing doubles partners based on, 344
  defined, 410
  using, 348

Tip icon, 3

topspin
  achieving, 114
  defined, 410
  dropping with, 275–276
  generating in serves, 273
  racquetball compared with pickleball, 86

touch
  basketball compared with pickleball, 90
  as a skill transferred from soccer to pickleball, 93

Tourna Hot Glove, 59

Tournament Director (TD), 410

tournaments
  about, 329–330
  changing partners, 350–351
  choosing doubles partners, 343–344
  coaches, 342–343
  defined, 410
  double elimination, 331–333
  expectations for players, 338–339
  formats and types, 330–334
  line judges, 339–341
  maintaining mental focus, 346–348
  official skill-rating definitions, 335–336
  player ratings, 334–338
  playing, 329–351
  rating systems for, 336–338
  referees, 339–341
  reflecting after, 349–350
  roles and expectations, 338–343
  round robins, 331, 360–361
  sanctioned vs. non-sanctioned, 333–334
  self-rating for, 337
  setting expectations for, 345–346
  single elimination with consolation, 333
  spectators, 342–343
  tips for your first, 343–350
  using time-outs, 348
  what to bring, 344–345

track stance, 103

traditional/standard/volley serve, 410

training, 365–366, 373–375

transition zone, 103, 410

transitioning
  to the kitchen phase, for singles points, 247–248
  to the line phase, of doubles points, 195–197
  from other sports, 81–95

trash talk, 410

traveling, pickleball and, 362–366

triangles, as a skill transferred from soccer to pickleball, 92

trick shots, 174–175

trunk rotation, basketball compared with pickleball, 90

tube-style ball collectors, 59

tweener, 174, 410

two and out, 331–333, 410

Two-Bounce Rule, 20, 129, 214, 396, 410

two-handed backhands, 133, 161

two-person drills, 310–313

Two-Touch drill, 311

About the Authors

Mo Nard is a former national racquetball champion x 2 (Women's 19 and under doubles) turned certified pickleball teaching pro. She's cofounder of Positive Dinking pickleball instruction and has played pickleball at the local, regional, and national level. She is also a part of the *I Used to be Somebody* podcast, for which she is a contributing writer and the "Mo" in "Pickleball Life Lessons with Mo" on the podcast. She is a sponsored player for Head/Penn Pickleball. Mo is happiest when she is on the court teaching pickleball!

Reine Steel is a certified pickleball teaching pro and Head/Penn–sponsored tournament player. She is the cofounder of Positive Dinking, a pickleball instruction company based in Sacramento, California. One of the founding board members of Sunrise Pickleball Club, she has been actively involved in the community since 2016, volunteering as a USA Pickleball Ambassador, running tournaments and events, and advising for new facilities. Reine is also the creator of the PlayTime Scheduler website used daily by more than 120,000 pickleball players around the world (and counting!).

Diana Landau was a corporate marketing director for 20 years before finding her calling as a writer and editor for blogs and newsletters, most recently as Content Wrangler for Pickleball Media. When she's not writing or having typo nightmares, she finds every excuse to play pickleball.

Carl Landau is an entrepreneur and founder of Pickleball Media. He has started and sold three successful media companies, published five magazines, and now hosts the popular podcast *I Used to be Somebody*, inspiring 50-plus-year-olds how to build their (un)retirement good life, including, of course, the virtues of the game we love — pickleball.

Dedication

From Mo: To Stephanie Wilson, for your unwavering support and patience.

From Reine: To the memory of my mom, Helissa Penwell.

From Diana: To Carl Landau, whose encouragement and faith in me never seems to waiver.

From Carl: To my wonderful bride, Diana, and our family.

Authors' Acknowledgments

We would like to thank all the people who helped us make this book a reality, including Acquisitions Editor Jennifer Yee for guiding the book's development; our supportive, enthusiastic Project Editor Susan Christophersen, who fostered our creativity while showing us the Wiley Way (and also loves pickleball as much as we do); and for Wiley's exceptional production staff.

We'd also like to thank technical editor Mike Branon for his thoughtful insights and his love of pickleball; Aniko Kiezel, not only for her photography but for her positivity and encouragement; and Rio Del Oro/SpareTime Sports Clubs for allowing us to take over the courts for the photo shoots. We also thank our stunning and patient models: Melissa Suchomel (cover model); Kasha Ra; Tom Burkhart; Karen and John House; John Ivanusich; Patty Nicholas, DVM; Charlene McGhee; Hal Gordon; Gigja Hollyday; Stacy Turner; Nancy Cummings; Mary Richison; Julian Robinson; Trisha Pollock; and Christie Lammi. And finally, we thank the athletes who provided insights for Chapter 5: Robyn Penwell; Jennifer Fritz; Byron Lee; Thuy Washburn; Julie Klinger; Alex Chan; Kasha Ra; Nicolas De Francesco; Kelly Andrews; and Dawnita LiaBraaten.

Mo also thanks all the wonderful students I've worked with over the years; my amazing friends and family; my beloved dogs; my mom, who always encouraged me to play any sport I wanted and was proud of me, win or lose; Head/Penn Pickleball; Sarah Ansboury; Mark Renneson; Andrea Mayorga; Courtside Tennis; and my sister, Lisa Ryan, who got me out on a pickleball court the very first time (and Kate Lahti, who started an amazing trickle-down pickleball legacy). A special thanks to Reine Steel for being such a great partner in crime and a true friend.

Reine also thanks, first and foremost, Kasha Ra, for being the Best Boo in the History of Boos. Thanks to my friends and family, especially my big sister, Robyn Penwell, for always encouraging me to try scary new things, and my dad, Mark Penwell, for modeling strength and gratitude during tough times. Thanks to all our Positive Dinkers who make our job fun every day; Head/Penn Pickleball; and coaching mentors Sarah Ansboury and Mark Renneson. Huge thank you to Kate Lahti for not only teaching me how to play pickleball but also introducing me to my future PBFF and business partner. Mo, our friendship has led us places I've never dreamed possible — thanks for being you.

Diana also thanks my supportive family, friends, and the Coffee & Ink Writers' Group, who never let me know they were tired of hearing me talk about writing this book. To my buddies on the court: You've taught me so much. Thank you for welcoming me in and for your encouragement and patience. A special shout-out to Rio Del Oro and McKinley Village players!

Carl also thanks Bob Franceschelli, a board member of USA Pickleball and a true pickleball aficionado; Laura Gainor and the entire USA Pickleball Association; Anna Copley, cofounder of Pickleball Central; and Corky Logue, for being Corky. Thanks also to Katie Purdum Mohr, who introduced us to Wiley and the good people who run the *For Dummies* series, and to photographers David Tedoni, Darrel Dey, Steve Taylor, Bruce Yeung, Morgan Handy, and Michael Cummo. Thanks to Bekah Darksmith, for helping me out (once again) due to my dyslexic brain. A big thank you to the loyal listeners of our *I Used to be Somebody* podcast. Finally, thanks to my pickleball buddies at Rio Del Oro who occasionally let me win.

Publisher's Acknowledgments

Acquisitions Editor: Jennifer Yee

Project and Copy Editor: Susan Christophersen

Technical Editor: Mike Branon

Production Editor: Tamilmani Varadharaj

Cover Image: Courtesy of Desert Champions/ Michael Cummo

Take dummies with you everywhere you go!

Whether you are excited about e-books, want more from the web, must have your mobile apps, or are swept up in social media, dummies makes everything easier.

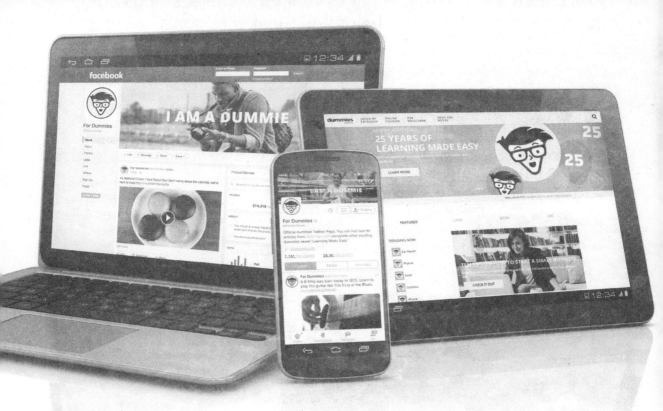

Find us online!

dummies.com

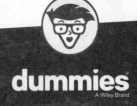
dummies
A Wiley Brand

Leverage the power

Dummies is the global leader in the reference category and one of the most trusted and highly regarded brands in the world. No longer just focused on books, customers now have access to the dummies content they need in the format they want. Together we'll craft a solution that engages your customers, stands out from the competition, and helps you meet your goals.

Advertising & Sponsorships

Connect with an engaged audience on a powerful multimedia site, and position your message alongside expert how-to content. Dummies.com is a one-stop shop for free, online information and know-how curated by a team of experts.

- Targeted ads
- Video
- Email Marketing
- Microsites
- Sweepstakes sponsorship

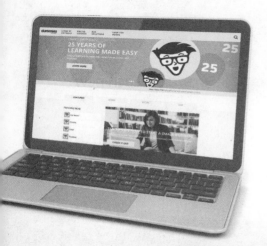

20 MILLION
PAGE VIEWS
EVERY SINGLE MONTH

15 MILLION UNIQUE
VISITORS PER MONTH

43%
OF ALL VISITORS
ACCESS THE SITE
VIA THEIR MOBILE DEVICES

700,000 NEWSLETTER SUBSCRIPTIONS
TO THE INBOXES OF
300,000 UNIQUE INDIVIDUALS EVERY WEEK

# of dummies

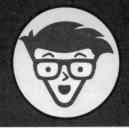

Custom Publishing

Reach a global audience in any language by creating a solution that will differentiate you from competitors, amplify your message, and encourage customers to make a buying decision.

- Apps
- Books
- eBooks
- Video
- Audio
- Webinars

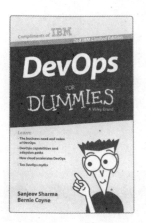
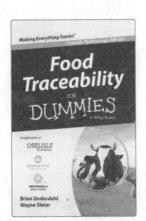
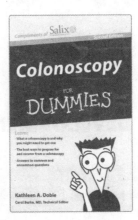
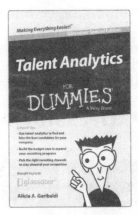

Brand Licensing & Content

Leverage the strength of the world's most popular reference brand to reach new audiences and channels of distribution.

For more information, visit **dummies.com/biz**

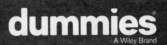

PERSONAL ENRICHMENT

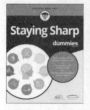

Staying Sharp
9781119187790
USA $26.00
CAN $31.99
UK £19.99

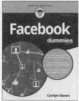

Facebook
9781119179030
USA $21.99
CAN $25.99
UK £16.99

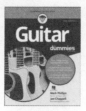

Guitar
9781119293354
USA $24.99
CAN $29.99
UK £17.99

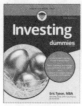

Investing
9781119293347
USA $22.99
CAN $27.99
UK £16.99

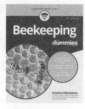

Beekeeping
9781119310068
USA $22.99
CAN $27.99
UK £16.99

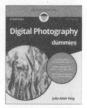

Digital Photography
9781119235606
USA $24.99
CAN $29.99
UK £17.99

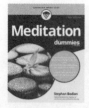

Meditation
9781119251163
USA $24.99
CAN $29.99
UK £17.99

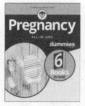

Pregnancy
9781119235491
USA $26.99
CAN $31.99
UK £19.99

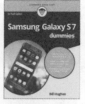

Samsung Galaxy S7
9781119279952
USA $24.99
CAN $29.99
UK £17.99

iPhone
9781119283133
USA $24.99
CAN $29.99
UK £17.99

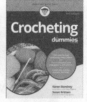

Crocheting
9781119287117
USA $24.99
CAN $29.99
UK £16.99

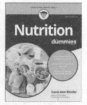

Nutrition
9781119130246
USA $22.99
CAN $27.99
UK £16.99

PROFESSIONAL DEVELOPMENT

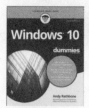

Windows 10
9781119311041
USA $24.99
CAN $29.99
UK £17.99

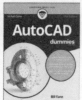

AutoCAD
9781119255796
USA $39.99
CAN $47.99
UK £27.99

Excel 2016
9781119293439
USA $26.99
CAN $31.99
UK £19.99

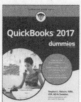

QuickBooks 2017
9781119281467
USA $26.99
CAN $31.99
UK £19.99

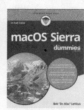

macOS Sierra
9781119280651
USA $29.99
CAN $35.99
UK £21.99

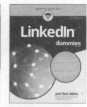

LinkedIn
9781119251132
USA $24.99
CAN $29.99
UK £17.99

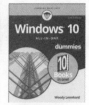

Windows 10 All-in-One
9781119310563
USA $34.00
CAN $41.99
UK £24.99

SharePoint 2016
9781119181705
USA $29.99
CAN $35.99
UK £21.99

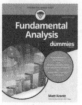

Fundamental Analysis
9781119263593
USA $26.99
CAN $31.99
UK £19.99

Networking
9781119257769
USA $29.99
CAN $35.99
UK £21.99

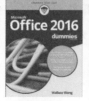

Office 2016
9781119293477
USA $26.99
CAN $31.99
UK £19.99

Office 365
9781119265313
USA $24.99
CAN $29.99
UK £17.99

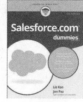

Salesforce.com
9781119239314
USA $29.99
CAN $35.99
UK £21.99

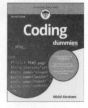

Coding
9781119293323
USA $29.99
CAN $35.99
UK £21.99